New Paradigms in Urology

New Paradigms in Urology

Editor: Ezra Martin

AMERICAN
MEDICAL PUBLISHERS
www.americanmedicalpublishers.com

AMERICAN
MEDICAL PUBLISHERS
www.americanmedicalpublishers.com

Cataloging-in-Publication Data

New paradigms in urology / edited by Ezra Martin.
p. cm.
Includes bibliographical references and index.
ISBN 979-8-88740-336-6
1. Urology. 2. Genitourinary organs--Diseases. 3. Urinary organs--Diseases. I. Martin, Ezra.
RC871 .N49 2023
616.6--dc23

American Medical Publishers,
41 Flatbush Avenue,
1st Floor, New York,
NY 11217, USA

ISBN 979-8-88740-336-6 (Hardback)

Contents

Preface

This book aims to highlight the current researches and provides a platform to further the scope of innovations in this area. This book is a product of the combined efforts of many researchers and scientists, after going through thorough studies and analysis from different parts of the world. The objective of this book is to provide the readers with the latest information of the field.

Urology is the branch of medicine that is concerned with the pathologies of the male and female urinary and reproductive tracts consisting of kidneys, ureters, bladder and urethra. It also deals with the conditions or disorders of male reproductive organs such as penis, testes, scrotum and prostate gland. Major sub-specialties of urology include pediatric urology, urologic oncology, kidney transplant, male fertility, urinary tract stones, female urology and neurourology. The discipline of urology is involved in the treatment of diseases such as adrenal gland cancer, bladder diseases, erectile dysfunction, kidney diseases, testicular diseases, penile cancer, upper urinary tract cancer, and urethral cancer. This book includes contributions of international experts and scientists which will provide novel insights into the field of urology. Various studies that are constantly contributing towards advancing techniques and the evolution of this field have been examined in detail. Researchers and students actively engaged in the study of urology will find this book full of crucial and unexplored concepts.

I would like to express my sincere thanks to the authors for their dedicated efforts in the completion of this book. I acknowledge the efforts of the publisher for providing constant support. Lastly, I would like to thank my family for their support in all academic endeavors.

Editor

1

Expression of mRNA vascular endothelial growth factor in hypospadias patients

Prahara Yuri[1*], Gunadi[2], Rahmadani P. Lestari[1], Firly P. Fardilla[1] and Ishandono Dachlan[3]

Abstract

Background: Hypospadias is a relatively common genital anomaly in humans, usually followed by inelastic dartos that causes penile chordee. Vascular endothelial growth factor (*VEGF*) is strongly linked to the viscoelasticity of tissues and their elastic phase. This study aimed to evaluate *VEGF* expressions in (1) fascia dartos between hypospadias and controls and (2) chordee severity.

Methods: This prospective cohort study involved 65 specimens from patients with hypospadias and ten specimens from controls. The samples were analyzed by quantitative real-time polymerase chain reaction (qPCR) for *VEGF* expression.

Results: The expressions of *VEGF* were not different between proximal and distal hypospadias patients and controls (fold change: distal − 0.25; fold change: proximal − 0.2; $p = 0.664$). The scaled expressions related to chordee severity were mild − 0.1; moderate 0.1; severe − 0.25 ($p = 0.660$).

Conclusions: *VEGF* expressions might not affect the severity of hypospadias and chordee, implying the pathogenesis is complex involving many growth factors. Further study with a larger sample size is necessary to clarify and confirm our findings.

Keywords: Hypospadias, *VEGF*, Dartos tissue, Elasticity, Chordee, Penile curvature

Introduction

Hypospadias, a relatively common human genital abnormality, is a urethral opening disorder that is not positioned correctly at the tip of the penis. Hypospadias is the second most common congenital anomaly in boys and the most common type of penis deformity [1, 2]. Molecular processes are needed in the occurrence of hypospadias, but the relationships and functions of these two elements are still unknown [3]. The exact cause of hypospadias has been identified in about 20% of cases, especially in the most challenging conditions [1].

Hypospadias may be related to an abnormality of the dartos fascia. However, this hypothesis is not supported by solid evidence from histopathology. There are contrasting studies of histopathological aspects of connective tissue in patients with hypospadias. The dartos fascia of hypospadias had abnormal tissue that gave it the thick and inelastic character [4, 5]. Inelastic dartos fascia tissue in patients diagnosed with hypospadias is a pathological tissue [4, 6, 7].

VEGF regulates elastic modulus and increases matrix stiffness in cardiomyocytes [8]. It is strongly associated with tissue viscoelasticity and the elastic cervix phase shortening [9]. *In addition, VEGF* plays a pivotal part in endothelial cells' proliferation, migration, and differentiation [10]. *VEGF* induces α1β1 and α2β1 integrins expression in microvascular endothelial cells [11], endothelial cell migration, and proliferation [12, 13]. *VEGF* is not retained intra-cellularly but attaches to the cell surface or

*Correspondence: prahara.yuri@ugm.ac.id; prahara.yuri@gmail.com
[1] Division of Urology, Department of Surgery, Faculty of Medicine, Public Health and Nursing, Universitas Gadjah Mada/Dr. Sardjito Hospital, Jl. Kesehatan No.1, Yogyakarta 55281, Indonesia
Full list of author information is available at the end of the article

extracellular membrane (ECM) and other matrix metalloproteinases (MMPs) [14]. However, the role of *VEGF* on dartos tissue remains unknown. Hence, this study aimed to investigate the impact of *VEGF* modulated dartos on tissue elasticity.

Methods

Patients

A prospective cohort study was performed in 65 patients who underwent repair of hypospadias with chordee without DSD, and ten patients underwent circumcision as controls between 2018 and 2020. The samples were then divided into three groups: distal hypospadias, proximal hypospadias, and controls. We used periurethral dartos tissues collected during excision of chordee. The Ethical Committee of our university approved this study(KE/0287/03/2020), and written informed consent to participate in this study was obtained from all the parents.

qPCR analysis

All dartos tissue of each patient was placed in a single tube. All samples were homogenized. Total RNA was extracted using Hybrid-R™ Isolation Kit, and cDNA was extracted from 200 ng of total RNA using NEXpro™ qRT-PCR Kit. Gene expression analysis by Quantitative PCR has been used for *VEGF* (F: 5'-CCCACTGAG GAGTCCAACAT-3′ and R: 5′-AAATGCTTTCTCCGC TCTGA-3′), and GAPDH (F: 5′-GCATCCTGGGCT ACACTGAG-3′ and R: 5′-TCCACCACCCTGTTGCTG TA-3′) used as internal control. Conditions for amplification consisted of an initial denaturing phase at 95 °C for 10 min, proceeded by 40 cycles at 95 °C for 20 secs, at 56 °C for 40 secs, and 72 °C for 60 secs. Extension done at 72 °C for 5 min. The qPCR amplified samples were analyzed by the BiONEER Exicycle™ 96 (BioNEER, Daejeon, South Korea). The Livak method was used to measure fold change between the three groups [15].

Statistical analysis

The Kruskal–Wallis test was used to compare VEGF expressions in control, distal and proximal hypospadias' tissues. Post hoc analysis used Mann–Whitney U test for comparison of each group. Values were considered statistically significant with $p < 0.05$.

Results

The age mean was 6.24 ± 4.36 years. Our study consisted of 24 (32%) distal hypospadias, 41 (54.7%) proximal hypospadias, and ten (13.3%) controls. Furthermore, five (6.7%) patients had penoscrotal transposition, and 70 (93.3%) patients were without penoscrotal transposition. Penile curvature in hypospadias was grouped into four groups: mild (< 30 degrees), moderate (30–60 degree), severe (> 60 degrees), and normal with each group number respectively: 19 (25.3%), 15 (20%), 23 (30.7%) and 18 patients (24%) (Table 1).

The qPCR analyses showed decreasing of *VEGF* expression in both distal and proximal (− 1.05 (− 0.1–(− 1.9)); − 1 (− 0.2–(− 2.3))) hypospadias compared with the control group − 0.8 (− 0.4–(− 1.1)), however were not significantly different. The fold change of VEGF expression in proximal and distal hypospadias and controls was not significantly different (mean fold change: hypospadias distal − 0.25; mean fold change: hypospadias proximal − 0.2; $p = 0.664$). Meanwhile, fold change expressions of *VEGF*-related chordees were scaled as follows: (mild − 0.1; moderate 0.1; severe − 0.25; $p = 0.660$) (Table 2).

Discussion

In almost every organ, the biomechanical properties of connective tissues perform essential physiological roles. Biochemical and biophysical properties of ECM are responsible for migration, adhesion, the integrity of

Table 1 Clinical characteristics of patients in our institution

Variable	
All groups (n = 75)	
Age, yr. # mean	6.24 ± 4.36
VEGF, Median (min–max) *	− 0.9 (− 0.1–(− 2.3)
Hypospadias Patients (n = 65)	
Hypospadias Type, n (%)	
Distal	24 (32)
Glandular	5 (20.8)
Subcoronal	5 (20.8)
Midshaft	14 (58.4)
Proximal	41 (54.7)
Penoscrotal	27 (65.)
Scrotal	13 (31.7)
Perineal	1 (2.4)
Penile curvature, n (%)	
Mild (< 30 degree)	12 (16)
Moderate (30–60 degree)	15 (20)
Severe (> 60 degree)	38 (50.7)
Normal	10 (13.3)
Penoscrotal transposition	
Yes	7 (9.3)
No	68 (90.7)
Bifid Scrotum	
Yes	7 (9.3)
No	68 (90.7)

VEGF, vascular endothelial growth factor

*Kolmogorov–Smirnov $p > 0.05$

[#] Kolmogorov–Smirnov $p > 0.05$

Table 2 Analysis based on hypospadias type and penile curvature severity

Variable	VEGF[#]	Fold change	*p*
Hypospadias type			
Distal hypospadias	− 1.05 (− 0.1–(− 1.9))	3.07	0.664
Proximal hypospadias	− 1 (− 0.2–(− 2.3))	2.96	
Control	− 0.8 (− 0.4–(− 1.1))		
Penile curvature severity			
Mild	− 0.9 (− 0.2–(− 1.4))	4.60	0.660
Moderate	− 0.7(− 0.1–(− 1.6))	0.723	
Severe	− 1.05 (− 0.1–(− 2.3))	2.03	

VEGF, vascular endothelial growth factor

[#] Kruskal–Wallis test;

individual cells, nutrition and differentiation of cells, angiogenesis, and intracellular contact formation [16]. ECM consists of collagenous (different types of collagen) and non-collagenous proteins, such as fibronectin, elastin, laminin, and other components. Elastin, collagen, and proteoglycans are essential factors in the mechanical properties of tissues [17].

Collagen remains possibly the essential component responsible for preserving the structural stability of the tissue. However, the viscoelasticity of biological tissue does not only involve the amount of components' biomechanical properties. It is the product of a dynamic relationship between cells, angiogenic cytokines, and the ECM, such as *VEGF*, which maintains the elasticity and integrity of normal tissues [17]. *VEGF* is a family of closely related growth factors, including several splice variants with numerous biological effects [18]. The production of particular cytokines, including fibroblast growth factor 2 (FGF-2) and *VEGF*, facilitate cell migration and neovascularization in freshly formed scar tissue [19].

Several studies have proved inelastic dartos tissue in hypospadias. The abnormal findings were found in smooth muscle fiber [20], collagen I and VI [4], total collagen, elastin, and reticulin [6]. Even though dartos tissue has abnormal development of some ECM structure, this study found that dartos tissue has well vascularization.

The present study showed a similar expression of *VEGF* in patients with hypospadias compared to the control group. *VEGF* is significantly correlated with the tissue viscoelasticity and the elastic shortening in some organs, such as the cervix. It does not work alone in the elastic mechanism because of crucial tissue mechanical properties such as collagen, elastin, and decorin [9]. A study shows similar blood vessels in the dartos fascia in patients with hypospadias and normal penis [6]. There is strong evidence that this family plays a fundamental role in the growth and differentiation of vascular and lymphatic endothelial cells, but the mechanism remains unclear [9, 18].

VEGF is an angiogenic peptide made from macrophages, endothelial cells, and many other cells [21]. It mediates angiogenesis and facilitates the survival of endothelial cells [10]. Integrin β1 acts as a signal transducer to regulate the mechanical environment during this process. Integrin consists of two subunits of transmembrane that modify conformational structures in response to extracellular force [22]. Previous studies identified integrin as a major mechanoreceptor for extracellular signal sensing [23]. Mechanical stimulation enables integrin subunits to be nucleated and clustered to support the maturation of focal adhesions, such as FAK phosphorylation [24].

Pressure overload, particularly integrin β1, can upregulate and activate integrins [25–27]. Interestingly, FAK activation was dispensable in angiogenic response mediated by the elastic modulus [9]. Instead, an elevated elastic module upregulated integrin β1 expression in H9c2 cells and activated its Talin-dependent downstream targets, Akt and PI3K. Activating PI3K/Akt signaling resulted in *VEGF* being upregulated by its primary transcriptional regulator, HIF-1α [28]. Hypoxia-inducible factor-1 (HIF-1) is a primary transcriptional mediator of the O2 homeostasis hypoxic response. Its master regulator consists of two separate subunits, α, and β [29]. HIF-1 (hypoxia-inducible factor-1) is a key transcriptional mediator of the response to hypoxic conditions [30]. Hypoxia is the primary stimulus for VEGF release [31]. Hypoxia also reduces the power of the tissue and predisposes it for rupture [9]. Increased *VEGF* and paracrine are affected by the elevated ECM stiffness in cardiomyocytes. It subsequently stimulates cardiac angiogenesis and the development of *VEGF*, which can be modulated during cardiac hypertrophy through the elastic modulus of the ECM [8]. Accordingly, Wingate also reported that mesenchymal stem cells in soft *VEGF* matrices display more mature endothelial cell markers than MSC on soft non-*VEGF* matrices [32].

However, this study has several limitations, including small sample size and unequal control allocation, a heterogeneous study cohort with both proximal and distal hypospadias. In addition, the tissue studied is the periurethral dartos collected during the excision of the chordee. Most of the distal hypospadias do not require chordee correction or excision. Moreover, VEGF expression needs to be checked in other tissues before a definite conclusion is drawn.

Conclusions

VEGF expressions might not affect the severity of hypospadias and chordee, implying the pathogenesis is complex involving many growth factors. Further study with a larger sample size is necessary to clarify and confirm our findings.

Acknowledgements
We thank all staffs and nurses who have taken care of patients in our Hospital.

Authors' contributions
PY collected the patient data, and PY, G, and ID analyzed and interpreted data. PY, RP, and FP performed qPCR analysis. PY, G, and ID were major contributors in writing the manuscript. All authors' read and agreed to the final manuscript.

Competing interests
The authors declared no potential conflicts of interest concerning this article's research, authorship, and/or publication.

Author details
[1]Division of Urology, Department of Surgery, Faculty of Medicine, Public Health and Nursing, Universitas Gadjah Mada/Dr. Sardjito Hospital, Jl. Kesehatan No.1, Yogyakarta 55281, Indonesia. [2]Pediatric Surgery Division, Department of Surgery, Faculty of Medicine, Public Health and Nursing, Universitas Gadjah Mada/Dr. Sardjito Hospital, Yogyakarta, Indonesia. [3]Division of Plastic, Aesthetic and Reconstructive Surgery, Department of Surgery, Faculty of Medicine, Public Health and Nursing, Universitas Gadjah Mada/Dr. Sardjito Hospital, Yogyakarta, Indonesia.

References

1. Kalfa N, Sultan C. Hypospadias: etiology and current research. Urol Clin N Am. 2010;37(2):159–66. https://doi.org/10.1016/j.ucl.2010.03.010.
2. Yuri P, Heriyanto DS, Rodjani A, Hutasoit YI, Hutahaean AYA, Rahman MR, et al. expression of mrna mastermind-like domain-containing 1, androgen receptor, and estrogen receptor in patients with hypospadias. Open Access Maced J Med Sci. 2020;8:543–7.
3. Zhuang L, Bai M, Zhou W, Yu Y, Wang J. MAMLD1 gene mutation in the incidence of hypospadias in the Chinese population. J Med Biochem. 2014;33(4):341–6.
4. Yuri P, Gunadi, Lestari RP, Fardilla FP, Setyaningsih WAW, Arfian N, et al. The impact of COL1A1 and COL6A1 expression on hypospadias and penile curvature severity. BMC Urol. 2020;20(1):1–5.
5. Makovey I, Higuchi TT, Montague DK, Angermeier KW, Wood HM. Congenital penile curvature: update and management. Curr Urol Rep. 2012;13(4):290–7.
6. Atmoko W, Shalmont G, Situmorang GR, Wahyudi I, Tanurahardja B, Rodjani A. Abnormal dartos fascia in buried penis and hypospadias: evidence from histopathology. J Pediatr Urol. 2018;14(6):536.e1-536.e7.
7. Devine CJ, Horton CE. Chordee without hypospadias. J Urol. 1973;110(2):264–71. https://doi.org/10.1016/S0022-5347(17)60183-6.
8. Shen J, Xie Y, Liu Z, Zhang S, Wang Y, Jia L, et al. Increased myocardial stiffness activates cardiac microvascular endothelial cell via VEGF paracrine signaling in cardiac hypertrophy. J Mol Cell Cardiol. 2018;122:140–51. https://doi.org/10.1016/j.yjmcc.2018.08.014.
9. Sfakianaki AK, Buhimschi IA, Ravishankar V, Bahtiyar MO, Dulay AT, Buhimschi CS. Relationships of maternal serum levels of vascular endothelial growth factor and tensile strength properties of the cervix in a rat model of chronic hypoxia. Am J Obs Gynecol. 2008;198(223):e1-7.
10. Leung DW, Cachianes G, Kuang W, Goeddel DV, Ferrara N. Vascular endothelial growth factor is a secreted angiogenic mitogen. Science. 1989;246:4935.
11. Senger DR, Claffey KP, Benes JE, Perruzi CA, Sergiou AP, Detmar M. Angiogenesis promoted by vascular endothelial growth factor: regulation through α1 β1 and α2 β1 integrins. Proc Natl Acad Sci. 1997;94:13612–7.
12. Senger DR, Ledbetter SR, Claffey KP, Papadopoulos-sergiou A. Stimulation of endothelial cell migration by vascular permeability factor / vascular endothelial growth factor through cooperative mechanisms involving the a bf3 integrin. Am J Pathol. 1996;149(1):293–305.
13. Wang S, Li X, Parra M, Verdin E, Bassel-duby R, Olson EN. Control of endothelial cell proliferation and migration by VEGF signaling to histone deacetylase 7. Proc Natl Acad Sci. 2008;105(22):7738–43.
14. Lee S, Jilani SM, Nikolova GV, Carpizo D, Iruela-arispe ML. Processing of VEGF-A by matrix metalloproteinases regulates bioavailability and vascular patterning in tumors. J Cell Biol. 2005;169(4):681–91.
15. Livak KJ, Schmittgen TD. Analysis of relative gene expression data using real-time quantitative PCR and the 2- CT method. Methods. 2001;25:402–8.
16. Koláčná L, Bakešová J, Varga F, Áková E, Plánka L, Necas A, et al. Biochemical and biophysical aspects of collagen nanostructure in the extracellular matrix. Physiol Res. 2007;56:S51-60.
17. Gelse K, Po E, Aigner T. Collagens-structure, function, and biosynthesis. Adv Drug Deliv Rev. 2003;55:1531–46.
18. Ferrara N. Role of vascular endothelial growth factor in regulation of physiological angiogenesis. Am J Physiol Cell Physiol. 2001;280:1358–66.
19. Stroncek JD, Reichert WM. Overview of wound healing in different tissue types. In: Indwelling neural implants. CRC Press, Boca Raton; 2008. 1–37 p.
20. Spinoit AF, Van Praet C, Groen LA, Van Laecke E, Praet M, Hoebeke P. Congenital penile pathology is associated with abnormal development of the dartos muscle: a prospective study of primary penile surgery at a tertiary referral center. J Urol. 2015;193(5):1620–4. https://doi.org/10.1016/j.juro.2014.10.090.
21. Ferrara N. VEGF: an update on biological and therapeutic aspects napoleone ferrara. Curr Opin Biotechnol. 2000;11(6):617–24.
22. Jin M, Andricioaei I, Springer TA. Conversion between three conformational states of integrin i domains with a C-terminal pull spring studied with molecular dynamics. Structure. 2004;12:2137–47.
23. Puig M, Lugo R, Gabasa M, Alicia G, Velasques A. Matrix stiffening and beta1 integrin drive subtype-specific fibroblast accumulation in lung cancer. Mol Cancer Res. 2015;13(1):161–73.
24. Butcher DT, Alliston T, Weaver VM. A tense situation : forcing tumour progression. Nat Rev Cancer. 2009;9(2):108–22.
25. Fan D, Takawale A, Shen M, Samokhvalov V, Basu R, Patel V, et al. A disintegrin and metalloprotease-17 regulates pressure overload-induced myocardial hypertrophy and dysfunction through proteolytic processing of integrin β 1. Hypertention. 2016;68(4):937–48.
26. Israeli-rosenberg S, Manso AM, Okada H, Ross RS, Israeli-rosenberg S, Manso AM, et al. Integrins and integrin-associated proteins in the cardiac myocyte. Circ REs. 2014;114:572–86.
27. Li R, Wu Y, Manso AM, Huang MS, Dalton ND, Peterson KL, et al. β1 integrin gene excision in the adult murine cardiac myocyte causes defective mechanical and signaling responses. AM J Pathol. 2012;180(3):952–62.
28. Lee JS, Yi J-K, An SY, Heo JS. Increased osteogenic differentiation of periodontal ligament stem cells on polydopamine film occurs via activation of integrin and PI3K signaling pathways. Cell Physiol Biochem. 2014;34:1824–34.
29. Bardos JI, Ashcroft M. Negative and positive regulation of HIF-1: a complex network. Biochim Biophys Acta. 2005;1755(2):107–20.
30. Zimna A, Kurpisz M. Hypoxia-inducible factor-1 in physiological and pathophysiological angiogenesis : applications and therapies. Biomed Res Int. 2015;2015:1–13.
31. Barrientos S, Stojadinovic O, Golinko MS, Brem H, Tomic-canic M. Growth factors and cytokines in wound healing. Wound Repair Regen. 2008;16(5):585–560.
32. Wingate K, Floren M, Tan Y, Ou P, Tseng N, Tan W. Synergism of matrix stiffness and vascular endothelial growth factor on mesenchymal stem cells for vascular endothelial regeneration. Tissue Eng Part A. 2014;20(17–18):2503–12.

2

The Resonance and the Allium ureteral stents in the treatment of non-malignant refractory ureterostenosis

Wei Gao, Tianying Xing and Tongwen Ou*

Abstract

Background: Refractory non-malignant ureterostenosis is challenging to treat. The experience to treat the stenosis primarily cause by retroperitoneal fibrosis with the Resonance and Allium metallic stent is still limited. We aim to evaluate the efficacy and safety of these two stents and provide alternative treatment options.

Methods: A retrospective study was conducted for patients with non-malignant ureterostenosis and treated with the Resonance and Allium stents from March 2011 to September 2020 in our department. The efficacy was evaluated by the change of serum creatinine, glomerular filtration rate (GFR), the proportion of GFR of the affected side and hydronephrosis grade. The safety was evaluated by postoperative presence of moderate or severe overactive bladder (OAB), recurrent urinary infection, pain, stent displacement, encrustation and re-obstruction.

Results: 33 patients were eligible for the study, including 18 cases treated by the Resonance stents and 15 patients treated by the Allium stents. The patients of two groups had similar age and gender proportion. The cause of ureterostenosis was mainly retroperitoneal fibrosis in both groups but the Resonance group had more idiopathic cases. Follow-up time was significantly longer in the Resonance group than the Allium group (36.2 ± 24.0 vs 9.4 ± 5.0 months, $p < 0.001$). Both groups showed improvement or maintenance of serum creatinine level, GFR, the GFR proportion of the affected side and hydronephrosis grade after treatment. The Resonance group presented significant higher incidence of moderate or severe OAB, recurrent urinary infection and pain, while the Allium group showed significant more cases of re-obstruction.

Conclusion: Both the Resonance and Allium stent can relieve the non-malignant refractory ureterostenosis effectively. The Resonance stent may cause more irritable symptoms while the Allium stent may have a higher rate of re-obstruction. The long term efficacy and safety of the Allium stent in treating non-malignant refractory ureterostenosis requires further study.

Keywords: Ureterostenosis, Retroperitoneal fibrosis, Resonance stent, Allium stent, Efficacy, Safety

Introduction

A ureteral stent can drain the upper urinary tract and preserve kidney function, thereby providing time for further treatment and improving the patient's quality of life. However, the conventional plastic or polymeric stents may become occluded after several months and require frequent change. Importantly, a typical plastic or polymeric ureteral stent often fail to relieve the hydronephrosis and provide insufficient resistance to the traction displacement of the ureter secondary to some refractory conditions, such as primary or metastatic retroperitoneal

*Correspondence: outongwen@sohu.com
Department of Urology, Xuanwu Hospital, Capital Medical University, Beijing 100053, China

malignancies [1]. Thus, metallic ureteral stents are widely used.

Currently, there are two common types of commercial metallic stents: the Resonance Metallic Ureteral Stent and Allium Ureteral Stent. The Resonance stent has potent tensile strength and provides good drainage. In addition, it is resistant to extrinsic compression and occlusion. These properties allow longer dwelling time and less frequent stent exchanges. Thus, this stent provided a long-term renal protective effect and might be more cost-effective [2]. Allium stent is a self-expanding stent made of a super elastic nitinol skeleton and with biocompatible polymeric cover. The metal component provides radial and longitudinal strength, while the polymer bio-inertness prevents tissue ingrowth into the lumen and early encrustation. Both two stents have shown good efficacy in treating malignant ureteral strictures [3, 4].

Several benign disorders may cause refractory ureteral obstruction, including idiopathic retroperitoneal fibrosis (IRPF) and secondary retroperitoneal fibrosis (SRPF), iatrogenic injury during ureteral lithotripsy. Retroperitoneal fibrosis is rare and characterized by extensive fibrosis and inflammation in the retroperitoneal region, frequently causing extrinsic compression of the ureter. Ureterolysis and nephrostomy are the treatment options, but they may be time-consuming, risky and impact quality of life [5, 6]; less invasive but effective treatment ways are in urgent need. Meanwhile, traditional stents may fail to relieve the obstruction because of insufficient strength. Although metallic stents are suitable for malignant obstruction, their efficacy and safety for the treatment of non-malignant ureteral strictures still needs further evaluation. Thus, we reviewed patients with non-malignant ureterostenosis (primarily retroperitoneal fibrosis) treated by Resonance and Allium, and compared the efficacy and safety of the two different groups.

Methods

Study design

A retrospective study was conducted in patients with non-malignant cause of ureterostenosis treated by Resonance or Allium stent from March 2011 to September 2020 at Department of Urology, Xuanwu Hospital, Capital Medical University, Beijing, PR China. Inclusion criteria included 1. patients underwent traditional stents placement due to non-malignant ureteral stenosis but still had aggravated hydronephrosis or worse renal function; 2. Resonance (COOK, Bloomington, IN, USA) or Allium (Allium, Caesarea, Israel) stent was placed; 3. the placement of stents was performed by a single surgeon (Gao). Since radiotherapy in the corresponding area may cause urethral stricture in patients with history of malignancy, and the stricture is caused by SRPF secondary to radiation but not the malignancy itself, these patients were also included in the study if they have no evidence of tumor recurrence. Exclusion criteria included 1. patients with malignant tumors history who had radiation-caused SRPF ureteral stricture but showed evidence of recurrence or required further chemotherapy or radiotherapy; 2. patients with nephrostomy; 3. intraoperative placement failure and subsequent replacement with a different type of stent. This research was approved by the Ethics Committee of Xuanwu Hospital, Capital Medical University and conducted in accordance with the declaration of Helsinki. Each patient provided informed consent.

Clinical practice

Before each operation, the patient underwent routine preoperative evaluation, including urine analysis, serum creatinine, abdominal Computed Tomography (CT) scan to evaluate hydronephrosis and renography (using Tc-99m-DTPA as the tracer) to evaluate glomerular filtration rate (GFR). Intraoperative placement of ureteral stents was usually under fluoroscopic guidance. For Resonance stents, 24 cm ones were chosen for patients shorter than 165 cm, 26 cm for patients between 165 and 175 cm, and 28 cm for patients taller than 175 cm, mostly referring to the previous literature but adjust for Asian population [7]. For Allium stents, the length and perimeter of the stent were selected according to the length and degree of the stenosis assessed by imaging. The availability of Allium stent was much later than the Resonance stent. When both stents were available and alternative, the use of the stent was mainly according to the patient's selection after considering the potential benefit, side effects and cost. On the first day after surgery, X-rays were used in the postoperative settings to confirm placement. Follow-up was conducted postoperatively at 1 month, 3 month and 6 months and 1 year (with time range due to patients' compliance), and the patient underwent urine analysis, blood creatinine, abdominal CT scan and renogram. For patients with good response and tolerance, the Resonance stents were replaced yearly.

Efficacy and safety evaluation

For efficacy evaluation, blood creatinine, GFR and hydronephrosis grade at last follow up were compared with their preoperative values. Hydronephrosis grade was divided into 5 grades (0–IV) according to the CT images [8]. For safety evaluation, presence of recurrent urinary tract infection, moderate or severe overactive bladder symptom and flank pain were documented. Recurrent urinary infection was defined as 2 times urinary infection in the past 6 months and 3 times in the past year. Moderate or severe overactive bladder symptom was evaluated by Overactive Bladder Symptom Score (OABSS) with score equal or greater than 6. Also, complications discovered by CT images was recorded, including stent displacement, encrustation around the stent and re-obstruction.

Statistical analysis

Continuous variables were described as mean ± standard deviation, and categorical variables was described as frequency or median. For patients' demographics, the difference between the Resonance and Allium groups were examined by student *t* test for continuous variables, and Fisher's exact test or Mann–Whitney U test were used for categorical variables. Paired t test or Mann–Whitney U test were used to examine the changes of efficacy parameters before and after treatment in each group. Fisher's exact test was used to compare safety parameters. All tests were two-sided. *P* value < 0.05 was regarded as statistically different. SPSS 22.0. software was used for all statistical analysis.

Results

Patient demographics

We reviewed 128 patients who were treated with metallic ureteral stents for ureteral strictures during the study period. 33 of them met the inclusion criteria. Patient demographics were summarized in Table 1.

Table 1 Patients demographics

	Resonance stent	Allium stent	*P* value
Number of patients	18	15	
Age (years)	55.7 ± 13.4	52.5 ± 12.5	0.487
Gender			
Male	12	9	0.731
Female	6	6	
Follow-up time (months)	36.2 ± 24.0	9.4 ± 5.0	< 0.001
Causes of stenosis			
IRPF	14	5	0.013
SRPF	4	6	
Ureteroscope lithotripsy	0	4	

IRPF idiopathic retroperitoneal fibrosis, *SRPF* secondary retroperitoneal fibrosis

Among the patients, 18 cases received the Resonance stents, and 15 patients received the Allium stents. The mean age and gender proportion of the two groups did not show significant difference. The treatment duration was 36.2 ± 24.0 months for the Resonance group, which was significantly longer than 9.4 ± 5.0 months for the Allium group. The cause of ureterostenosis included IRPF, SRPF (after radiotherapy) and ureteroscope lithotripsy. But the proportion of each cause was significantly different between the two groups: the Resonance group had more IRPF patients, while obstruction secondary to ureteroscope lithotripsy only existed in the Allium group.

Efficacy and safety

Efficacy was evaluated by comparison of serum creatinine, GFR, GFR proportion of the affected side and hydronephrosis grade before operation and at last follow-up (Table 2). Both groups showed improved creatinine level and GFR, although they did not reach significant difference. The GFR proportion of the affected side increased in the Resonance group, but dropped minimally in the Allium group. The level of hydronephrosis relieved significantly in both groups. In general, Both the Resonance and the Allium group showed good efficacy to protect renal function and relieve hydronephrosis. However, Allium stents showed short term good efficacy as the follow-up time was significantly shorter in the Allium group.

For the safety parameter, regarding to the patients' complaint, the Resonance group showed a higher frequency of the presence of moderate to severe OAB, recurrent urinary infection and pain than the Allium group (all $p < 0.05$). Via CT scan, the Allium group revealed significant higher rate of re-obstruction and more cases of displacement. However, encrustation was more common in the Resonance group, but did not show significant difference (Table 3).

Table 2 Efficacy evaluation of the Resonance and Allium stent

	Resonance stent			Allium stent		
	Preoperative	Postoperative	*P* value	Preoperative	Postoperative	*P* value
Serum creatinine (μmol/L)	213.7 ± 268.8	89.8 ± 22.3	0.065	96.3 ± 52.8	84.3 ± 27.6	0.349
GFR (ml/min)	28.4 ± 15.1	30.4 ± 13.7	0.422	33.0 ± 15.8	35.3 ± 15.7	0.414
Affected side GFR proportion[a] (%)	49.0 ± 24.5	50.5 ± 25.6	0.455	44.7 ± 16.1	44.1 ± 17.1	0.693
Hydronephrosis grade (median)	3	2	0.004	2	1	0.001

[a] Affected side GFR proportion calculated as affected side GFR/affected side GFR + contralateral GFR

Table 3 Safety evaluation of the Resonance and Allium stent

	Resonance stent	Allium stent	*P* values
Moderate to severe OAB	7	0	0.009
Recurrent urinary tract infection	7	1	0.046
Pain	7	1	0.038
Displacement	1	4	0.152
Encrustation	11	1	0.255
Reobstruction	0	5	0.013

OAB overactive bladder

Discussion

Compared with the ureteral obstruction caused by extrinsic compression of malignancies, non-malignant refractory ureterostenosis is rarer. It is challenging for urologists not only because of deteriorating renal function but also difficulty in choosing the appropriate treatment plan for the individual. Traditional silicone or plastic ureteral stents are most commonly used and cost-effective. Despite their advantages, they have shown a relatively high failure rate when used to treat some chronic ureteral stenosis, especially in patients with retroperitoneal fibrosis or iatrogenic injury. In our study, we reviewed patients treated by the Resonance or the Allium metallic stents for ureterostenosis caused by non-malignant reasons (primarily retroperitoneal fibrosis). Both two types of stents showed good efficacy to protect renal function from deterioration. The Resonance stents caused more irritative complications while the Allium stent had higher frequency of displacement and re-obstruction.

The majority of our cases were retroperitoneal fibrosis, including 18 IRPF and 11 SRPF. IRPF is related to autoimmune diseases and characterized by chronic non-specific inflammation of the tissues around the retroperitoneal aorta with progressive hyperplasia of fibrous tissue. The factors of SRPF include drug side effects, infection, trauma, dissection, radiation therapy, malignant tumors [9–12]. Fibrous tissue surrounds and compresses its adjacent structure with the ureters involved especially. In our study, IRPF cases were diagnosed by rheumatologists, and SRPF cases were caused by radiotherapy. Although SRPF patients had history of cancer, most of them underwent 18F-FDG-Positron Emission Tomography to rule out malignant ureteral obstruction, reinforcing the accuracy of SRPF diagnosis [13]. Although percutaneous nephrostomy or ureterolysis can drain the upper urinary tract and relieve the stenosis, it reduces the patients' quality of life or confronts great operative difficulty. Metallic stents become promising ways to treat RPF in some refractory cases.

The Resonance metal stent has a special coil structure and alloy composition, making it resistant to external compression and the ingrowth of proliferative tissue. The usage of Resonance metal stents has been reported in patients with benign ureteral stenosis primarily due to ureteropelvic junction obstruction or benign stricture, showing good drainage and good tolerance in most of the patients [14–17]. Benson et al. reported no stent failure in 15 patients with benign obstruction after a median follow-up time of 14 months. López-Huertas et al. [16] reported that the Resonance stents succeeded in 92% of the patients with benign obstruction. Both of these studies included 1 case of IRPF without stent failure. The Allium stent is a self-expanding, large-caliber ureteral stent to treat benign or malignant ureteral stenosis. It displayed good efficacy in some benign conditions like post ureteroscope lithotripsy stricture. Moskovitz used Allium stents to treat benign urinary stricture after endoscopic lithotripsy, urinary diversion and renal transplant. All stents were patent except from 1 case of endoscopic ureteral lithotripsy after 11 months [18]. The data regarding to RPF was still lacking. Our study compared the efficacy of the Resonance and the Allium stents in benign cases, primarily RPF. The result was favorable in protecting the renal function and reliving the hydronephrosis. This was expectable as both the two stents had greater tensile strength than traditional stents. Although the creatinine level and GFR did not increased significantly, both stents could improve the renal function or protect renal function from deteriorating. However, besides the successful cases in our study, we also experience 2 intraoperative failure when placing the Allium stents for two SRPF patients. The stent distorted and failed to dilate the stricture after self-expansion. This had not happened for the Resonance stent yet, suggesting the Resonance had more intensity against foreign force and were more suitable in severe ischemic fibrosis stenosis conditions secondary to radiation.

During follow-up, the Allium group showed 4 cases of displacement, accounting for 26% of the group cases. Among them, 2 cases were SRPF, 1 case was IRPF, and 1 case was post-lithotripsy stenosis. 2 of 4 patients received replacement of the thicker Allium stents; 1 patient received the Resonance stent replacement; 1 patient received observation. The rate was higher than previous literature, where 7 out of 49 (14.2%) stents migrated [18]. Meanwhile, only 1 patient with the Resonance stent had migration, but not necessary for intervention.

Stent occlusion was not rare for both the two types of stents. Moskovitz el at reported 1 occlusion case out of 49 Allium stent placements. Lopez et al. showed a high success rate of the Resonance stent in treating benign ureteral obstruction, with only 1 failed case because of the extremely tortuous ureter. Wang et al. reported a higher re-obstruction rate (22.7%) of the Resonance stent, but the failure mainly happened in the malignant cases with radiotherapy history. In our study, the Allium group had significant higher rate of postoperative re-obstruction, mostly in SRPF cases. Thus, close follow-up is necessary to discover the position changes or occlusion especially after the Allium stent placement. And the Resonance stents might be a safer choice for SRPF secondary to radiotherapy. During follow-up of RPF cases, images like plain X-ray help to understand whether the ureters and the stents are shifted to the midline and to decide whether to replace or remove the stents.

Irritable lower urinary tract symptoms are common complications of indwelling catheters. Likewise, moderate to severe OAB happened frequently in the Resonance group but not the Allium group. Some patients even requested to remove the Resonance stent due to disturbing OAB. Also, patients with the Resonance stents had significantly higher chance of recurrent urinary infection. On the contrary, the Allium stents were well tolerated. Those patients who had the Resonance stent withdrawn and replaced by the Allium stent were also satisfied with the relief of irritable symptoms. The Resonance stent is a full ureteral stent which is connected from the renal pelvis to the bladder, which may impair the peristaltic function of the ureter and leaves a "foreign body" inside the bladder. The Allium stent is segmental and only expands the narrowed ureter without affecting the peristalsis of other segments of the ureter. These reasons might contribute to the higher frequency of irritation and infection in the Resonance group. Although more patients with the Resonance stents had encrustation formed on the bladder and lower ureteral stents, the blood creatinine, GFR and CT images showed no signs of aggravated obstruction.

Some researcher proposed that metal stents are not suitable for benign ureteral obstruction, especially when ureteral stricture was caused by proliferation into the ureteral lumen. Careful selection of suitable cases before surgery and close follow-up after surgery are critical to the success of metal stent implantation [7]. In our study, there were 4 patients with refractory stenosis after ureterolithiasis surgery. The problem was completely solved by inserting Allium stent because the structure of the stent is a metal stent with double layers of polymer attached to the inside and outside of the metal mesh stent. The hydrophilic walls prevent the problem of the proliferation into the ureteral lumen. Also, according to our early experience, we placed tandem ureteral stents (TUS) in 3 patients with RPF but all stents failed at 3-month follow-up. Although studies showed TUS had good efficacy in benign conditions like ureteral stricture or severe stone disease [19], their efficacy in treating refractory cases with RPF needs further study.

In summary, both the Resonance and Allium stents could effectively protect the renal function. The Resonance stents showed higher frequency of irritable symptoms, while the Allium stents had more possibility of re-obstruction. The main limitation of the study is it small samples, mostly due to the rarity of non-malignant ureterostenosis like RPF. To evaluate the quality of life with ureteral stents, Ureteral Stent Symptom Questionnaire should be the most proper method. But we did not apply this questionnaire as it was not valid in the Chinese language at the early study period. Also, because the Resonance stents were introduced much earlier in our hospital, the follow-up time of the Resonance group was significantly longer than the Allium group. This bought bias to our study as the long-time efficacy and safety of the Allium stents were not possible to evaluate. For the same reason, more patients with IRPF were treated with the Resonance stents especially at the early stage of the study period. This bought bias to the disease consistency at baseline. The long-time efficacy and safely of the Allium stents to treat non-malignant ureterostenosis needs further study.

Conclusion

Both the Resonance metallic stent and Allium stent can be applied to treat non-malignant refractory ureterostenosis with good efficacy and safety. However, the Resonance stent causes more irritative complications, and the Allium stent has higher possibility of re-obstruction. The efficacy and safety of the Allium stent still requires long term close follow-up.

Abbreviations

IRPF: Idiopathic retroperitoneal fibrosis; SRPF: Secondary retroperitoneal fibrosis; CT: Computed tomography; GFR: Glomerular filtration rate; OAB: Overactive bladder; OABSS: Overactive bladder symptom score; TUS: Tandem ureteral stents.

Acknowledgements

Not applicable.

Authors' contributions

Gao performed all the operations, followed up the patients, analyzed the data and wrote the manuscript. Xing revised the manuscript. Ou checked the data and revised the manuscript. All authors read and approved the final manuscript.

Competing interests

The authors declare that they have no competing interests.

References

1. Christman MS, L'esperance JO, Choe CH, Stroup SP, Auge BK. Analysis of ureteral stent compression force and its role in malignant obstruction. J Urol. 2009;181(1):392–6.

2. Blaschko SD, Deane LA, Alfred Krebs BSF, et al. In-vivo evaluation of flow characteristics of novel metal ureteral stent. J Endourol. 2007;21:780–4.
3. Christman MS, L'esperance JO, Choe CH, et al. Analysis of ureteral stent compression force and its role in malignant obstruction. J Urol. 2009;181:392–6.
4. Oderda M, Lacquaniti S, Fasolis G. Allium stent for the treatment of a malignant ureteral stenosis: a paradigmatic case. Urologia. 2018;85(2):87–90.
5. Duchene DA, Winfield HN, Cadeddu JA, Clayman RV, Gomella LG, Kavoussi LR, Mikhail AA, Park S, Permpongkosol S, Shalhav AL. Multi-institutional survey of laparoscopic ureterolysis for retroperitoneal fibrosis. Urology. 2007;69(6):1017–21.
6. Stifelman MD, Shah O, Mufarrij P, Lipkin M. Minimally invasive management of retroperitoneal fibrosis. Urology. 2008;71(2):201–4.
7. Liatsikos E, Kallidonis P, Kyriazis I, et al. Ureteral obstruction: is the full metallic double-pigtail stent the way to go? Eur Urol. 2010;57:480–7.
8. Ito Y, Kikuchi E, Tanaka N, Miyajima A, Mikami S, Jinzaki M, Oya M. Preoperative hydronephrosis grade independently predicts worse pathological outcomes in patients undergoing nephroureterectomy for upper tract urothelial carcinoma. J Urol. 2011;185(5):1621–6.
9. Vaglio A, Salvarani C, Buzio C. Retroperitoneal fibrosis. Lancet. 2006;367(9506):241–51.
10. Vaglio A, Maritati F. Idiopathic retroperitoneal fibrosis. J Am Soc Nephrol. 2016;27(7):1880–9.
11. Oshiro H, Ebihara Y, Serizawa H, et al. Idiopathic retroperitoneal fibrosis associated with immunohematological abnormalities. Am J Med. 2005;118(7):782–6.
12. Neild GH, Rodriguez-Justo M, Wall C, Connolly JO. Hyper-IgG4 disease: report and characterisation of a new disease. BMC Med. 2006;6(4):23.
13. Fernando A, Pattison J, Horsfield C, D'Cruz D, Cook G, O'Brien T. [^{18}F]-fluorodeoxyglucose positron emission tomography in the diagnosis, treatment stratification, and monitoring of patients with retroperitoneal fibrosis: a prospective clinical study. Eur Urol. 2017;71(6):926–33.
14. Benson AD, Taylor ER, Schwartz BF. Metal ureteral stent for benign and malignant ureteral obstruction. J Urol. 2011;185:2217–22.
15. Polcari AJ, Hugen CM, López-Huertas HL, et al. Cost analysis and clinical applicability of the resonance metallic ureteral stent. Expert Rev Pharmacoecon Outcomes Res. 2010;10:11–5.
16. López-Huertas HL, Polcari AJ, Acosta-Miranda A, et al. Metallic ureteral stents: a cost-effective method of managing benign upper tract obstruction. J Endourol. 2010;24:483–5.
17. Wang HJ, Lee TY, Luo HL, et al. Application of resonance metallic stents for ureteral obstruction. BJU Int. 2011;108(3):428–32.
18. Moskovitz B, Halachmi S, Nativ O. A new self-expanding, large-caliber ureteral stent: results of a multicenter experience. J Endourol. 2012;26(11):1523–7.
19. Elsamra SE, Motato H, Moreira DM, et al. Tandem ureteral stents for the decompression of malignant and benign obstructive uropathy. J Endourol. 2013;27(10):1297–302.

3

Feasibility, technique and accuracy of ultrasound-guided transurethral injections into the urinary sphincter of female cadavers: Proof of concept

Florian A. Schmid[1], Dominic Gascho[2], Niklaus Zoelch[2], Jenny A. Prange[1], Giovanni Colacicco[3] and Daniel Eberli[1]*

Abstract

Background: The injection of muscle precursor cells (MPC) into the external urinary sphincter muscle (EUS) is a promising therapeutic option for regenerative treatment of stress urinary incontinence (SUI). The objective of the present project was to conduct a pre-clinical trial to investigate the feasibility and accuracy of ultrasound (US) guided, transurethral injections into the EUS of female cadavers.

Methods: This is a prospective, anatomical, interventional and radiological cadaveric laboratory investigation. Two urologists performed transurethral US-guided injections to deliver nano-iron particles into the EUS. The intervention was performed in three unfixed, fresh female cadavers. Each cadaver received MRI before and CT as well as MRI of the pelvis after the injections.

Results: The precision and accumulation of nano-iron particles in the EUS was compared using a rating scale to evaluate left versus right and anterior versus posterior distribution in axial and sagittal orientation with US, MRI and CT. The accuracy of our US-guided injections into the anterior target region yielded 4 points on the rating scale. Adequate precision and accumulation of particles in the left versus right EUS were also demonstrated (3 vs. 3.33 points, respectively). Signal intensity in MRI revealed a mean ratio of 0.33 before and after injection. CT scans showed no relevant artefacts impairing the assessment.

Conclusion: US-guided, transurethral injection into the EUS is feasible and imaging reveals a precise accumulation in the target region. Our method provides an appropriate approach to deliver MPC in the EUS muscle for a regenerative treatment of SUI in the near future.

Keywords: Transurethral injection, Urinary sphincter, Ultrasound-guided, MRI, Female

Background

Stress Urinary Incontinence (SUI) is a disease affecting almost 200 million people worldwide and is twice as common in women as in men [1]. The quality of life in these patients is markedly decreased due to reduced activity, unpleasant sensation and odor as well as recurrent urinary tract infections caused by wet pads [2, 3]. Several therapeutic options exist in the treatment of SUI: Besides physiotherapy of the lower pelvis, various medical, mechanical and surgical approaches can be discussed with the patients [4–8]. However, all of these therapies have limitations and new solutions with long-term effects are needed. The regenerative approach, administering

*Correspondence: daniel.eberli@usz.ch
[1] Department of Urology, University Hospital of Zurich, University of Zurich, Frauenklinikstrasse 10, 8091 Zurich, Switzerland
Full list of author information is available at the end of the article

muscle precursor cells (MPC), is a promising new strategy to strengthen the external urinary sphincter muscle (EUS) in a sustainable manner in patients with SUI [9–11]. Pursuing the ultimate goal of treating the cause rather than the symptom was already convincing in the animal model, and the translation of this therapy into humans demonstrated first promising results in the past [12, 13]. However, particularly the precise deliverance of MPCs into the target region is a challenging endeavor. Stem cells are highly influenced by the microenvironment and therefore an accurate injection into the external EUS is required. The aim of the present study was to prove the feasibility and precision of a new ultrasound (US) guided transurethral injection technique into the EUS.

Methods

In this prospective, anatomical, interventional and radiological cadaveric laboratory investigation, we included three unfixed, fresh female cadavers for research purposes between May 2019 and January 2020. As initial baseline investigation, a radiological technologist performed magnetic resonance imaging (MRI) of the lower pelvis at the Institute of Forensic Medicine shortly after arrival of the cadaver. Before, the cadaveric bodies were stored at 4 °C for a maximum of 72 h. After imaging, we transported the bodies to the "Skills Laboratory" of the Institute of Anatomy and put them into lithotomy position. The lower pelvis was investigated by initial vaginal US carried out by two urologists, performing a 3D block of the lower pelvis. This allowed the identification of important anatomical landmarks and the location of the EUS in mid-urethral position as a hypoechoic structure. The next step was the insertion of a transurethral indwelling bladder catheter (12 French) and the filling of the catheter balloon with 10 ml (ml) of saline solution. Further, a urethral therapy (stainless steel) shaft was attached to the catheter outside of the urethral meatus. After filling of the bladder with 100 ml of saline solution, we attached a Kochers' clamp at the rear of the catheter to prevent outflow. Further, this assured fixation of the catheter balloon at the bladder neck as an anatomical reference structure. We then reassured a good position of the vaginal US probe and double-checked image quality. Thereafter, the urethral therapy shaft was inserted into the urethral meatus in Seldinger technique along the transurethral catheter until mid-urethral position and then linked to the vaginal ultrasound probe. This led to a signal loss in the distal part of the US image. After bringing in a puncture cannula through the therapy shaft, the tip of the needle was identified in the target region at 12 o'clock position. The needle was then adapted to a syringe with a cooled solution of 4 ml nano-iron particles (Endorem®, Guerbet AG, dextran-coated SPIO nanoparticles, size distribution 120–180 nm, iron-content 11.2 mg/ml), that was transported to the facility of the Anatomical Institute in a refrigerated box. For the injection in cadaver 1, the nano iron-particles were used in the above-mentioned, original dosage. Due to a massive extinction signal in cadaver 1 (Additional file 1: Appendix, Figs. 4 and 5), we diluted the particles in a 1:100 manner with saline solution for cadavers 2–3 (Additional file 1: Appendix, Figs. 4 and 5). Further, the nano-iron particles were mixed with a collagen solution. Collagen changes its viscosity with increasing temperature and turns into a jelly composition. Therefore, an out- or backflow of the injection mixture through the puncture canal can be minimized in living humans. However, because the cadavers had to be stored in the fridge at 4 °C, this effect was only minimal. We started with the first injection at the 12 o'clock position and changed the angle gradually to the right or to the left for each of the subsequent injections. It was our intention to focus mainly on anterior injection, since the EUS has an inverse "horseshoe" configuration. At the end of the procedure, all of the instruments were removed. Back at the Institute of Forensic Medicine, each of the female corpses received a second MRI of the pelvis in order to compare the acquired images to those before the injection. Further, a computer tomography (CT) examination was performed to exclude artefacts in the region of interest, such as the presence of air bubbles caused by the injection. Air bubbles would alter the signal-intensity (SI) in MRI, whereas the quality of evaluation would be limited.

MRI and CT scanning protocol

The MRI examination was performed using a 3 T MRI unit (Achieva 3.0 TX, Philips Medical System, Best, The Netherlands) and a 16 elements phased-array SENSE XL Torso coil. The scan protocol included a T1-weighted turbo-spin-echo (TSE) sequence (orientation: transversal; TR: 578 ms; TE: 6.8 ms; acquisition voxel size [mm]: $0.7 \times 0.7 \times 2.5$), T2-weighted TSE sequences (orientation: transversal/coronal/sagittal; TR: 3765/3464/1958 ms; TE: 60 ms; acquisition voxel size [mm]: $0.8 \times 0.8 \times 2.5$), and T2*-(susceptibility-) weighted fast-field-echo (FFE) sequences (orientation: transversal/coronal; TR: 1117 ms; TE: 16 ms; acquisition voxel size [mm]: $0.9 \times 1.2 \times 2.5$). The same MRI scanning protocol was used before and after the injection of the nano-iron particles.

The CT scans were performed using a 128-slice CT (SOMATOM Definition Flash, Siemens Healthcare, Forchheim, Germany). First, a CT scan over the entire pelvis was performed. The scan parameters were 120 kVp, 800 mAs, and a pitch of 0.35. The raw data were reconstructed using a slice thickness of 0.6 with a hard kernel (B60) and a soft kernel (B30). Second, a high-resolution

CT over the region of the sphincter was performed using 120 kVp, 330 mAs, and a pitch of 0.35. Reconstructions were calculated using small field-of-view (50 × 50 mm; pixel spacing (in-plane voxel): 0.098 mm) with a slice thickness of 0.4 mm and a hard kernel (U70) [14].

Evaluation of imaging

Baseline MRI and an US 3D-block of the lower pelvis assessed the status quo and the exact anatomy before injection (Fig. 1a, b). US was then used as guidance and documentation of the whole injection procedure (Figs. 1c, d, 2a). The MRI and the additional CT scan after the injections were performed for the analysis of injection precision (Fig. 2b–d). With three different imaging modalities (US, MRI and CT), we were able to compare injection accuracy in an objective and qualitative way. We rated the precision of our injections according to a rating scale from 1–4 points: 1 = center (diameter/distance = 5 mm), 2 = inner ring/line (diameter/distance = 10 mm), 3 = middle ring/line (diameter/distance = 15 mm), 4 = outer ring/line (diameter/distance > 15 mm). For the evaluation, images were divided into left/right in axial as well as anterior/posterior in sagittal orientation (Fig. 2c, d). With this scoring system, the accuracy of injections through imaging was evaluated by the consensus of two independent raters (radiological

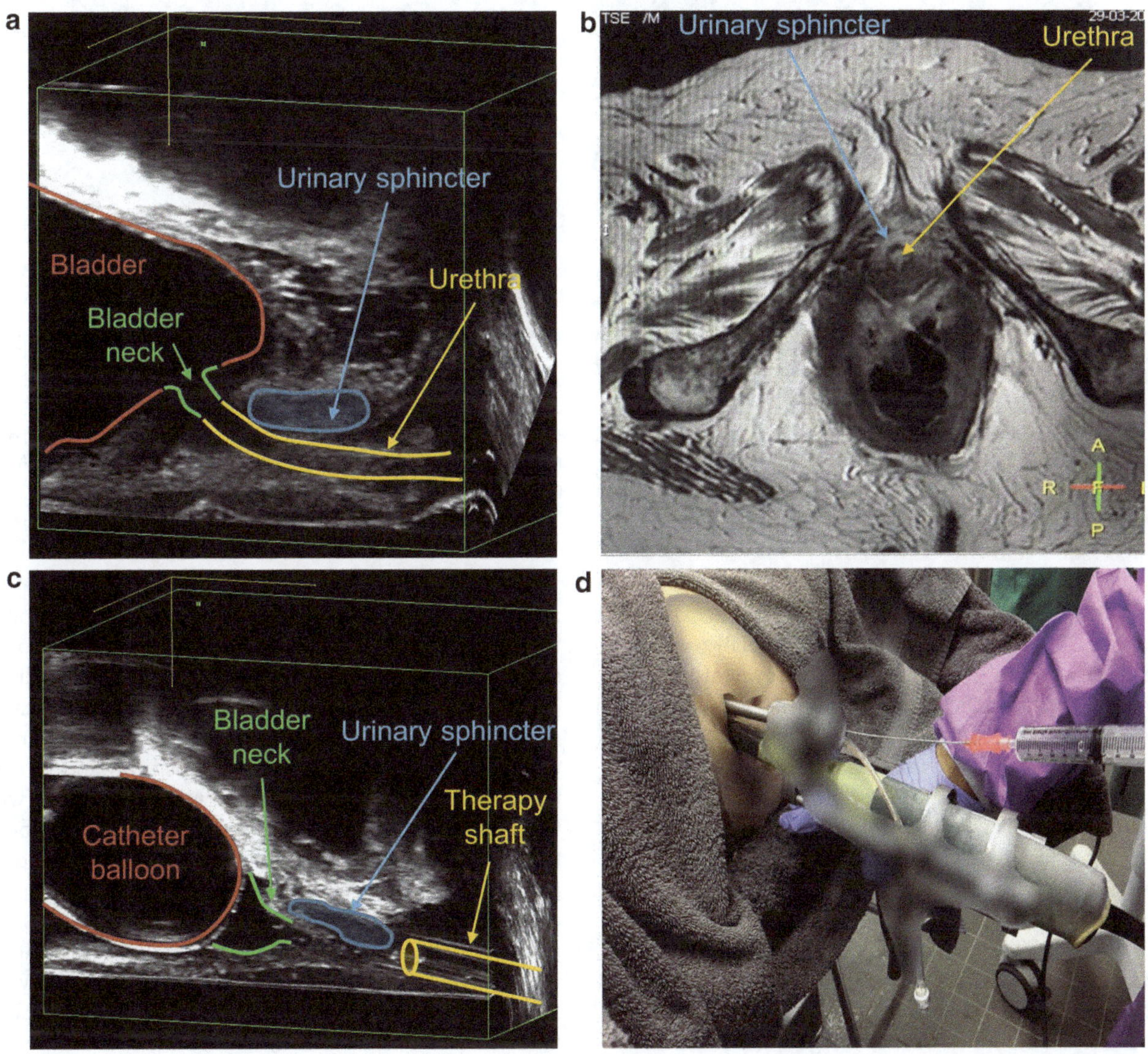

Fig. 1 **a** Anatomy of the lower female pelvis in 3D US with transversal view and **b** MRI T2 sequence in axial view. **c** Setting before transurethral injection of nano-iron particles. Extracorporeal setup, where vaginal US probe and urethral therapy shaft are linked together. **d** Needle puncture and injection are performed through the therapy shaft

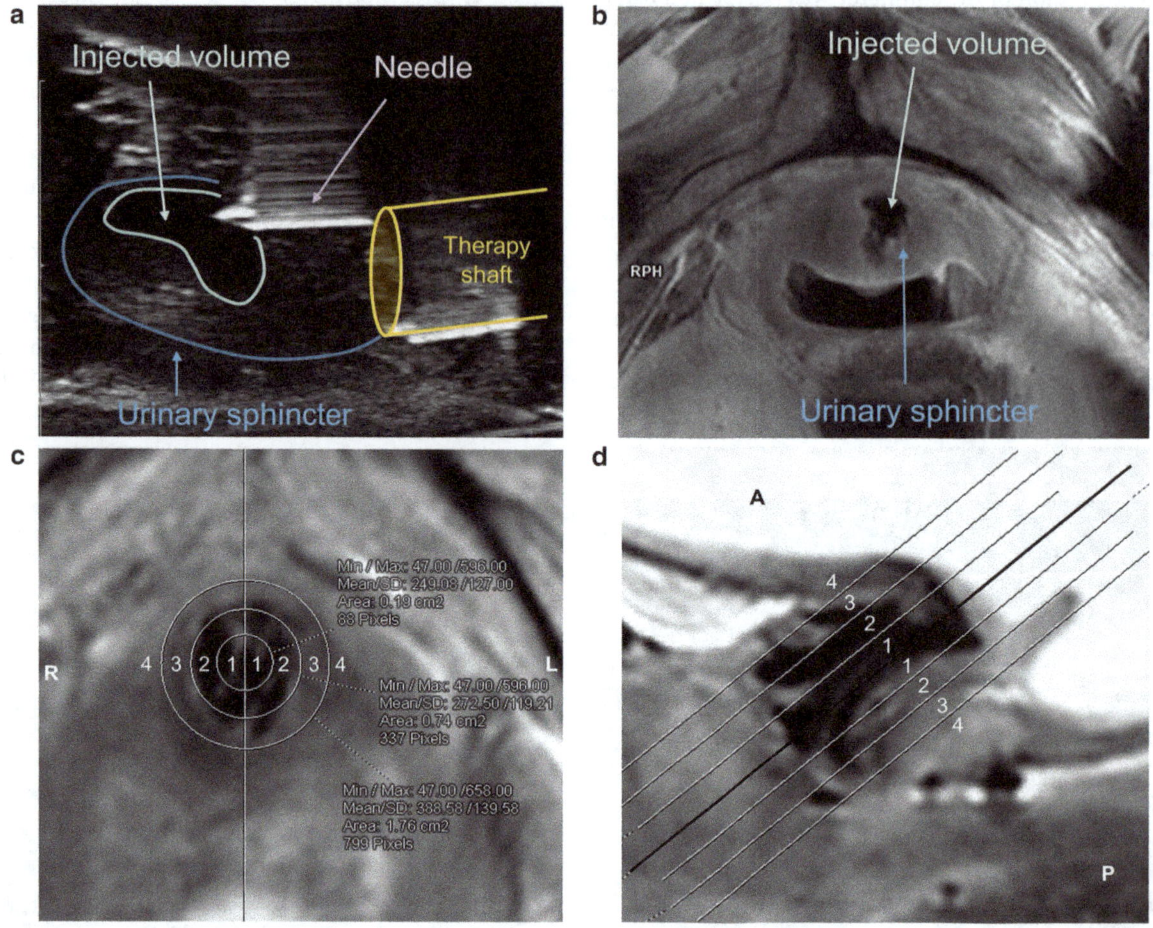

Fig. 2 **a** US image in sagittal orientation during transurethral injection. **b** MRI image in axial orientation after injection of nano-iron particles. **c, d** Scoring of injection defined on a rating scale from 1 to 4 points according to extinction signal of injected iron nano-particles in MRI images. **c** Axial orientation with division into right and left, **d** sagittal orientation with division into anterior and posterior. Diameter and distances in (**a**) and (**b**), respectively: 1 = 5 mm, 2 = 10 mm, 3 = 15 mm, 4 > 15 mm

technologist and urologist). The cumulative extinction signal in both orientations (sagittal and axial) was calculated as 3D-volumes. Additionally, we evaluated signal-intensity changes in MRI: According to signal-intensity curves (Fig. 3a, b, Additional file 1: Appendix Figs. 6 and 7), the ratio before and after injection of diluted nano-iron particles was calculated for the EUS region. To do so, standard protocols were used.

Results

In each of the cadavers, all three imaging modalities—US, MRI and CT—were applied. In MRI, we have qualitatively evaluated the sharpness and details of the images for the inspection and extension of small muscle structures, such as the EUS muscle. Image quality was evenly distributed among all of the cadavers, except for artefacts in cadaver 2 due to bilateral hip prosthesis. However, these artifacts did not impede measurements on the rating sale; thus, this cadaver was not excluded. Further, the fixation of an US-probe to the therapy shaft and the subsequent imaging quality was of relevance and did not differ among cadavers. Additionally, it was important to evaluate the impact of ventral artefacts after inserting the urethral therapy shaft (metal composition) and to assess whether the needle could still be tracked precisely, which was the case in all three interventions. As described in the methods section, our injectable solution of nano-iron particles and collagen needed to be diluted with saline after the first procedure, due to strong extinction signals in cadaver 1 (Additional file 1: Appendix, Figs. 4 and 5). However, since the center of the extinction signal was in the right anatomical location, cadaver 1 was not excluded from the analysis. In total, the MRI revealed the location of our injections precisely at intended mid-urethral and anterior position (Additional file 1: Appendix, Figs. 4 and 5). CT scans additionally assured the absence of air

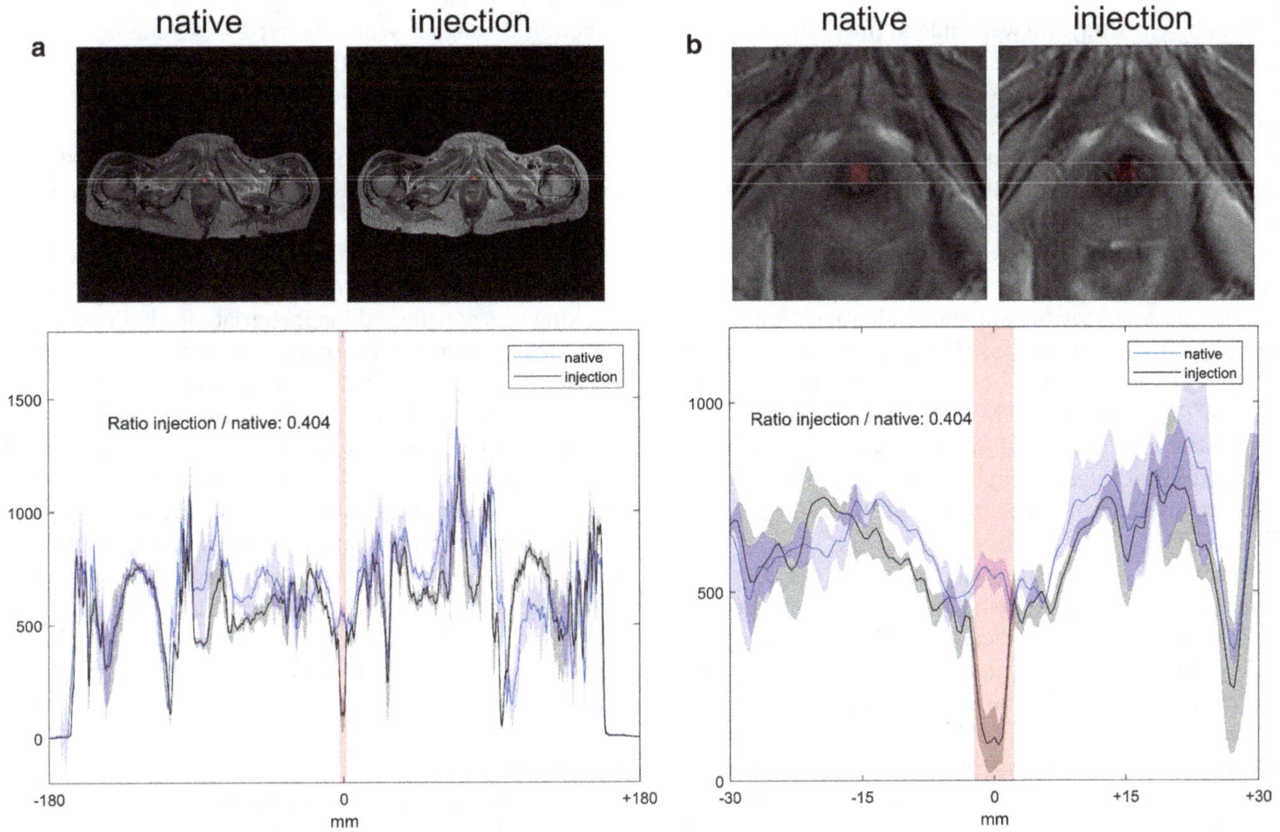

Fig. 3 Evaluation of the ratio of signal intensity in the EUS muscle in MRI. Measured differences due to extinction before and after injection of nano-iron particles in Cadaver 3. The red area marks the EUS in all parts of the figure. **a** Overall, **b** zoom

bubbles in the area of injection (Additional file 1: Appendix, Figs. 4 and 5). The handling of the needle, assuring the correct depth of puncture and the equal distribution of the 4 ml solution through all the intended injections spots were feasible at all times. The assessment of injection location revealed a maximum score of 4 points on the rating scale in anterior orientation and comparable results regarding division of the injection volume were obtained left vs. right (3 vs. 3.33 points). The lowest amount was seen in the posterior region with a mean rating score of 2.67 points. The mean injection volume calculated by the MRI was 1.75 cm^3 (Table 1). The measurement of the MRI extinction signal revealed a signal-intensity (SI) curve with a consistent ratio of less than a half (mean SI-ratio = 0.33) before and after injection of nano-iron particles into the EUS (reference SI: air ≈ 0, purefat ≈ 1500) (Table 1).

Table 1 Scores per cadaver on the rating scale according to extinction signal in MRI image in axial (left, right) and sagittal (anterior, posterior) orientation

Cadaver	Axial left	Axial right	Sagittal anterior	Sagittal posterior	Overall mean	Radius (mm)	Area (mm^2)	Volume measured in MR (cm^3)	SI-ratio
1	4	4	4	4	4	2.5	19.6	3.82	0.055
2	2	4	4	1	2.75	5.0	78.5	0.32	0.526
3	3	2	4	3	3	7.5	176.7	1.11	0.404
Column mean	3	3.33	4	2.67	3.25	5	91.60	1.75	0.33

Measured radius, area and volume of injection. Signal-intensity ratio before and after injection in the EUS

SI signal-intensity, *MR* magnetic resonance

Discussion

In the present study, we were able to prove that our technique for transurethral injections into the EUS under US guidance is feasible and yields good precision as seen in subsequent imaging proof. The signal decrease in pelvis MRI demonstrates a mean ratio of 0.33 when comparing intensities before and after the injection of nano-iron particles into the EUS. The indication for the use of nano-iron particles (SPIO = superparamagnetic iron oxide) in clinical MRI became broad over the last years, but was initially intended for the enhanced identification of focal malignant liver lesions [15]. For our purpose of a local injection, the signal alterations due to enhanced susceptibility in T2*-sequences in MRI was ideal and additionally not visible in CT scans. Our investigation showed that the anatomical reference in T2*-weighted imaging shows adequate mid-urethral accumulation in the target region (EUS).

Substantial research has looked into the feasibility, adverse effects and outcome of different interventions to treat SUI in women. Recently, a Cochrane systematic review compared different urethral injection therapies and concluded that the current evidence remains insufficient to guide practice [16]. They reported a similar outcome of periurethral versus transurethral outcomes regarding symptoms of SUI, whereas early complications tended to be higher in the periurethral group. The cost-effectiveness of urethral bulking agents compared to sling surgery was doubted during a longer follow-up period of 15 months. Burdzinska and colleagues compared the accuracy between the transurethral and periurethral route of intrasphincteric injections of autologous cellular suspensions in goats [17]. Their investigation revealed that 2/3 of all injections could be located in the urethral wall, while less than 1/5 were found inside EUS muscle structures. The main difference to our investigation was the fact that transurethral injections were performed under endoscopic but no US guidance, which could be an explanation for the lower accuracy. American researches evaluated transurethral injections of bulking agents (Macroplastique®) by 3D endo-vaginal US to describe location and distribution after the intervention [18]. By using US, they reported good precision at 3 and 9 o'clock position of the EUS, but highly variable distances from the urethro-vesical junction. Blaganje et al. demonstrated, that transurethral injections of autologous myoblasts through US guidance are feasible and reveals improvement of symptoms in combination with functional electrical stimulation in more than 75% of female patients suffering from SUI [19]. Interestingly, Aicher and his group recently published a needle-free technique using a novel waterjet injection to deposit mesenchymal stromal cells into the EUS of fresh porcine urethrae [20]. The yield of viable cells was significantly higher than by injection through a William's needle while assuring similar accuracy. Therefore, this novel approach could be a promising technique to deposit viable cells into the EUS in the future.

A limitation of this proof of concept is the post-mortem character of our investigation. The injection and imaging in female cadavers may differ from in-vivo procedures and therefore results need to be interpreted with caution. Further, the use of nano-iron particles for MPC tracking was considered inappropriate for living humans, since macrophages tend to uptake and evacuate MPCs previously stained with iron oxide [21]. In addition, the two independent raters (radiological technologist and urologist) were not blinded to the treatment method, which could potentially induce assessor bias. However, the evaluation with the rating scale was performed in reference to the urethra as an anatomical structure and was the same in all three cadavers. Therefore, and according to our imaging series, the approach and the technique may be reliably used for the accurate deposition of injectables through the transurethral route under US guidance.

Conclusion

Our US-guided injection technique for EUS application is feasible and shows an adequate as well as precise accumulation of nano-iron particles in the desired target region, as confirmed by MRI. It may be applied as a simple approach to accurately deliver MPCs in the EUS for the regenerative treatment of female SUI in the near future.

Acknowledgements

We thank Sebastian Pilz and Prof. Dr. Caroline Maake from the Anatomical Institute of the University Zurich for their organizational support and their help in realizing this cadaveric investigation. We also thank Prof. Dr. Michael J. Thali, the director at the Institute of Forensic Medicine at the University of Zurich, to render possible the collaboration as research partners and enable post-mortem imaging.

Authors' contributions

Contributions to the conception: FAS, GC and DE; Design of the work: FAS and DE; The acquisition: FAS, DG, GC; Analysis or interpretation of data: FAS, DG, NZ, JAP and DE; Drafted the work: FAS; Revised the manuscript: DG, NZ, JAP, GC and DE. All authors read and approved the final manuscript.

Competing interests

The authors declare that they have no competing interests.

Author details

[1] Department of Urology, University Hospital of Zurich, University of Zurich, Frauenklinikstrasse 10, 8091 Zurich, Switzerland. [2] Institute of Forensic Medicine, University of Zurich, Zurich, Switzerland. [3] Institute of Anatomy, University of Zurich, Zurich, Switzerland.

References

1. Irwin DE, Kopp ZS, Agatep B, Milsom I, Abrams P. Worldwide prevalence

estimates of lower urinary tract symptoms, overactive bladder, urinary incontinence and bladder outlet obstruction. BJU Int. 2011;108(7):1132–8.
2. Lukacz ES, Santiago-Lastra Y, Albo ME, Brubaker L. Urinary incontinence in women: a review. JAMA. 2017;318(16):1592–604.
3. Mota RL. Female urinary incontinence and sexuality. Int Braz J Urol. 2017;43(1):20–8.
4. Nambiar AK, Bosch R, Cruz F, Lemack GE, Thiruchelvam N, Tubaro A, et al. EAU guidelines on assessment and nonsurgical management of urinary incontinence. Eur Urol. 2018;73(4):596–609.
5. Ptak M, Brodowska A, Ciecwiez S, Rotter I. Quality of life in women with stage 1 stress urinary incontinence after application of conservative treatment—a randomized trial. Int J Environ Res Public Health. 2017;14(6):577.
6. Kobashi KC, Albo ME, Dmochowski RR, Ginsberg DA, Goldman HB, Gomelsky A, et al. Surgical treatment of female stress urinary incontinence: AUA/SUFU guideline. J Urol. 2017;198(4):875–83.
7. Fusco F, Abdel-Fattah M, Chapple CR, Creta M, La Falce S, Waltregny D, et al. Updated systematic review and meta-analysis of the comparative data on colposuspensions, pubovaginal slings, and midurethral tapes in the surgical treatment of female stress urinary incontinence. Eur Urol. 2017;72(4):567–91.
8. Lemack GE, Xu Y, Brubaker L, Nager C, Chai T, Moalli P, et al. Clinical and demographic factors associated with valsalva leak point pressure among women undergoing burch bladder neck suspension or autologous rectus fascial sling procedures. Neurourol Urodyn. 2007;26(3):392–6.
9. Garriboli M, Radford A, Southgate J. Regenerative medicine in urology. Eur J Pediatr Surg. 2014;24(3):227–36.
10. Hart ML, Izeta A, Herrera-Imbroda B, Amend B, Brinchmann JE. Cell therapy for stress urinary incontinence. Tissue Eng B Rev. 2015;21(4):365–76.
11. Zhou S, Zhang K, Atala A, Khoury O, Murphy SV, Zhao W, et al. Stem cell therapy for treatment of stress urinary incontinence: the current status and challenges. Stem Cells Int. 2016;2016:7060975.
12. Vinarov A, Atala A, Yoo J, Slusarenco R, Zhumataev M, Zhito A, et al. Cell therapy for stress urinary incontinence: present-day frontiers. J Tissue Eng Regen Med. 2018;12(2):e1108–21.
13. Williams JK, Dean A, Badlani G, Andersson KE. Regenerative medicine therapies for stress urinary incontinence. J Urol. 2016;196(6):1619–26.
14. Gascho D, Thali MJ, Niemann T. Post-mortem computed tomography: technical principles and recommended parameter settings for high-resolution imaging. Med Sci Law. 2018;58(1):70–82.
15. Winter TC 3rd, Freeny PC, Nghiem HV, Mack LA, Patten RM, Thomas CR Jr, et al. MR imaging with i.v. superparamagnetic iron oxide: efficacy in the detection of focal hepatic lesions. AJR Am J Roentgenol. 1993;161(6):1191–8.
16. Kirchin V, Page T, Keegan PE, Atiemo KO, Cody JD, McClinton S, et al. Urethral injection therapy for urinary incontinence in women. Cochrane Database Syst Rev. 2017;7:CD003881.
17. Burdzinska A, Dybowski B, Zarychta-Wisniewska W, Kulesza A, Hawryluk J, Graczyk-Jarzynka A, et al. Limited accuracy of transurethral and periurethral intrasphincteric injections of cellular suspension. Neurourol Urodyn. 2018;37(5):1612–22.
18. Yune JJ, Quiroz L, Nihira MA, Siddighi S, O'Leary DE, Santiago A, et al. The location and distribution of transurethral bulking agent: 3-dimensional ultrasound study. Female Pelvic Med Reconstr Surg. 2016;22(2):98–102.
19. Blaganje M, Lukanovic A. Ultrasound-guided autologous myoblast injections into the extrinsic urethral sphincter: tissue engineering for the treatment of stress urinary incontinence. Int Urogynecol J. 2013;24(4):533–5.
20. Jager L, Linzenbold W, Fech A, Enderle M, Abruzzese T, Stenzl A, et al. A novel waterjet technology for transurethral cystoscopic injection of viable cells in the urethral sphincter complex. Neurourol Urodyn. 2020;39(2):594–602.
21. Azzabi F, Rottmar M, Jovaisaite V, Rudin M, Sulser T, Boss A, et al. Viability, differentiation capacity, and detectability of super-paramagnetic iron oxide-labeled muscle precursor cells for magnetic-resonance imaging. Tissue Eng C Methods. 2015;21(2):182–91.

4

Congenital midureteral stenosis in children: A 13-year retrospective study based on data from a large pediatric medical center

Zhaoyi Meng, Defu Lin, Guannan Wang, Yanchao Qu and Ning Sun*

Abstract

Background: Midureteral stenosis is very rare in children and can cause congenital hydronephrosis. We report our experience treating children with congenital midureteral stenosis at our center, focusing on the differences in preoperative diagnosis and treatment compared with other congenital obstructive uropathies.

Methods: We retrospectively reviewed the medical records of 26 children diagnosed with congenital midureteral stenosis at our center between January 2007 and December 2020, such as preoperative examination methods, intraoperative conditions, and postoperative follow-up results.

Results: Of the 1625 children treated surgically for ureteral narrowing, only 26 (1.6%) were diagnosed with midureteral stenosis, including 15 infants and 11 children. Eighteen (69.2%) were boys, 13 (50%) were affected on the left side, and 23 (88.5%) had isolated ureteral stenosis. Overall, 13 (50%) of the children presented with prenatal hydronephrosis, and 13 (50%) presented with abdominal pain or a mass. All the children had undergone urinary ultrasound and intravenous urography preoperatively; the diagnostic rate of ultrasound was 92.3%. Only 7 (26.9%) children had undergone pyelography. All the children had undergone surgery. The ureteral stenotic segment was less than 1 cm long in 25 (96.2)% of the children. The mean follow-up duration was 22 months (range: 6–50 months). One child developed anastomotic strictures. Urinary tract obstruction was relieved in the other children without long-term complications.

Conclusions: Congenital midureteral stenosis is rare, accounting for 1.6% of all ureteral obstructions, and its diagnosis is crucial. Urinary ultrasound has a high diagnostic rate and should be the first choice for midureteral stenosis. Retrograde pyelography can be used when the diagnosis is difficult, but routine retrograde pyelography is not recommended. Congenital ureteral stenosis has a relatively short lesion range, largely within 1 cm. The treatment is mainly resection of the stenotic segment and end-to-end ureteral anastomosis, with a good prognosis.

Keywords: Midureteral stenosis, Hydronephrosis, Congenital, Obstruction, Children

Background

Congenital midureteral stenosis is characterized by a narrowing that occurs between the two ends of the ureter and is a very rare cause of hydronephrosis and dilatation of the upper ureter in children. In general, most upper urinary tract obstruction lesions are located at either the proximal or distal end of the ureter, such as ureteropelvic junction obstruction (UPJO), ureterovesical junction

*Correspondence: doctorsn@163.com
Department of Urology, Beijing Children's Hospital Affiliated With Capital Medical University, National Center for Children's Health, No. 56 Nanlishilu Rd, West District, Beijing 100045, China

obstruction (UVJO) and nonrefluxing megaureter, and stenosis in the main length of the ureter is extremely rare. Campbell reported that, in an autopsy of a sequence of 12,080 children, 72 children had ureteral stenosis, 34% at the UVJ and 62% at the UPJ, and only 4% (3 children) had middle ureteral stenosis [1]. However, according to our statistics, middle ureteral stenosis accounts for only 1.6% of all ureteral strictures.

Because this condition is relatively rare, the diagnosis may be confused with UPJO or UVJO, particularly when ureteral dilation above the stenotic segment is not evident. Previous studies in the literature have reported low rates of preoperative midureteral stenosis diagnosis; this condition is usually found intraoperatively or by retrograde pyelography after anesthesia. Because our center is a large children's medical center in northern China, many children with midureteral stenosis have been treated at our center over the past decade. We observed a relatively high rate of preoperative diagnosis of this condition, so we hypothesized that preoperative ultrasound and intravenous urography (IVU) are of great help to the diagnosis of midureteral stenosis. In this study, we describe our experience in treating children with midureteral stenosis, focusing on the preoperative diagnosis, surgical management and posttreatment outcomes.

Table 1 Patient clinical characteristics

Age (years)	
Infant	1.99 ± 0.72
Children	8.9 ± 2.9
Sex	
Male	18 (69.2%)
Female	8 (30.8%)
Side	
Left	13 (50%)
Right	13 (50%)
Stenosis	
Isolated	23 (88.5%)
Multiple	3 (11.5%)
Symptoms	
Prenatal hydronephrosis	13 (50%)
Abdominal/flank pain	11 (42.3%)
Abdominal mass	2 (7.7%)
Prior surgery	
Nephropyeloplasty	3 (11.5%)
Bilateral ureter reimplantation	1 (3.8%)
Nephrostomy	1 (3.8%)
Associated anomalies	
Contralateral multicystic dysplastic kidney	3 (11.5%)
Isolated kidney	2 (7.7%)
Dysrotation of renal axis	2 (7.7%)
Ipsilateral UPJO	2 (7.7%)

Methods

We reviewed the clinical records of children diagnosed with midureteral stenosis at Beijing Children's Hospital from January 2007 to December 2020 (The basic characteristics of the children are shown in Table 1). Urinary ultrasound examination was performed by a professional sonographer with more than 5 years of working experience. Before all ultrasound examinations, the children fasted for 6–8 h and then drank sufficient water (more than 500 ml) over 30 min to induce diuresis and dilate the renal pelvis and ureter to enhance the detection of ureteral obstruction. At the time of examination, the child was first placed in the supine position and then on the side in the decubitus position. When the ureter showing expansion suddenly narrowed or was suddenly interrupted, careful observation was made to determine whether thickening of the ureteral wall or external oppression occurred in this position. Children with abdominal distension were treated with laxative suppositories to stimulate exhaust defecation to reduce the interference of intestinal flatulence. After the examination, the sonographer marked ureteral stenosis at the projection point on the body surface. Intravenous urography (IVU) was performed 10, 20 and 40 min after the contrast agent was injected.

Magnetic resonance urography (MRU) was performed in 3 children, and computed tomography urography (CTU) was performed in 7 children. In children suspected of having multiple or long stenotic segments without obvious dilation of the proximal ureter and without a thick-thin junction of the ureter across the iliac vessels and in other cases with an unclear diagnosis, we performed preoperative retrograde pyelography after anesthesia. Iohexol and 0.9% saline at a ratio of 1:1 were selected for retrograde pyelography. If the child had a nephrostomy at another hospital, we used a direct renal fistula tube for antegrade pyelography. Voiding cystourethrography (VCUG) was performed to rule out vesicoureteral reflux (VUR) in 4 children with ultrasound or IVU indicating distal ureteral dilation or a history of fever that was not determined to be caused by urinary tract infection. Radioisotopic diethylenetriamine pentaacetic acid (DTPA) was used to calculate relative renal function and assess the degree of obstruction in 10 children (Table 2).

The surgeries were performed by 5 pediatric urologists with 10 years of clinical experience. The open surgery used a transverse incision on the outer edge of the rectus abdominis muscle of the lower abdomen to expose the ureter and iliac vessels using an extraperitoneal approach. After removing the narrow segment, the distal end of

Table 2 Preoperative imaging studies

	Total	Positive	Negative
Urinary ultrasound (US)	26 (100%)	24 (92.3%)	2 (7.7%)
Intravenous urography (IVU)	26 (100%)	20 (76.9%)	6 (23.1%)
Computerized tomography urography (CTU)	7 (26.9%)	6 (85.7%)	1 (14.3%)
Magnetic resonance urography (MRU)	3 (11.5%)	3 (100%)	0 (0%)
Pyelography (antegrade or retrograde)	7 (26.9%)	7 (100%)	0 (0%)

the ureter was explored and a catheter was inserted into it for the water injection test to observe whether resistance was evident in the distal ureter. After confirming no obstruction at the distal end, ureteroureterostomy was performed. Laparoscopic surgery used a transperitoneal three-port laparoscope to remove the narrow ureter and perform an intracorporeal suture. All the resected segments were sent for pathological examination, and the diagnosis of ureteral stenosis was based on intraoperative observation and histological examination. Follow-up protocols included ultrasound every three months in the first postoperative year, every six months in the second, and every one to two years thereafter; intravenous pyelography or dynamic nuclide renal imaging was performed at 6 and 12 months postoperatively.

Results

Over the past 13 years, 1625 children had received surgical treatment for ureteral obstruction at our center. Only 26 (1.6%) cases of hydronephrosis were caused by midureteral stenosis. Of these children, 18 (69.2%) were boys, 13 (50%) were affected on the left side, and 23 (88.5%) had isolated stenosis. Additionally, 15 were infants, with an average age of 1.99 ± 0.72 years and presenting primarily with prenatal hydronephrosis; 11 were children, with an average age of 8.9 ± 2.9 years and presenting primarily with intermittent abdominal pain or an abdominal mass. Among them, 5 children had received surgical treatment at another hospital and were referred to our hospital because of failure of the treatment to relieve the urinary obstruction. One of them was an 11-year-old girl who had bilateral hydroureter and was diagnosed at another hospital with right ectopic ureterocele and left side grade III VUR. She had undergone bilateral ureteral reimplantation. Six months after surgery, her right kidney hydroureter still existed, and she still had intermittent abdominal pain. The remaining 4 children had undergone pyeloplasty because of hydronephrosis, and the ureter was still obstructed after surgery. The renal fistula was maintained for 6 to 20 months when referred to our hospital and was not removed postoperatively. One of four children had undergone a second pyeloplasty and still had ureteral obstruction. No cases of urinary infection were found. According to the Society of Fetal Urology classification, 21 children had grade 3 hydronephrosis, 5 had SFU grade 4 hydronephrosis and obvious ipsilateral upper urinary tract obstruction, which was confirmed on DTPA imaging in 10 children and on IVU in the remaining 16, showing severe dilation of the renal pelvis and calyces. VCUG examination revealed contralateral grade I VUR in one child and grade III VUR in another.

Preoperative assessment was performed in all children using IVU and urinary ultrasound. Preoperative ultrasound revealed 24 cases of midureteral stenosis and 2 cases of UVJO, for a diagnostic rate of 92.3%. Midureteral stenosis was confirmed in 9 cases by ultrasound and IVU, in 9 cases by MRU or CTU, in 7 cases by antegrade or retrograde pyelography (1 case through a renal fistula, 2 cases by percutaneous pyelography and 4 cases by retrograde pyelography), and in 1 case by intraoperative diagnosis (Figs. 1, 2 and 3; Table 2).

While open surgery was used in most of our cases, laparoscopic surgery was performed in 3 cases (Fig. 4). In 23 (88.5%) cases, the stenotic site was located at or near the level of the iliac vessels. The stenotic segment was less than 1 cm long in 25 (96.2%) of the children, and no stenotic segments were longer than 2 cm. Therefore, for a single site of ureteral stenosis, 22 (84.6%) patients had undergone ureteroureterostomy. Tension-free anastomosis was achieved in these children. A 10-year-old boy was diagnosed with middle ureteral stenosis and ipsilateral multicystic dysplastic kidney (MCDK). Preoperative renal dynamic imaging showed that the differential renal function was approximately 9%, and the proximal ureter was expanded by approximately 2.5 cm, but the middle ureter was not significantly expanded. Because of suspected multiple ureteral stenoses, retrograde pyelography was performed after anesthesia, and multiple ureteral stenoses were confirmed in the upper and middle ureters. The child had undergone nephroureterectomy after approval was obtained from his parents. The 11-year-old girl's ureteral stenosis was approximately 1.5 cm in length. After this stenosed segment

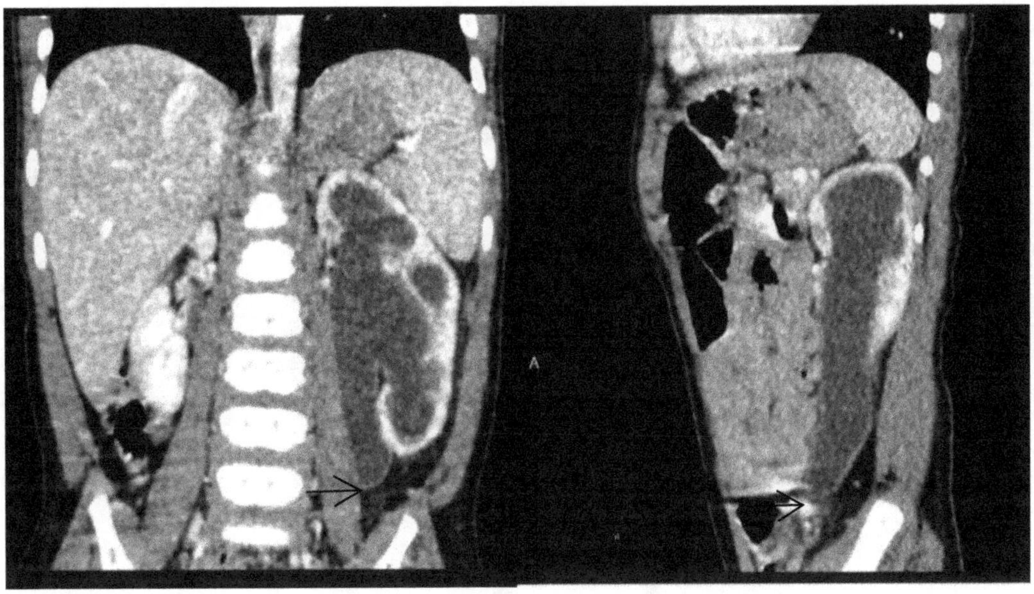

Fig. 1 A 12-month-boy, CTU images on coronal and sagittal show dilation of the proximal ureter and midureteral stricture (arrow)

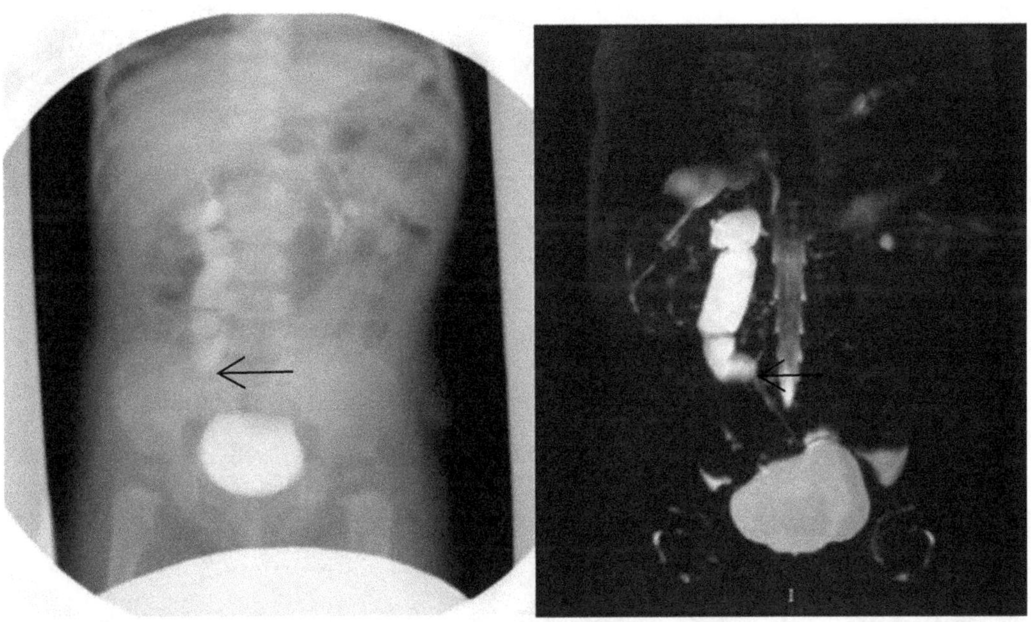

Fig. 2 A 8-year-old boy with midureteral stenosis (arrow), IVP and MRU images show the left proximal ureter turning medial and tapering, with proximal ureter dilation

was removed, anastomosis of the two broken ends of the ureter could not be completed. The proximal end of the ureter was measured to be approximately 5 cm from the bladder, so a Boari flap was used for anastomosis. Ileal ureteral replacement was used in two children with multiple ureteral strictures. The stenotic ureter was replaced with 12 cm and 15 cm isoperistaltic ileum intestinal segments. The characteristics of the stenotic segment and surgical methods are shown in Table 3.

Pathologically, the ureter was shaped similar to an umbrella or dumbbell on gross observation, with a narrow lumen in the middle through which the probe could pass but not urine. Microscopic examination of the stenotic area suggested submucosal fibrous tissue hyperplasia

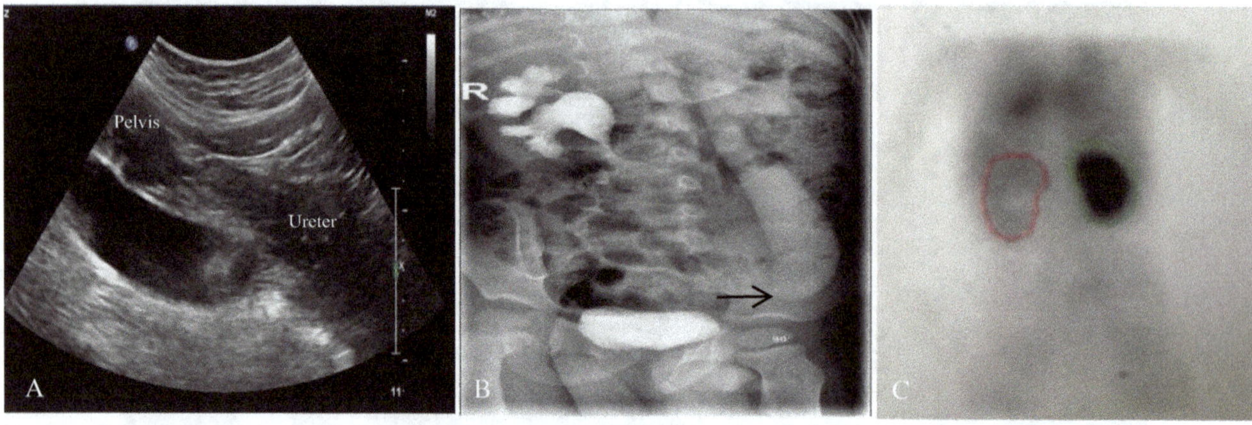

Fig. 3 A 1.2-year-old boy. **a** Ultrasound of the affected kidney shows hydronephrosis and hydroureter. **b** IVU reveals the left midureteral stenosis (arrow); **c** preoperative DTPA renography demonstrated delayed drainage of the left kidney

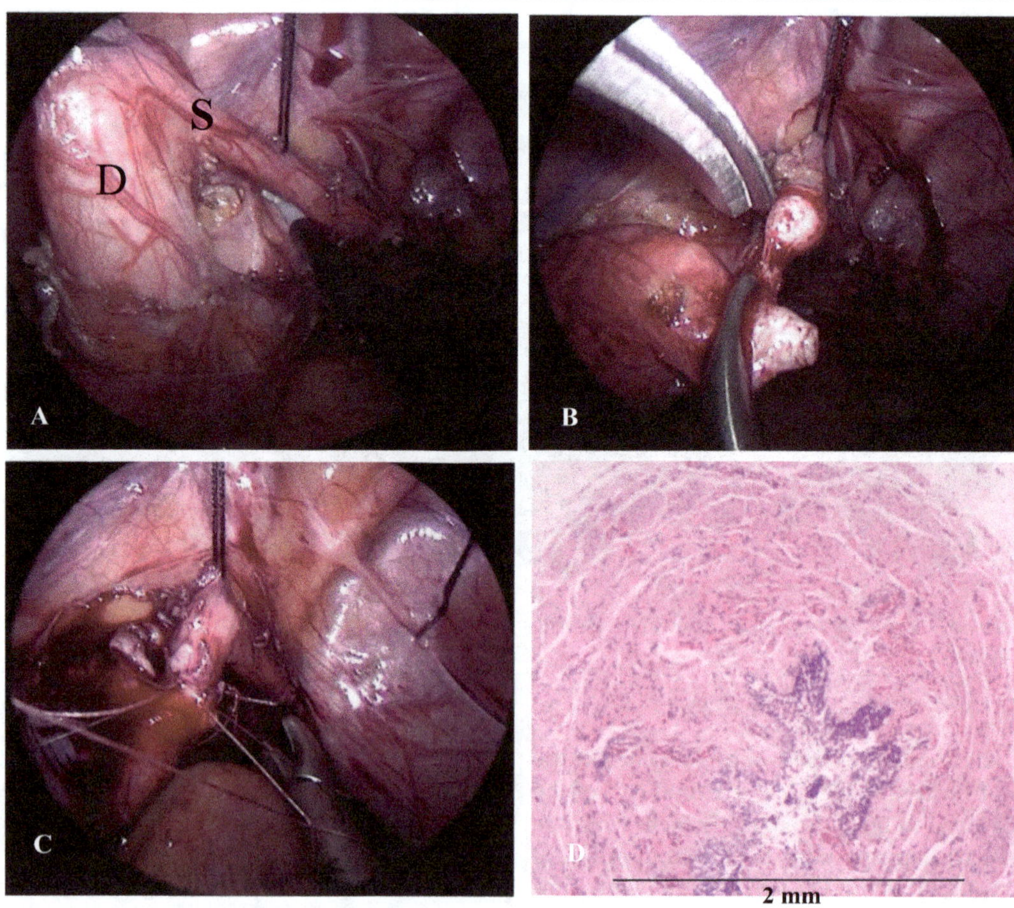

Fig. 4 A 3-year-old boy. **a** Congenital midureteral stenosis (S) and dilated proximal ureter (D). **b** Ureterectomy of the stenosed segment. **c** Ureteroureterostomy. **d** Pathology of the resected segment showing ureteral lumen stenosis

Table 3 Characteristics of and surgical technique used for the stenosis segment

Stenosis location	
At or near the iliac vessels	23 (88.5%)
Scattered multiple stenosis	3 (11.5%)
Length of the stenosed segment	
L ≤ 5 mm	17 (65.4%)
5 mm < L ≤ 10 mm	8 (30.8%)
> 10 mm	1 (3.8%)
Surgical technique	
Ureteroureterostomy	22 (84.6%)
Boari bladder flap	1 (3.8%)
Ileal ureteral replacement	2 (7.7%)
Nephroureterectomy	1 (3.8%)

with scattered lymphocytic infiltration and muscularis thickening with muscle fiber degeneration (Fig. 4). All cases of ureteral stenosis were considered congenital, without an intrinsic or extrinsic pathology, and all the specimens were positive on Masson staining. Ureteral valves or folds were not identified in the longitudinal sections of specimens from any of the children. Associated anomalies were observed in 8 children, such as MCDK in 3 cases, an isolated kidney in 2 cases, ipsilateral UPJO in 2 cases, and concomitant ipsilateral dysrotation of the renal axis in two cases. The details of the clinical characteristics of all the patients are shown in Table 1.

The total follow-up period ranged from 6 to 50 months (mean: 22 months). All 26 children were followed up by telephone, and 20 of them regularly visited our hospital for ultrasound examination. All the children were relieved of their symptoms, and none had palpable masses, abdominal pain or urinary infections. Postoperative ultrasound evaluation during the follow-up period showed a significant decrease in hydronephrosis in all the children. The average anteroposterior diameter of the renal pelvis (APD) of all the children was reduced postoperatively. Among them, 21 children with hydronephrosis SFU3 showed a decrease in the APD from 3.12 ± 0.05 mm before the operation to 2.35 ± 0.09 mm, and four children with SFU4 showed a decrease in the APD from 4.15 ± 0.19 mm preoperatively to 2.96 ± 0.16 mm. IVU showed no obstruction in the urinary tract of all the children. Eight children had undergone dynamic renal nuclide imaging, indicating that split renal function improved or stabilized after surgery. No electrolyte disturbances or VURs were found in the two children who had undergone ileal ureteral replacement. The contralateral kidney function of the boy who underwent nephroureterectomy was normal. The child who had undergone Boari flap replacement of the ureter developed anastomotic stricture one year after surgery that was resolved after a third surgical procedure. No other complication occurred.

Discussion

Congenital middle ureteral stenosis is a rare cause of hydroureteronephrosis. To date, few studies have investigated the incidence of ureteral stenosis, and the previously reported incidence is based on a large-scale autopsy of children. We reviewed the clinical data of 1625 children who had undergone surgical treatment because of an obstructive hydroureter in the past 13 years. Among them, 26 had congenital midureteral stenosis, accounting for approximately 1.6%, which was lower than that reported in the literature. However, our statistical data were based on actual clinical data and were more representative. The pathogenesis of this condition is unclear, and many theories attribute it to abnormal embryonic development, including abnormal fetal vessel compression, intrauterine inflammation, incomplete ureteral recanalization, ischemia due to abnormal branches of blood vessels and localized developmental arrest [1–5]. A review of the previous literature has revealed that in children, congenital midureteral stenosis is often associated with urological anomalies, such as contralateral renal agenesis or atrophy, VUR, UPJO, crossed renal ectopia, solitary kidney and contralateral blind-ending ureter [6–8], suggesting the possibility of bilateral aberrant renal and ureteral development and indicating that ureteral stenosis may be a mild manifestation of unilateral hypoplasia. In the present study, one case of contralateral MCDK with systemic growth retardation and two cases of contralateral renal axis malrotation were found.

Pathologically, ureteral stenosis is a mechanical obstruction due to structural abnormalities in the wall that are distinct from the neurogenic and myogenic mechanisms of UPJO. Two etiologies of ureteral stenosis exist: ureteral valves and true ureteral stenosis. Ureteral valves are anatomically demonstrable transverse folds of ureteral mucosa, potentially containing bundles of smooth muscle fiber covered with normal urothelium [9]. In the present study, no ureteral valves were found in any of the children after careful observation of the pathological specimens. Studies on the ultrastructure of ureteral stenosis found that the stenotic ureter did not deviate fundamentally from its pattern, and only quantitative changes in its composition were observed. These changes included lumen shrinkage and relative or absolute loss of smooth muscle with a normal, altered or disorganized arrangement, with or without connective tissue changes [1–8]. Our pathological specimens exhibited smooth muscle hyperplasia and fibrous tissue degeneration. A low level of chronic inflammatory cell infiltration was observed in the narrow segment, a finding that is consistent with that reported in the literature.

Midureteral stenosis occurs at the level of the bifurcation of the common iliac vessels, also a site of physiological ureteral narrowing. In this study, stenosis in this region accounted for 88% of cases. Ninety-six percent of the stenotic segments were within 1 cm in length, and upper ureteral stenosis was more common in patients with multiple stenotic sites and was rarely isolated. Additionally, ureters with multiple ureteral stenotic sites were generally poorly developed and small in appearance. Previous literature has demonstrated that at sites of stenosis, the ureter lumen usually shrinks by approximately 60% and significantly impedes urine delivery [6]. However, clinically, we found that compared with UPJO, children with midureteral stenosis had relatively mild hydronephrosis and a later onset of symptoms. In this study, 12 children were older than 5 years when they developed symptoms. Midureteral stenosis has also been diagnosed at 15 and 20 years of age [10, 11]. The upper ureteral dilation in some children was not very severe, likely because of absorption by ureteral lymphoid tissue and the buffering effect of the ureter on the urine during low stenosis. Murnaghan speculated that the narrow segment transmitted peristaltic waves when the urine flow was low, allowing smooth passage; when the urine flow load exceeded a critical value, the narrow segment decompensated, resulting in clinical symptoms [12].

Midureteral stenosis results in dilatation of the ureter above the stenotic site, usually with dilatation of the renal pelvis. The ureter may also stretch, curl and droop clinically similar to that of UVJ malformation. However, these two diseases are very different. Midureteral stenosis comprises an obstruction at a certain distance from the bladder; in intramural ureteral lesions, the ureter is usually dilated next to the bladder. Previous studies have shown that the preoperative diagnosis of midureteral stenosis is relatively difficult because of its symptomatic and radiographic similarity to intrinsic UVJO or UPJO. Most cases are diagnosed intraoperatively or by retrograde pyelography, and the rate of diagnosis on preoperative ultrasound is low. Many scholars have considered ultrasound to have limited value in distal ureteral obstruction localization. Hawang et al. believed that children with hydronephrosis and megaureter should routinely undergo retrograde pyelography unless the distal ureter is well demonstrated on other tests [1]. MRU is recommended to be routinely performed in children with ureteral dilatation because MRU provides excellent anatomic and functional details of the collection system, allowing the accurate diagnosis and treatment of ureteral stenosis [13]. However, routine retrograde pyelography in children with congenital hydronephrosis is controversial. It is an invasive examination with the risks of ureteral injury, urinary tract infection, and iatrogenic obstruction of the UVJ. Ruston pointed out that retrograde pyelography or contrast visualization of the ureter before pyeloplasty is rarely necessary in children [14]. Previously, Cockrell et al. reported that the secondary abnormalities found by retrograde pyelography were in the surgical field where they would be detected and managed normally [15]. The main purpose of RGP or MRU examination is to clearly show the shape of the ureter and clarify the location and number of ureteral stenoses. However, performing RGP or MRU is not required routinely but is critical for secondary surgery and in children with unclear diagnoses.

With the development of ultrasound techniques for ureteral examination and improvements in the diagnostic rate, ultrasound can serve as a noninvasive and repeatable effective method to diagnose ureteral stenosis or stricture. Ultrasound can be used to determine the location of a ureteral obstruction according to the degree of ureteral dilation and morphological changes, as well as to determine the etiology and extent of stenosis according to differences in the acoustic images of the stenosis site. At our center, the diagnosis of ureteral stenosis mainly relies on ultrasound, IVU and CTU, while MRU and retrograde pyelography are performed irregularly. The accuracy of the ultrasound examination is highly dependent on the personal experience of the examiner. Notably, our rate of preoperative midureteral stenosis diagnosis is higher than that reported in the literature, with the diagnostic rate of ultrasound reaching 96%. As early as 10 years ago, related reports in the domestic literature demonstrated rates of coincident lesion location diagnosis and quantitative ureteral stricture diagnosis by ultrasound of 96.6% and 91.5%, respectively [16]. The ultrasound examination and diagnosis at our center were completed by sonographers with certain clinical experience in urology. It is a real-time dynamic examination accompanied by parents. Before the examination, the children had fasted for approximately 6 h and drank adequate water to maintain a state of bladder filling. In the state of holding urine, the prone sites of ureteral stenosis were examined emphatically and repeatedly—namely, the ureteropelvic junction, vicinity of ureter crossing iliac vessels and vesicoureteral junction. Ureteropelvic junction obstruction combined with ureterovesical junction obstruction and iliac ureteral vessel stenosis is very rare; but for children with hydronephrosis, exploring the ureter repeatedly by ultrasound is necessary, particularly the three common sites of ureteral stenosis and those with hydronephrosis. Next, after allowing the child to urinate, another examination was performed and compared with the first examination. Because of the sound window of the kidney and bladder, the UPJ and terminal ureter adjacent to the bladder were well displayed; however, the ureter in the middle segment was deep, and the ureter did not dilate behind the bladder in many cases. Therefore, ureteral stenosis can be missed or a dilated bowel can be mistaken for a ureter. To avoid these situations, we prepared the bowel sufficiently to reduce interference with intestinal contents and gases. When necessary, the children were placed in the prone position and padded with cotton pads with a height of approximately 15 cm on the upper abdomen to naturally increase abdominal pressure and then checked again. We believe that the false-negative rate is due to limited experience; an experienced sonographer can diagnose most cases of midureteral stenosis.

IVU is a common and accurate visual examination to diagnose ureteral stenosis. If children have good renal function, IVU can often clearly show the degree of ureteral hydronephrosis and shape and location of ureteral stenosis, and the accuracy of ureteral stenosis localization is high. Long-term obstruction causes poor renal function, which must be extended to approximately 1 h to improve the positive rate of diagnosis. Therefore, we do not recommend preoperative MRU or retrograde pyelography in children with suspected midureteral stenosis but instead propose ultrasound and IVU for routine preoperative evaluation. When ureteral dilatation is not obvious, the distal ureter is not clearly displayed, or the diagnosis is unclear, such as suspected cases of multiple stenotic sites, MRU, CTU or retrograde pyelography will be performed to confirm the diagnosis.

Preoperative ultrasound localization is an essential reference surgical approach selection. The surgical method is considerably affected by the location and number of stenotic segments. Most single stenotic segments are short. Thus, resection of the stenotic segment and ureteroureterostomy are feasible. For upper ureteral stenosis combined with UPJO, pyeloplasty can be performed directly. In two children with multiple left ureteral stenoses, because the stenosis was relatively dispersed and the distance was longer, we adopted ileal ureteral replacement. Technically, replacing the left ureter with the appendix is challenging because the appendix in children is short and the mesoappendix length is limited. Thus, the cecum and even the ascending colon must be moved to provide a sufficient vascular pedicle length, which is prone to postoperative complications such as poor blood transport, appendix necrosis, anastomotic stenosis, and intestinal obstruction. We did not use the appendix for left ureteral replacement. Laparoscopic and robotic technology has been successfully used to treat ureteral stenosis. Compared with open surgery, minimally invasive surgery has the advantages of less postoperative pain, a shorter hospitality stay, less scarring, and less parental anxiety. In the future, more children will undergo treatment with laparoscopic and robotic surgery. The prognosis of the patients in the present study was very good; the symptoms resolved on long-term follow-up, ultrasound examination suggested that hydronephrosis was relieved or resolved, the urinary tract was unobstructed, and IVU examination showed no obstruction.

The present study has some limitations. Because of the single-center retrospective design over a long period, the preoperative and postoperative clinical data of some children cannot be followed up, especially the treatment information of the 5 referred children in other hospital. Additionally, the renal dynamic imaging technology and level were limited, the postoperative follow-up of the children was primarily performed using IVU and ultrasound, and an accurate assessment of renal function was lacking. Additionally, the ultrasound examination technology introduced must be further summarized and promoted and does not apply to all hospitals.

Conclusion

Congenital midureteral stenosis is a rare cause of hydronephrosis. A precise preoperative diagnosis is manda tory for successful surgical management. Ultrasound should be the first choice to examine ureteral stenosis in children. The combination of ultrasound and IVU has complementary advantages to improve the diagnostic accuracy. When a diagnosis is challenging or uncertainty in the ultrasound or IVU, further MRU or retrograde paragraph examination is necessary.

Acknowledgements
Not applicable.

Authors' contributions
ZM (first author): protocol development, data analysis, manuscript writing. DL (co-first author): protocol development, data analysis, manuscript editing. GW: data collection. YQ: data analysis. NS (corresponding author): manuscript editing. All authors read and approved the final manuscript.

Competing interests
The authors declare that there are no competing interests.

References

1. Hwang AH, McAleer IM, Shapiro E, et al. Congenital mid ureteral strictures. J Urol. 2005;174:1999–2002.
2. Ayyat FM, Adams G. Congenital midureteral strictures. Urology. 1985;26:170–2.
3. Docimo SG, Lebowitz RL, Retik AB, et al. Congenital midureteral obstruction. Urol Radiol. 1989;11:156–60.
4. Gitlin J, Kaefer M. Congenital mid ureteral stricture presenting as prenatal hydronephrosis. J Urol. 2002;168:1154–5.
5. Smith BG, Metwalli AR, Leach J, et al. Congenital midureteral stricture in children diagnosed with antenatal hydronephrosis. Urology. 2004;64:1014–9.
6. Cauchi JA, Chandran H. Congenital ureteric strictures: an uncommon cause of antenatally detected hydronephrosis. Pediatr Surg Int. 2005;21:566–8.

7. Kannaiyan L, Karl S, Mathai J, et al. Congenital ureteric stenosis: a study of 17 children. Pediatr Surg Int. 2009;25:513–7.
8. Alhazmi H, Fouda NA. Congenital mid-ureteral stricture: a case report of two patients. Bmc Urol. 2018;18:108.
9. Maizels M, Stephens FD. Valves of the ureter as a cause of primary obstruction of the ureter: anatomic, embryologic and clinical aspects. J Urol. 1980;123:742.
10. Bhandarkar DS, Lalmalani JG, Shah VJ. Laparoscopic resection and ureteroureterostomy for congenital midureteral stricture. J Endourol. 2005;19:140.
11. Thiel DD, Badger WJ, Winfield HN. Robot-assisted laparoscopic excision and ureteroureterostomy for congenital midureteral stricture. J Endourol. 2008;22:2667–70.
12. Murnaghan GF. The mechanism of congenital hydronephrosis with reference to the factors influencing surgical treatment. Ann R Coll Surg Engl. 1958;23:25–46.
13. Lu L, Bi Y, Wang X, et al. Laparoscopic resection and end-to-end uretero-ureterostomy for midureteral obstruction in children. J Laparoendosc Adv S. 2017;27:197–202.
14. Rushton HG, Salem Y, Belman AB, et al. Pediatric pyeloplasty: is routine retrograde pyelography necessary? J Urol. 1994;152:604–6.
15. Cockrell SN, Hendren WH. The importance of visualizing the ureter before performing a pyeloplasty. J Urol. 1990;144(588–592):593–4.
16. Wang Z, Yu J, Ding Z, Li Q. The location and qualitative diagnosis of ultrasonography in ureterostenosis. Chin J Med Ultrasound (Electronic Edition). 2010;06:941–7.

5

RNA-sequencing profiling analysis of pericyte-derived extracellular vesicle–mimetic nanovesicles-regulated genes in primary cultured fibroblasts from normal and Peyronie's disease penile tunica albuginea

Guo Nan Yin[1†], Shuguang Piao[2†], Zhiyong Liu[2], Lei Wang[2], Jiyeon Ock[1], Mi-Hye Kwon[1], Do-Kyun Kim[3], Yong Song Gho[4], Jun-Kyu Suh[1*] and Ji-Kan Ryu[1*]

Abstract

Background: Peyronie's disease (PD) is a severe fibrotic disease of the tunica albuginea that causes penis curvature and leads to penile pain, deformity, and erectile dysfunction. The role of pericytes in the pathogenesis of fibrosis has recently been determined. Extracellular vesicle (EV)–mimetic nanovesicles (NVs) have attracted attention regarding intercellular communication between cells in the field of fibrosis. However, the global gene expression of pericyte-derived EV–mimetic NVs (PC–NVs) in regulating fibrosis remains unknown. Here, we used RNA-sequencing technology to investigate the potential target genes regulated by PC–NVs in primary fibroblasts derived from human PD plaque.

Methods: Human primary fibroblasts derived from normal and PD patients was cultured and treated with cavernosum pericytes isolated extracellular vesicle (EV)–mimetic nanovesicles (NVs). A global gene expression RNA-sequencing assay was performed on normal fibroblasts, PD fibroblasts, and PD fibroblasts treated with PC–NVs. Reverse transcription polymerase chain reaction (RT-PCR) was used for sequencing data validation.

Results: A total of 4135 genes showed significantly differential expression in the normal fibroblasts, PD fibroblasts, and PD fibroblasts treated with PC–NVs. However, only 91 contra-regulated genes were detected among the three libraries. Furthermore, 20 contra-regulated genes were selected and 11 showed consistent changes in the RNA-sequencing assay, which were validated by RT-PCR.

Conclusion: The gene expression profiling results suggested that these validated genes may be good targets for understanding potential mechanisms and conducting molecular studies into PD.

Keywords: Peyronie's disease, Pericytes, Nanovesicles, Gene expression, RNA-sequencing

Background

Peyronie's disease (PD) is caused by excessive fibrosis and scar tissue formation in the tunica albuginea (TA), resulting in penile pain, abnormal curvature, and erectile dysfunction (ED) [1, 2]. Although the existence of PD has been known for a long time, the

*Correspondence: jksuh@inha.ac.kr; rjk0929@inha.ac.kr
†Guo Nan Yin and Shuguang Piao have contributed equally to this work
[1] Department of Urology and National Research Center for Sexual Medicine, Inha University School of Medicine, 7-206, 3rd St, Shinheung-Dong, Jung-Gu, Incheon 22332, Republic of Korea
Full list of author information is available at the end of the article

pathophysiology of PD has not been studied as widely as fibrosis in other organs, such as the kidneys, liver, or lungs. Currently, the most available medical therapy is collagenase and interferon injection and surgical intervention [3, 4]. However, these treatments can cause glandular hypoesthesia and a high risk of new onset ED [5]. Therefore, the identification of novel therapeutic targets related to PD fibrosis is required.

Pericytes play a fundamental role in vascular contractility and stability, regulation of vascular development, and as a storage vault of mesenchymal stem cells [6, 7]. In vitro studies have shown that pericytes exhibit fibrogenic potential [8, 9] and transition to myofibroblasts [10]. Moreover, the inhibition of angiogenesis may be effective in the suppression of fibrosis [11]. However, recently studies have shown that the inhibition of angiogenesis may aggravate fibrosis [12, 13]. These findings suggest that different antiangiogenic and molecular targets produce different results in the treatment of fibrosis. We recently reported in a mouse model of diabetic ED that pericyte-derived angiogenic factor restored erectile function by enhancing cavernous angiogenesis [14, 15].

Extracellular vesicles (EVs) were previously believed to be cell excretions. However, a number of studies have shown that EVs contain proteins, lipids, and RNA, which can affect the physiological and pathological communications between cells [16, 17]. Many studies regarding the potential role of EVs have been conducted for human diseases, including strokes [18], tumor metastasis [19], and kidney disease [20]. Therefore, clarifying the role of EVs in fibrosis would be beneficial to aid in the understanding of fibrosis mechanisms. However, one of the major limitations of EVs is the low production yield [21]. Therefore, to maximize the production of vesicles, we used a mini extruder system and extracted more than 100-fold greater EV–mimetic NVs from pericytes. The cell-derived EV–mimetic NVs showed similar characteristics to the natural EVs [22]. We recently demonstrated that intracavernous injection of PC–NVs induced penile angiogenesis and rescued erectile function in a mouse model of cavernous nerve injury [15]. Along with potential relationship between angiogenesis and suppression of tissue fibrosis [11–13], the angiogenic potential of pericytes and PC–NVs led us to investigate the potential role of PC–NVs in the fibrogenic process of PD.

Gene expression profiling analysis in physiological and pathological conditions can provide a foundation for studying the mechanisms of fibrosis in PD. In the present study, we performed an RNA-sequencing assay on normal fibroblasts, PD fibroblasts, and PD fibroblasts treated with PC–NVs.

Methods

Ethics statement and study design

All TA tissues and animals used in this study were approved by the Institutional Review Board (IRB No: 2007-730) and the Institutional Animal Care and Use Committee of our University (approval number: 171129-527), respectively. The plaque tissue of a patient with PD (48 years old) and the normal TA tissue from control patients (undergoing penoplasty for congenital curvature, 21 years old) were used for the human fibroblast culture study. In addition, 10 adult male C57BL/6J mice (8 weeks old, Orient Bio, Korea) were used for the mouse cavernous pericytes (MCPs) primary culture.

Primary culture and characterization of human fibroblasts

The TA tissues were used for the primary fibroblast culture as described previously [23, 24]. Briefly, PD plaque and normal TA tissues were maintained in sterile vials with Hank's balanced salt solution (HBSS, Gibco, Carlsbad, CA, USA) and washed three times with phosphate-buffered saline (PBS). The TA tissues were cut into 1–2 mm sections and incubated in 12.5 mL Dulbecco's modified Eagle's medium (DMEM, Gibco) supplemented with 0.06% collagenase A (Sigma-Aldrich, St. Louis, MO, USA) at 37 °C for 1 h in a 5% CO_2 atmosphere. The cells and tissue fragments were collected by centrifugation (400 g for 5 min), washed with fresh culture medium, and placed in 100 mm cell culture dishes (Falcon-Becton Dickinson Labware, Franklin Lakes, NJ, USA) with DMEM containing 10% fetal bovine serum (FBS), penicillin (100 U/mL), and streptomycin (100 μg/mL) at 37 °C in a 5% CO_2 atmosphere. Media were changed every 2 days and the cells were characterized as previously described [23, 24]. Passages 5 to 8 were used for the experiments.

To determine cell type, the cells were cultured on sterile cover glasses, placed into 12-well plates and grown until nearly confluent. The cells were stained with antibody to CD90 (fibroblast marker, R&D Systems Inc., Minneapolis, MN, USA; 1:100), Vimentin (fibroblast marker, R&D Systems Inc., 1:50), NG2 chondroitin sulfate proteoglycan (NG2, pericyte marker, Millipore, San Francisco, CA, USA; 1:50), CD31 (endothelial cell marker, Chemicon, Temecula, CA, USA; 1:50), or DAPI (nucleus marker; Vector Laboratories Inc., Burlingame, CA, USA), as previously described [25]. Signals were visualized and digital images were obtained using a confocal fluorescence microscope (K1-Fluo, Nanoscope Systems, Inc., Daejeon, Korea).

Primary culture of MCPs

The primary cultures of MCPs were performed as described previously [26, 27]. Shortly, 8 weeks old male C57BL/6J mice were anesthetized with ketamine (100 mg/kg) and xylazine (5 mg/kg) intramuscularly, and sacrificed by cervical dislocation. Then, the penis tissues were harvested and maintained in sterile vials with HBSS (Gibco). After washing three times with PBS, the urethra and dorsal neurovascular bundle were removed, and only the corpus cavernosum tissues were used. The corpus cavernosum tissues were cut into approximately 1–2 mm sections and settled via gravity into collagen I-coated 35 mm cell culture dishes with 300 μL complement DMEM (GIBCO) at 37 °C for 20 min in a 5% CO_2 atmosphere. Thereafter, 900 μL of complement medium was added and incubated at 37 °C with 5% CO_2. The complement medium contained 20% FBS, 1% penicillin/streptomycin, and 10 nM human pigment epithelium-derived factor (PEDF; Sigma-Aldrich). The medium was changed every 2 days, and after approximately 10 days sprouting cells were sub-cultured into collagen I (Advanced BioMatrix, San Diego, CA, USA)-coated dishes. Cells from passages 2 to 3 were used for the experiments.

Preparation and characterization of MCP-derived EV–mimetic nanovesicles (NVs)

MCP-derived EV–mimetic NVs (PC–NVs) were prepared using a mini extruder system (Avanti Polar Lipids, Birmingham, AL, USA), as described previously [28, 29]. Briefly, MCPs were washed three times with PBS, detached with 0.25% Trypsin–EDTA (Invitrogen, Carlsbad, CA, USA) and re-suspended in 4-(2-Hydroxyethyl) piperazine-1-ethanesulfonic acid (HEPES)buffer solution (Gibco). The cell suspension was sequentially extruded 10 times across 10, 5, and 1 μm pore-sized polycarbonate membranes (Nuclepore, Whatman Inc., Clifon, NJ, USA), respectively. Next, ultracentrifugation was performed at 100,000 g for 2 h at 4 °C with a step gradient, which was formed with 50% iodixanol (1 mL; Axis-Shield PoC AS, Oslo, Norway) overlaid with 10% iodixanol (2 mL) and topside with the extruded samples (7 mL). PC–NVs were filtered with a 0.45 μm filter and stored at − 80 °C until further use. To quantify the PC–NVs, the EXOCET exosome quantitation assay kit (System Biosciences, Palo Alto, CA, USA) was used, and 1 μg/μL of the final concentration of the PC–NVs was prepared for all experiments.

Western blotting

For the immunoblot analyses of PC–NVs, equal protein amounts (10 μg) of purified PC–NVs and whole cells extracted using RIPA lysis buffer (Sigma-Aldrich) were separated by SDS-PAGE (12% gel) and transferred to polyvinylidene fluoride (PVDF) membranes. Each blot was blocked and incubated with antibodies to GM130 (BD Biosciences, San Jose, CA, USA; 1:1000), CD9 (Abcam, Cambridge, UK; 1:1000), CD81 (Novus Biologicals; 1:1000), or TSG101 (Novus Biologicals; 1:500).

RNA-sequencing assay

For the RNA-sequencing study, the normal and PD TA-derived fibroblasts were cultured and treated with PC–NVs (n = 4 per group). The RNA-sequencing assay was performed by E-Biogen Inc. (Korea). Briefly, total RNA was isolated 24 h after exposure to PC–NVs using TRIzol reagent (Invitrogen). RNA quality was assessed using an Agilent 2100 Bioanalyzer (Agilent Technologies, Amstelveen, The Netherlands), and RNA quantification was performed using an ND-2000 Spectrophotometer (Thermo Inc., DE, USA).

Library sequencing and data analysis

Libraries were prepared from total RNA using the SMARTer Stranded RNA-Seq Kit (Clontech Laboratories, Inc., USA). The isolation of mRNA was performed using the Poly(A) RNA Selection Kit (LEXOGEN, Inc., Austria). Indexing was performed using the Illumina indices 1–12. The enrichment step was performed using PCR. Subsequently, libraries were checked using the Agilent 2100 Bioanalyzer (DNA High Sensitivity Kit) to evaluate the mean fragment size. Quantification was performed using the library quantification kit using a StepOne Real-Time PCR System (Life Technologies, Inc., USA). High-throughput sequencing was performed as paired-end 100 sequencing using HiSeq 2500 (Illumina, Inc., USA).

Quality control of the raw sequencing data was performed using FastQC (https://www.bioinformatics.babraham.ac.uk/projects/fastqc/). Adapter and low-quality reads (< Q20) were removed using FASTX_Trimmer (http://hannonlab.cshl.edu/fastx_toolkit/) and BBMap (https://sourceforge.net/projects/bbmap/). Then, the trimmed reads were mapped to the reference genome using TopHat [30]. Gene expression levels were estimated using RC (read count) and FPKM (fragments per kb per million reads) values by BEDTools [31] and Cufflinks [32]. The expression values were normalized with the Quantile normalization method using EdgeR within R (https://www.r-project.org). Data mining and graphic visualization were performed using ExDEGA (E-Biogen, Inc., Korea). The datasets generated and/or analyzed during the current study are available in the Gene Expression Omnibus repository (www.ncbi.nlm.nih.gov/geo/query/acc.cgi?acc=GSE146500. Accession no. GSE146500).

Validation of sequencing data by RT-PCR

Total RNA was extracted from cultured cells using TRIzol (Invitrogen) following the manufacturer's protocols. Reverse transcription was performed using 1 μg of RNA in 20 μL of reaction buffer with oligo dT primer and AccuPower RT Premix (Bioneer Inc., Korea). The PCR reaction was performed with denaturation at 94 °C for 30 s, annealing at 60 °C for 30 s, and extension at 72 °C for 1 min in a DNA Engine Tetrad Peltier Thermal Cycler. For the analysis of PCR products, 10 μL of each PCR productwas electrophoresed on a 1% agarose gel and detected under ultraviolet light. GAPDH was used as an internal control [14].

All digital image, western blot, and PCR band densitometry analyses were performed using an image analyzer system (National Institutes of Health [NIH] ImageJ 1.34, http://rsbweb.nih.gov/ij/).

Statistical analysis

All data are expressed as means ± standard errors. Statistical analysis was performed using Student t-test. *p* values less than 0.05 were considered statistically significant.

Results

Identification of human fibroblasts

The fibroblasts were isolated from human normal and PD plaque tissues. Representative images showed high positive staining for CD90 and Vimentin (fibroblast markers) of more than 95%, but not for pericyte (NG2) or endothelial cell (CD31) markers (Fig. 1A, B).

PC–NV preparation and characterization

PC–NVs were prepared from MCPs according to previous methods [28]. Western blot analysis showed that PC–NVs displayed positive exosomes markers, including

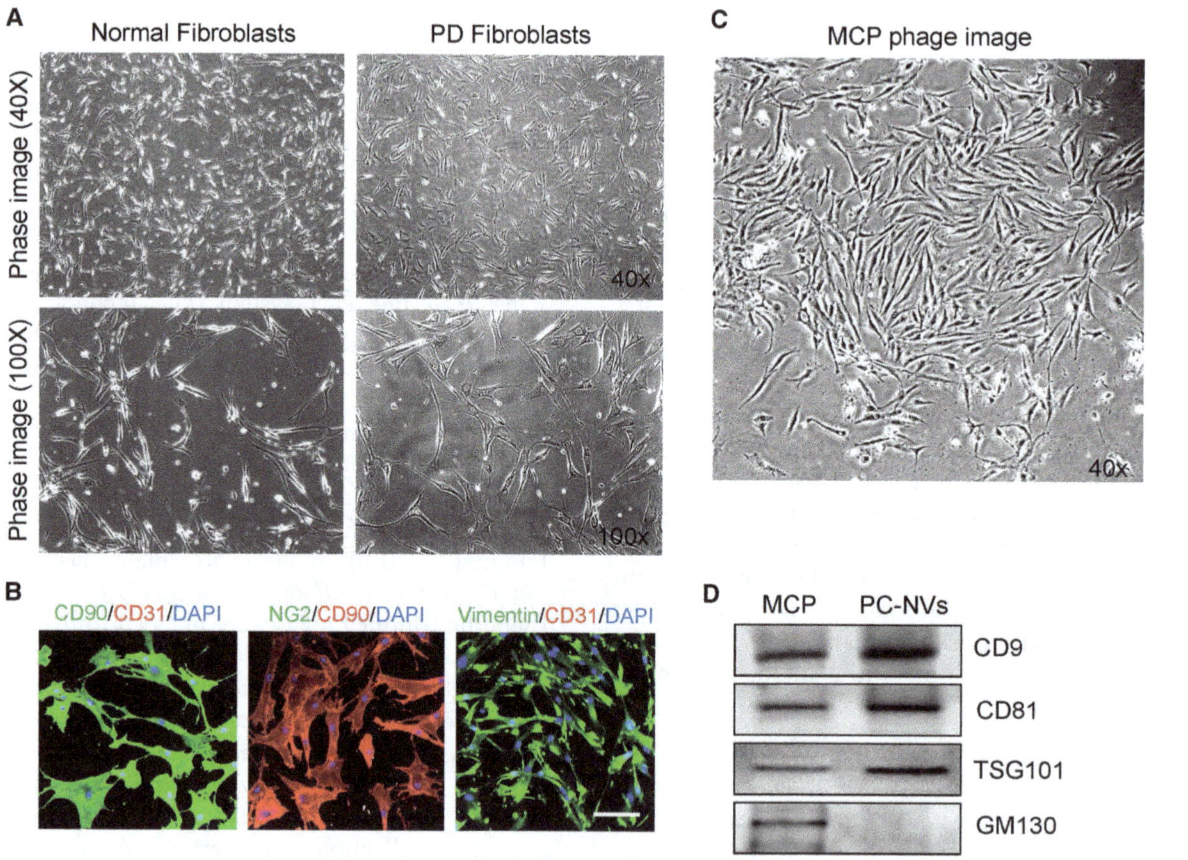

Fig. 1 Isolation and characterization of fibroblasts from human tunica albuginea (TA) and extracellular vesicle (EV)–mimetic nanovesicles (NVs) from mouse cavernous pericytes (MCPs). **A** Representative phage images (screen magnification ×40 and ×100) of primary cultured fibroblasts from the TA tissues of healthy subjects and those with PD at passage 5. **B** Immunofluorescent staining of fibroblasts with antibodies against CD90 (fibroblast marker), Vimentin (fibroblast marker), NG2 (pericyte marker), and CD31 (endothelial cell marker). Nuclei were labeled with the DNA dye DAPI. Scale bar indicates 100 μm. DAPI = 4,6-diamidino-2-phenylindole. **C** Representative phage images (screen magnification ×40) of primary cultured mouse cavernous pericytes at passage 2. **D** Representative western blot for EV positive markers (CD9, CD81, and TSG101) or an EV negative marker (GM130) in MCPs and pericyte-derived EV–mimetic NVs

CD9, CD81, and TSG101, but not for negative marker GM130 (Fig. 1C, D).

Transcriptional profiling and gene ontology (GO) category analysis

For this study, three gene libraries for the normal fibroblast (NF), PD fibroblast (PF), and PC–NVs-treated PF (PFPC) groups were constructed for an RNA-sequencing assay (n = 4 for each group). In total, 25,737 genes were detected in three libraries. Significant gene selection was performed with three conditions: fold-change > 2.0, log2 > 4, and p value < 0.05. Among all detected genes, 3961 showed significant differential expression in the PF group compared with the NF group, and 174 were significantly differentially expressed in the PFPC group compared with the PF group (Fig. 2A–C). Only 91 contra-regulated genes (Additional file 1: Table S1) were detected between PF/NF and PFPC/PF through Venn diagram analysis (Fig. 2D).

To evaluate the GO categories, all significantly differentially expressed genes (DEGs) were classified in 16 GO categories by ExDEGA software (E-Biogen, Inc., Korea). Among these, extracellular matrix (33.61%), angiogenesis (32.33%), and fibrosis (31.07%) made up the largest proportion in the PF group compared with the NF group (Fig. 3A, B). However, fibrosis (3.88%), extracellular matrix (2.92%), and angiogenesis (2.59%) made up the largest proportion in the PFPC group compared with the PF group (Fig. 3C, D).

Validation of RNA-sequencing results by RT-PCR

To validate the RNA-sequencing results, we selected 20 genes (Additional file 1: Table S2) from 91 contra-regulated DEGs, and 11 (primers as shown in Additional

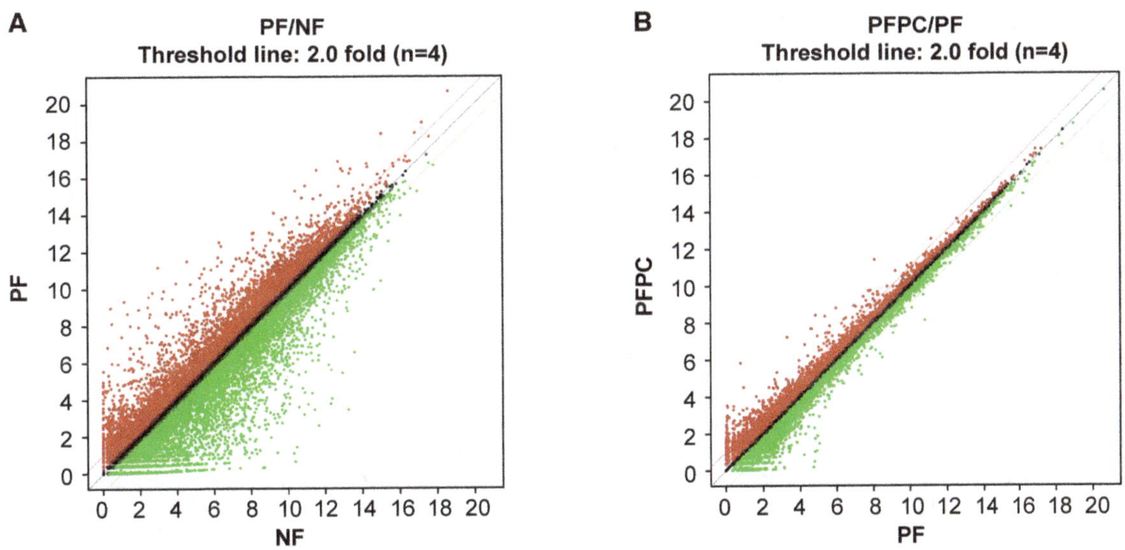

C

	Significant gene selection (Fold change > 2.0, Log2 > 4, and p-value < 0.05)		
	Total	Up-regulated	Down-regulated
PF/NF	3961	1543	2418
PFPC/PF	174	111	63

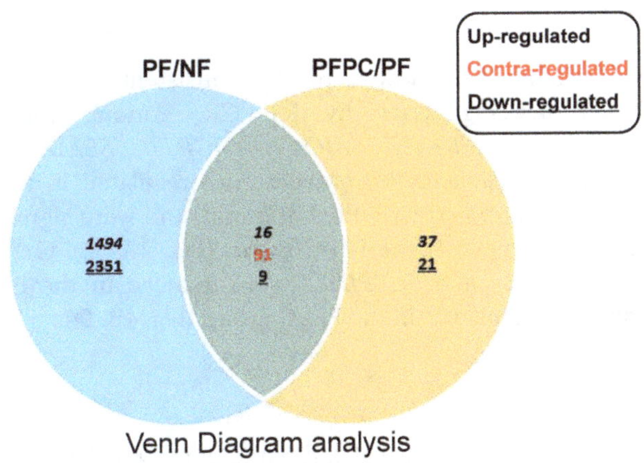

Fig. 2 Analysis of differentially expressed genes (DEGs) from three libraries. **A** Total gene expression of normal fibroblasts (NF) and PD fibroblasts (PF). **B** Total gene expression of PF and PC–NV-treated PF (PFPC) groups. **C** DEG analysis for significantly altered gene selection according to the conditions set: fold-change > 2.0, log2 > 4, and p value < 0.05. **D** Venn diagram analysis between PF/NF and PFPC/PF

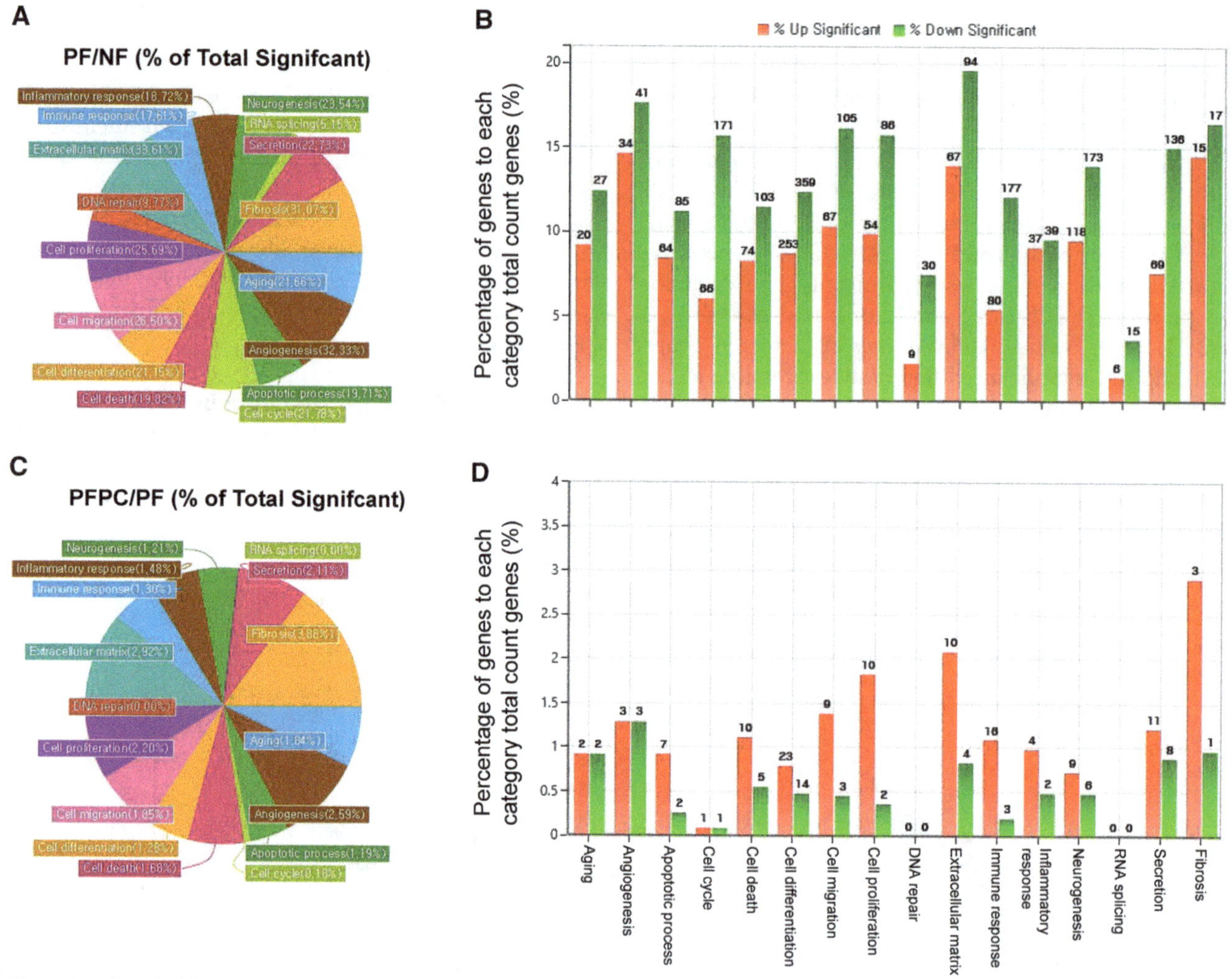

Fig. 3 Significantly differentially expressed genes (DEGs) of the RNA-sequencing data were distributed to gene ontology (GO) categories. **A**, **B** The distribution (**A** total percentage; **B** detailed percentage and numbers of upregulated and downregulated genes, respectively) of total significantly DEGs in 16 GO categories in the PD fibroblast (PF) group compared with the normal fibroblast (NF) group. **C**, **D** The distribution (**C** total percentage; **D** detailed percentage and numbers of upregulated and downregulated genes, respectively) of total significantly DEGs in 16 GO categories in the PC–NV-treated PF group compared with the PF group

file 1: Table S3) showed results consistent with the RNA-sequencing assay by RT-PCR. Among these genes, *MMP3, AKR1C1, SMOC1, ANGPTL2, SEMA3A, TRIM15, EGR1,* and *BMP2* were downregulated in the PF group compared with the NF group, and were significantly recovered in the PFPC group (Fig. 4A, C). Only *TFPI2, SFRP4,* and *SERPINE1* were induced in the PF group and recovered in the PFPC group (Fig. 4B, D).

Discussion

The accurate physiological and pathological mechanisms of PD remain poorly understood. To date, most gene expression studies have focused on human PD plaque at a tissue level in vivo [33, 34] but not at a cellular level in vitro. Therefore, to investigate the exact mechanisms and potential target genes for PD, we cultured human fibroblasts from human PD plaque and performed RNA-sequencing assays.

EVs display a potential role in kidney fibrosis and other fibrotic diseases [20, 35]; however, little is currently known regarding the detailed mechanisms. Considering the low yield of EVs, we extracted more than 100-fold greater EV–mimetic NVs from MCPs, which were primarily cultured from mouse corpus cavernosum tissues. Many previous studies have found that pericytes display diverse features in relation to fibrosis that are dependent on different molecular targets [8, 9, 11]. We used

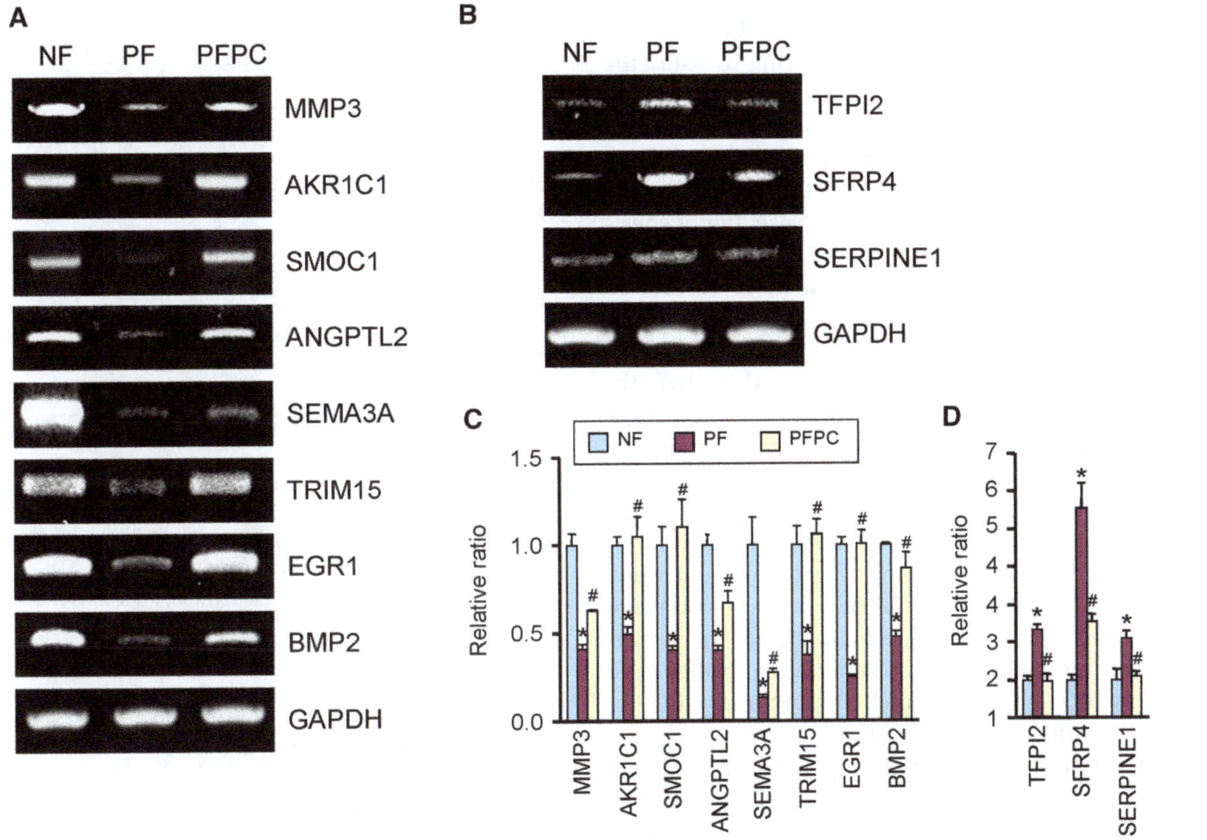

Fig. 4 RT-PCR validation of differentially expressed genes selected from the RNA-sequencing assay. **A**, **B** Eleven contra-regulated genes were found to be consistent with the RNA-sequencing result in normal fibroblast (NF), PD fibroblast (PF), and PC–NV-treated PF (PFPC) groups. **C**, **D** Each bar depicts the mean value (±standard error) from three separate experiments. $^{*}p<0.001$ compared with the NF group. $^{\#}p<0.05$ compared with the PF group

pericytes isolated from mouse cavernous tissue, but not a human tissue, because it was not easy to harvest human erectile tissue in a large quantity. Although there are animal models of PD by using intratunical injection of fibrin [36] or transforming growth factor-β1 [37, 38], these animal models cannot represent the complex pathophysiologic processes of the human PD. Meanwhile, we can easily obtain fibrotic plaque from the patients with PD during reconstructive surgery. In the present study, therefore, human PD fibroblasts exposed to mouse origin of PC–NVs were compared with human PD fibroblasts to investigate the regulation of gene expression by PC–NVs in PD.

From the RNA-sequencing assay, 3961 DEGs were detected, and the 16 top GO categories were assessed in this study. GO analysis showed that significantly altered genes were enriched in the extracellular matrix, angiogenesis, and fibrosis. The extracellular matrix is a driver of progressive fibrosis [39], and angiogenesis is closely associated with chronic liver fibrosis [20]. These data suggest that our DEG detection is credible. However, the molecular basis of PC–NVs in regulating the extracellular matrix or angiogenesis pathway in PD remains largely unknown. In this study, only 91 contra-regulated genes were identified from the three libraries (NF, PF, and PFPC). After precision screening, 20 genes were selected and validated by RT-PCR in same conditions. However, only 11 genes were validated to be consistent with the RNA-sequencing results as showed in Fig. 4. Through literature analysis, we found that most target genes have multiple roles, such as angiogenesis, extracellular matrix (ECM), and fibrosis. Some studies have shown that the *MMP3* attenuated the process of fibrosis by degrading α2-antiplasmin and ECM [40] and these enzymes inhibitors are up-regulated (*TFPI2*) [41]. Many studies have shown that fibrosis and angiogenesis have common characteristics. Wound healing is a typical example of the synergistic interaction between the molecular mechanisms of fibrosis and angiogenesis [42, 43]. Although some studies have shown that *AKR1C1* [44], *SMOC1* [45], *ANGPTL2* [46], *SEMA3A* [47], *TRIM15* [48], *EGR1* [49], *BMP2* [50], *SFRP4* [51], and *SERPINE1* [52] are related to angiogenesis or fibrosis, but the detailed mechanism of action of these genes is still unknown, and it will be interesting to study the network and pathway of these genes in fibrosis and angiogenesis in the future. Therefore, on the one hand, we hypothesized that pericytes might be releasing nanovesicles, which contain these target genes to directly affect nearby fibroblasts, such as increase angiogenesis and reducing excessive pathological ECM deposition during fibrosis. On the other hand, pericyte-derived nanovesicles might indirectly affect the expression of these target genes in fibroblasts through microRNA, and further research is needed to resolve these hypotheses. These genes may be the key to understanding how PC–NVs regulate the extracellular matrix, angiogenesis, and fibrosis mechanisms in PD.

To the best of our knowledge, this is the first study to demonstrate the systematic profiling of gene alterations in NF, PF, and PFPC. However, the present study has some limitations. First, a small number of cultured human fibroblast samples were used in target gene validation and age differences existed among groups, and need to collect more age-matched samples for further studies. It would be more appropriate to use healthy TA from an age-matched PD patient instead of using TA from a young patient with congenital penile curvature. Second, we were unable to demonstrate the network of these validated genes in the extracellular matrix, angiogenesis, and fibrosis pathways. Further studies are needed to document the function of each gene at cellular and molecular levels as well as in animal models of PD. Third, mouse corpus cavernous pericytes were used for EV–mimetic NVs isolation, and further research is needed to cultivate human corpus cavernous pericytes and isolate human PC–NVs and process them in human PD fibroblasts to study the detailed mechanism of these initial selected target genes.

Conclusion

In summary, we profiled the DEGs of human TA cultured fibroblasts in NF, PF, and PFPC groups. We hypothesize that these validated genes are good candidates for the study of the mechanism of PC–NVs in PD. Further studies exploring the effect of these target genes will be beneficial to further our understanding of the detailed mechanisms of the extracellular matrix, angiogenesis, and fibrosis in PD.

Abbreviations

PD: Peyronie's disease; EV: Extracellular vesicle; NVs: Nanovesicles; PC–NVs: Pericyte-derived EV–mimetic NVs; RT-PCR: Reverse transcription polymerase chain reaction; TA: Tunica albuginea; ED: Rrectile dysfunction; MCPs: Mouse cavernous pericytes; HBSS: Hank's balanced salt solution; PBS: Phosphate-buffered saline; DMEM: Dulbecco's modified Eagle's medium; FBS: Fetal bovine serum; PEDF: Pigment epithelium-derived factor; HEPES: 4-(2-Hydroxyethyl) piperazine-1-ethanesulfonic acid; PVDF: Polyvinylidene fluoride.

Acknowledgements

The manuscript is edited by a professional, native English-speaking editor at Editage (direct@editage.com; Vikas Narang, Chief Operating Officer, Editage).

Authors' contributions

GNY, SGP, JKS and JKR drafted and designed the research. GNY, SGP, JYO, MHK performed the experiments. GNY, SGP, ZYL, LW, JYO, DKK, analyzed the data. GNY, SGP prepared the figures and drafted the manuscript. YSG, JKS and JKR edited and revised the manuscript. GNY, SGP, ZYL, LW, JYO, MHK, DKK, YSG, JKS and JKR have read and approved the final version of the manuscript. All authors are accountable for all aspects of work. All authors read and approved the final manuscript.

Competing interests

The authors declare that they have no competing interests.

Author details

[1]Department of Urology and National Research Center for Sexual Medicine, Inha University School of Medicine, 7-206, 3rd St, Shinheung-Dong, Jung-Gu, Incheon 22332, Republic of Korea. [2]Department of Urology at Changhai Hospital Affiliated with the Naval Medicine University, Shanghai 200433, People's Republic of China. [3]Korea Zoonosis Research Institute, Jeonbuk National University, Iksan, Jeonbuk 54531, Korea. [4]Department of Life Sciences, Pohang University of Science and Technology, Pohang, Kyeongsangbuk-do 37673, Korea.

References

1. Gholami SS, Gonzalez-Cadavid NF, Lin CS, Rajfer J, Lue TF. Peyronie's disease: a review. J Urol. 2003;169:1234–41.
2. Hellstrom WJ, Bivalacqua TJ. Peyronie's disease: etiology, medical, and surgical therapy. J Androl. 2000;21:347–54.
3. Duncan MR, Berman B, Nseyo UO. Regulation of the proliferation and biosynthetic activities of cultured human Peyronie's disease fibroblasts by interferons-alpha, -beta and -gamma. Scand J Urol Nephrol. 1991;25:89–94.
4. Russo GI, Milenkovic U, Hellstrom W, Levine LA, Ralph D, Albersen M. Clinical efficacy of injection and mechanical therapy for Peyronie's disease: a systematic review of the literature. Eur Urol. 2018;74:767–81.
5. Levine LA, Greenfield JM, Estrada CR. Erectile dysfunction following surgical correction of Peyronie's disease and a pilot study of the use of sildenafil citrate rehabilitation for postoperative erectile dysfunction. J Sex Med. 2005;2:241–7.
6. Armulik A, Abramsson A, Betsholtz C. Endothelial/pericyte interactions. Circ Res. 2005;97:512–23.
7. Armulik A, Genove G, Betsholtz C. Pericytes: developmental, physiological, and pathological perspectives, problems, and promises. Dev Cell. 2011;21:193–215.
8. Crisan M, Yap S, Casteilla L, et al. A perivascular origin for mesenchymal stem cells in multiple human organs. Cell Stem Cell. 2008;3:301–13.
9. Cai X, Lin Y, Friedrich CC, et al. Bone marrow derived pluripotent cells are pericytes which contribute to vascularization. Stem Cell Rev Rep. 2009;5:437–45.
10. Lin SL, Kisseleva T, Brenner DA, Duffield JS. Pericytes and perivascular fibroblasts are the primary source of collagen-producing cells in obstructive fibrosis of the kidney. Am J Pathol. 2008;173:1617–27.
11. Yoshiji H, Kuriyama S, Yoshii J, et al. Vascular endothelial growth factor and receptor interaction is a prerequisite for murine hepatic fibrogenesis. Gut. 2003;52:1347–54.
12. Patsenker E, Popov Y, Stickel F, et al. Pharmacological inhibition of integrin alphavbeta3 aggravates experimental liver fibrosis and suppresses hepatic angiogenesis. Hepatology. 2009;50:1501–11.
13. Stockmann C, Kerdiles Y, Nomaksteinsky M, et al. Loss of myeloid cell-derived vascular endothelial growth factor accelerates fibrosis. Proc Natl Acad Sci U S A. 2010;107:4329–34.
14. Yin GN, Jin HR, Choi MJ, et al. Pericyte-derived Dickkopf2 regenerates damaged penile neurovasculature through an angiopoietin-1-Tie2 pathway. Diabetes. 2018;67:1149–61.

15. Yin GN, Park SH, Ock J, et al. Pericyte-derived extracellular vesicle–mimetic nanovesicles restore erectile function by enhancing neurovascular regeneration in a mouse model of cavernous nerve injury. J Sex Med. 2020;17:2118–28.
16. Colombo M, Raposo G, Thery C. Biogenesis, secretion, and intercellular interactions of exosomes and other extracellular vesicles. Annu Rev Cell Dev Biol. 2014;30:255–89.
17. Record M, Carayon K, Poirot M, Silvente-Poirot S. Exosomes as new vesicular lipid transporters involved in cell–cell communication and various pathophysiologies. Biochim Biophys Acta. 2014;1841:108–20.
18. Zhang ZG, Chopp M. Exosomes in stroke pathogenesis and therapy. J Clin Investig. 2016;126:1190–7.
19. Li K, Chen Y, Li A, Tan C, Liu X. Exosomes play roles in sequential processes of tumor metastasis. Int J Cancer. 2019;144:1486–95.
20. Zhang W, Zhou X, Zhang H, Yao Q, Liu Y, Dong Z. Extracellular vesicles in diagnosis and therapy of kidney diseases. Am J Physiol Renal Physiol. 2016;311:F844–51.
21. Kim OY, Lee J, Gho YS. Extracellular vesicle mimetics: novel alternatives to extracellular vesicle-based theranostics, drug delivery, and vaccines. Semin Cell Dev Biol. 2017;67:74–82.
22. Jang SC, Kim OY, Yoon CM, et al. Bioinspired exosome-mimetic nanovesicles for targeted delivery of chemotherapeutics to malignant tumors. ACS Nano. 2013;7:7698–710.
23. Piao S, Choi MJ, Tumurbaatar M, et al. Transforming growth factor (TGF)-beta type I receptor kinase (ALK5) inhibitor alleviates profibrotic TGF-beta1 responses in fibroblasts derived from Peyronie's plaque. J Sex Med. 2010;7:3385–95.
24. Ryu JK, Kim WJ, Choi MJ, et al. Inhibition of histone deacetylase 2 mitigates profibrotic TGF-beta1 responses in fibroblasts derived from Peyronie's plaque. Asian J Androl. 2013;15:640–5.
25. Yin GN, Ryu JK, Kwon MH, et al. Matrigel-based sprouting endothelial cell culture system from mouse corpus cavernosum is potentially useful for the study of endothelial and erectile dysfunction related to high-glucose exposure. J Sex Med. 2012;9:1760–72.
26. Neng L, Zhang W, Hassan A, et al. Isolation and culture of endothelial cells, pericytes and perivascular resident macrophage-like melanocytes from the young mouse ear. Nat Protoc. 2013;8:709–20.
27. Yin GN, Das ND, Choi MJ, et al. The pericyte as a cellular regulator of penile erection and a novel therapeutic target for erectile dysfunction. Sci Rep. 2015;5:10891.
28. Kwon MH, Song KM, Limanjaya A, et al. Embryonic stem cell-derived extracellular vesicle–mimetic nanovesicles rescue erectile function by enhancing penile neurovascular regeneration in the streptozotocin-induced diabetic mouse. Sci Rep. 2019;9:20072.
29. Oh K, Kim SR, Kim DK, et al. In vivo differentiation of therapeutic insulin-producing cells from bone marrow cells via extracellular vesicle–mimetic nanovesicles. ACS Nano. 2015;9:11718–27.
30. Trapnell C, Pachter L, Salzberg SL. TopHat: discovering splice junctions with RNA-Seq. Bioinformatics. 2009;25:1105–11.
31. Quinlan AR, Hall IM. BEDTools: a flexible suite of utilities for comparing genomic features. Bioinformatics. 2010;26:841–2.
32. Roberts A, Trapnell C, Donaghey J, Rinn JL, Pachter L. Improving RNA-Seq expression estimates by correcting for fragment bias. Genome Biol. 2011;12:R22.
33. Wang Z, Liu JF, Zhou ZH, et al. Gene expression profiles and effects of transforming growth factor-beta1 intervention in Peyronie's disease. Zhonghua Wai Ke Za Zhi. 2004;42:182–6.
34. Sampaio FJ. Comparison of gene expression profiles between Peyronie's disease and Dupuytren's contracture. Int Braz J Urol. 2004;30:349–50.
35. Asef A, Mortaz E, Jamaati H, Velayati A. Immunologic role of extracellular vesicles and exosomes in the pathogenesis of cystic fibrosis. Tanaffos. 2018;17:66–72.
36. Davila HH, Ferrini MG, Rajfer J, Gonzalez-Cadavid NF. Fibrin as an inducer of fibrosis in the tunica albuginea of the rat: a new animal model of Peyronie's disease. BJU Int. 2003;91:830–8.
37. El-Sakka AI, Hassoba HM, Chui RM, Bhatnagar RS, Dahiya R, Lue TF. An animal model of Peyronie's-like condition associated with an increase of transforming growth factor beta mRNA and protein expression. J Urol. 1997;158:2284–90.
38. Piao S, Ryu JK, Shin HY, et al. Repeated intratunical injection of adenovirus expressing transforming growth factor-beta1 in a rat induces penile curvature with tunical fibrotic plaque: a useful model for the study of Peyronie's disease. Int J Androl. 2008;31:346–53.
39. Bruno S, Porta S, Bussolati B. Extracellular vesicles in renal tissue damage and regeneration. Eur J Pharmacol. 2016;790:83–91.
40. Niwa H, Kanno Y, Shu E, Seishima M. Decrease in matrix metalloproteinase3 activity in systemic sclerosis fibroblasts causes alpha2antiplasmin and extracellular matrix deposition, and contributes to fibrosis development. Mol Med Rep. 2020;22:3001–7.
41. Hanahan D, Folkman J. Patterns and emerging mechanisms of the angiogenic switch during tumorigenesis. Cell. 1996;86:353–64.
42. Folkman J, Shing Y. Angiogenesis. J Biol Chem. 1992;267:10931–4.
43. Kalluri R, Sukhatme VP. Fibrosis and angiogenesis. Curr Opin Nephrol Hypertens. 2000;9:413–8.
44. Zhu H, Chang LL, Yan FJ, et al. AKR1C1 activates STAT3 to promote the metastasis of non-small cell lung cancer. Theranostics. 2018;8:676–92.
45. Awwad K, Hu J, Shi L, et al. Role of secreted modular calcium-binding protein 1 (SMOC1) in transforming growth factor beta signalling and angiogenesis. Cardiovasc Res. 2015;106:284–94.
46. Carbone C, Piro G, Merz V, et al. Angiopoietin-like proteins in angiogenesis, inflammation and cancer. Int J Mol Sci. 2018;19:431.
47. Chen G, Sima J, Jin M, et al. Semaphorin-3A guides radial migration of cortical neurons during development. Nat Neurosci. 2008;11:36–44.
48. Kornberg LJ, Shaw LC, Spoerri PE, Caballero S, Grant MB. Focal adhesion kinase overexpression induces enhanced pathological retinal angiogenesis. Investig Ophthalmol Vis Sci. 2004;45:4463–9.
49. Sheng J, Liu D, Kang X, Chen Y, Jiang K, Zheng W. Egr-1 increases angiogenesis in cartilage via binding Netrin-1 receptor DCC promoter. J Orthop Surg Res. 2018;13:125.
50. Yang YL, Ju HZ, Liu SF, et al. BMP-2 suppresses renal interstitial fibrosis by regulating epithelial–mesenchymal transition. J Cell Biochem. 2011;112:2558–65.
51. Muley A, Majumder S, Kolluru GK, et al. Secreted frizzled-related protein 4: an angiogenesis inhibitor. Am J Pathol. 2010;176:1505–16.
52. Wu J, Strawn TL, Luo M, et al. Plasminogen activator inhibitor-1 inhibits angiogenic signaling by uncoupling vascular endothelial growth factor receptor-2-alphaVbeta3 integrin cross talk. Arterioscler Thromb Vasc Biol. 2015;35:111–20.

6

Lactobacillus rhamnosus PL1 and *Lactobacillus plantarum PM1* versus placebo as a prophylaxis for recurrence urinary tract infections in children: A study protocol for a randomised controlled trial

Maria Daniel, Hanna Szymanik-Grzelak*, Agnieszka Turczyn and Małgorzata Pańczyk-Tomaszewska

Abstract

Background: Urinary tract infections (UTIs) are one of the most common bacterial infections in children. In children < 7 years of age, the prevalence of one episode of symptomatic UTI has been estimated at 3–7% in girls and 1–2% in boys, whereas 8–30% of them will have one or more episodes of UTI. The use of some probiotics appears to reduce the risk of recurrence of UTIs. Since the effects of probiotics are strain-specific, the efficacy and safety of each strain has to be assessed. The main aim of this study is to determine whether probiotics (containing *Lactobacillus rhamnosus PL1* and *Lactobacillus plantarum PM1)* therapy are effective in preventing UTI in children compared to placebo.

Method: A superiority, double-blind, randomised, controlled trial is being conducted. One hundred and six patients aged 3 to 18 years with recurrent UTIs in last year (defined as: ≥ 2 episodes of UTI with acute pyelonephritis/upper UTI; or 1 episode of UTI with acute pyelonephritis and ≥ 1 episodes of UTI with cystitis/lower UTI; or ≥ 3 episodes of UTI with cystitis/lower UTI) or children with ≥ 1 infection in the upper urinary tract and ≥ 1 of recurrent UTIs risk factors (congenital anomalies of the kidney and urinary tract, constipation, bladder dysfunction, myelomeningocele, sexual activity in girls) will be randomly assigned to receive a 90-day prophylaxis arm (probiotic containing *L. rhamnosus PL1* and *L. plantarum PM1*) or a 90-day placebo arm. The primary outcome measure will be the frequency of recurrence of UTI during the intervention and in the period 9 months after the intervention.

Discussion: The findings of this randomised controlled trial (RCT), whether positive or negative, will contribute to the formulation of further recommendations on prevention of recurrent UTIs in children.

Keywords: Recurrent UTI, Children, Probiotics, Prophylaxis, RCT, *Lactobacillus rhamnosus PL1*, *Lactobacillus plantarum PM1*

Backround

Urinary tract infections (UTIs) are one of the most common bacterial infections in children. In children < 7 years of age, the prevalence of one episode of symptomatic UTI has been estimated at 3–7% in girls and 1–2% in boys, with 8–30% of them will have one or more recurrences of a UTI [1–3].

*Correspondence: h.szymanik@interia.pl
Department of Paediatric Nephrology, Medical University of Warsaw, Żwirki i Wigury 63A, 02-091 Warsaw, Poland

In previously published European and global guidelines, there have been no clear recommendation for prohylaxis of UTIs. According to the current recommendations, including the Polish Society of Paediatric Nephrology, antibacterial prophylaxis should be considered in children with congenital anomalies of kidney and urinary tract (CAKUT) with a history of UTIs [1, 2, 4–7].

Some randomised studies found no beneficial effect of antibiotic prophylaxis in decreasing the frequency of UTIs or preventing renal scarring. Furthermore, the antibiotic prevention strategies was associated with bacterial resistance [3, 8].

In recent years, we have observed an increasing interest in alternative methods of UTIs prevention, such as immunotherapy and probiotic therapy [9–12]. Use of some probiotics appears to reduce the risk of UTIs. Lee and et al. conducted randomised trial in children with persistent primary vescioureteral reflux (VUR) and with history of recurrent UTIs [13] and in children with VUR < 1 year old having experienced pyelonephritis [14], comparing the effect of *L. acidophilus* to a low-dose trimethoprim and sulfamethoxazole therapy (TMP/SMX). The effect on recurrent UTIs of probiotic and antibiotic therapy did not significantly differ [13, 14]. There are also some published trials with probiotics and their influence on decreasing UTIs in adult women [15–17]. In the up-to-date research, the methodology used varied considerably [18, 19]. Since the effect of probiotics are strain specific, the efficacy and safety of each strain has to be assessed.

This study products contains a specific combination of two bacterial strains *L. rhamnosus PL1* and *L. plantarum PM1*.

It is suggested that lactobacilli bacteria had a natural ability to move along gastrointenstinal tract to the rectum and anus and from where they migrate to the urethra and vagina [20, 21]. Lactic acid-producing bacteria may positively affect the urogenital microflora due to the strong adhesion to the epithelial urogenitaly tracts and displacing uropathogenic microorganism [22, 23]. Moreover, probiotics may inhibit the growth of pathogenic microorganism by producing substances, such as lactic and acetic acid, and bacteriocins [24, 25]. They may also prevent infections by immunomodulation [23, 26]. Some intervention studies have been reported if the administration of specific *Lactobacillus* strains can prevent UTIs [27, 28].

Methods/design

Trial objectives and hypothesis

The investigators aim to assess the effect and safety of administration of probiotic containing: *L. rhamnosus* PL1 with *L. plantarum* PM1 in prevention of recurrent UTIs in children. We hypothesise that study product is more effective than placebo in prophylaxis of UTIs in children.

The trial is registered at ClinicalTrials.gov (NCT03462160) and any significant changes will be included there.

Trial design

This study is designed as a randomised, placebo-controlled, double-blind, superiority trial.

Settings and participants

The study will be performed in paediatric units of the paediatric hospital and the nephrology outpatient clinic of the Medical University of Warsaw. The recruitment started in July 2018 and should be completed within the following 3 years.

Eligibility criteria

Participants must fulfil all inclusion criteria to be recruited for the trial:

aged from 3 to 18 years; diagnosis of recurrent UTIs in the last year, defined as:

- ≥ 2 episodes of UTI with acute pyelonephritis/upper UTI
- 1 episode of UTI with acute pyelonephritis and ≥ 1 episodes of UTI with cystitis/lower UTI
- ≥ 3 episodes of UTI with cystitis/lower UTI [29].

or 1 infection in the upper urinary tract and ≥ 1 of UTIs risk factors: CAKUT, constipation, bladder dysfunction, myelomeningocele, sexual activity in girls; ≥ 1 episode of urinary tract infection in the last 6 months; signed informed consent.

Exclusion criteria

Will include the following: intake of probiotic preparations for ≥ 1 month in the last 3 months; antibiotic use within last month due to any reason, known allergy to the study products, immunosuppression therapy, disease with immune deficiency, central catheter and children with other coexisting infections, e.g. meningitis, sepsis, pneumonia, otitis.

Interventions

All participants will be provided with probiotics containing *L. rhamnosus PL1* with *L. plantarum PM1* or placebo. The placebo powder consists of a mixture of potato maltodextrin, glucose, arabic gum, pectin and silicon dioxide. The formulation is identical with the active products but without *L. rhamnosus PL1* and *L. plantarum PM1*. The appearance of the placebo will be comparable to the powder containing probiotics. Placebo as the gold standard for assessing the effectiveness of a new treatment was chosen as the comparator in our trial.

The study products (probiotic and placebo) will be manufactured and supplied by Miralex (Pila, Poland) free of charge. The manufacturer will not take part in conception and protocol preparation, design and conduct study, or in the process of analysing and interpretation of the data.

Study procedure

Oral and written information will be given to parents of each participants and children > 16 years old. Participants will be randomised during hospitalisation or visit at outpatient clinic. Eligible patients will receive *L. rhamnosus PL1* with *L. plantarum PM1* at a dose of 10^9 CFU (2 g) each or placebo, orally, once daily, in the evening during a meal, after dissolving the powder in lukewarm water. The probiotics or placebo will be administered for 90 days. Throughout the study period caregivers will record the UTI. Caregivers will have the right to withdraw a participating child from the study at any time and they will not be obliged to give reasons for this decision and this will not affect subsequent medical care.

In the event of UTI, the proper treatment will be implemented [6].

Follow-up

All study participants will be followed up directly after intervention and 3, 6 and 9 months after the intervention.

Compliance

Face-to-face interview with patients and/or caregiver and through daily patient's diary (prepared by researchers and returned upon completion of the intervention) will be conducted to assess compliance with the study. Based on previously published trials [11, 13, 14], it seems appropriate to consider those participants receiving < 75% of the recommended doses as being non-compliant.

Concomitant medications

The physician may consider discontinuation or modification of the UTI prophylaxis if needed.

Outcome measures

The primary outcome measures will be the frequency of UTIs during the intervention and during the 9 months period after the intervention. The secondary outcome measures are as follows: the frequency of hospitalization due to UTI, the number of days of antibiotic therapy due to UTI.

Participant timeline

The plan for the recruitment, intervention, evaluation and visits of participants is presented in Table 1.

Sample size

Based on data from previous studies [1–3], we assumed that the frequency of reccurences of UTIs will be 30% in the group of patients at similar age in one year. 88 patients are required to have a 90% chance of detection, as significant at the 5% level, a decrease in the primary outcome measure from 30% in the control group to 5% in the experimental group. Taking into account that 20% of the patients will be lost for follow-up, we have calculated that a total of 106 children will be needed.

A power and sample size calculator for the binary outcome superiority trial was used to estimate the study and control group.

Recruitment

The recruitment rates will be followed up monthly. Patient, recruiting clinician, the centre and the trial design will be evaluated in the event of slow and poor recruitment due to reasons at various levels.

Sequence generation

Randomisation list will be generated by the independent reasercher from Medical University of Warsaw. Block randomisation will be used, with a block size of 6. Randomisation codes will be revealed when all data will be collecting and final analysis will performed. Reaserchers and participants will not know the assignment to the group of patients during the study.

Allocation concealment

Allocation concealment will be processed with use of opaque, sealed, numbered envelopes. It will be implemented after getting informed consent and after entering essential, demografic information to the case report form (CRF). An independent person will assign the numbered study products in accordance with randomisation list generated by a computer.

Blinding

The probiotic and placebo will be packaged in identical sachets. Powder will look and taste similar. The sachets will be delivered by Miralex in sealed and sequentially numbered opaque envelopes. The intervention will be blinded for all participants and investigators by the end of the study.

Table 1 Timetable of activities planned during the study

	Study period					
	Enrolment and allocation	Post allocation				Close-out (after the end of follow-up period)
Time point	Day 1	Month 3	Month 6	Month 9	Month 12	
Enrolment						
Eligibility screen	X					
Informed consent	X					
Randomisation of the participant	X					
Study product distribution	X					
Interventions						
Probiotic						
Placebo						
Assessments						
Recurrence of UTI		X	X	X	X	X
Frequencies of hospitalization due to UTI		X	X	X	X	X
No of days of antibiotic therapy due to UTI		X	X	X	X	X
Return of patient's diary		X				
Return of non-used study products		X				
Telephone contact*			X	x	X	X

UTI Urinary tract infection

Data collection and management

All participants will be ensured about data confidentiality during workshop process. All study participants will be allocated to a study identification number. Data will be collected and stored in the electronic database protected by password. Only involved researchers will have access to all participants records, CFRs, all documents, laboratory data, etc.

Statistical analysis

Intension-to treat (ITT) analysis will be performed, including all randomly assigned participants whom outcomes will be approachable (including dropouts and withdrawals). A per protocol analysis on the primary and secondary outcomes will be processed. This analysis will include children who have completed the entire treatment protocol as originally planned, with availability 9 months after intervention. X^2 tests (Pearson's or Fisher's test) will be performed for binary outcome measures.

Harms

Although the occurrence of adverse events as a result of participation in the current trial is not expected, data on adverse events data will be collected. All serious adverse events will be immediately reported to the project leader who will be responsible for notifying the Ethics Committee, all participating investigators and the manufacturer of the study products.

Auditing

Auditing for this study was not required by the Bioethics Committee.

Ethics and dissemination

The Bioethics Committee of the Medical University of Warsaw reviewed and accepted the study protocol and template consent. If any modifications to the protocol have influence on the conducting of the study, they will be presented to the Committee. Verbal and written information about informal consent will be revealed to the caregivers. The informed consent forms will have to be singed by a parent or legal gardian prior to the randomisation. Patients may abandon from the study at any time without warring, as is documented and explained at the time of providing consent. The full protocol will be available freely due to open access publication. Abstracts will be submitted to relevant national and international conferences.

Discussion

A precise clinical question has been posed to fill a gap in knowledge as to whether administration of *L. rhamnosus PL1* and *L. plantarum PM1* are effective in the prevention of UTIs in children. The findings of this RCT, whether positive or negative, will contribute to the formulation of further recommendations on prevention of UTIs.

Abbreviations

UTI: Urinary tract infection; RCT: Randomised controlled trial; CAKUT: Congenital anomalies of kidney and urinary tract; VUR: Vescioureteral reflux; TMP/SMX: Trimethoprim and sulfamethoxazole; *L. rhamnosus PL1*: *Lactobacillus rhamnosus PL1*; *L. plantarum PM1*: *Lactobacillus plantarum PM1*; CRF: Case report form; ITT: Intention-to-treat.

Author's contributions

MD and HSG conceptualised the study. MD, HSG and AT developed the first draft of the manuscript. MD and AT prepared the checklist. MD, HSG, AT and MPT contributed to the development of the study protocol. All authors reviewed and were involved in writing up the final version of the manuscript prior to submission. All authors read and approved the final manuscript.

Competing interests

The Miralex company had no input into the design of the trial. The authors have no competing financial or no-financial interests.

References

1. Simões Silva AC, Oliviera EA. Update on the approach of urinary tract infection in childhood. J Pediatr (Rio J). 2015;91(6 Suppl 1):S2–10. https://doi.org/10.1016/j.jped.2015.05.003.
2. Hellström A, Hanson E, Hansson S, Hjälmås K, Jodal U. Association between urinary symptoms at 7 years old and previous urinary tract infection. Arch Dis Child. 1991;66:232–4.
3. Conway PH, Cnaan A, Zaoutis T, Brandon VH, Grundmeier RW, Keren R. Recurrent urinary tract infections in children risk factors and association with prophylactic antimicrobials. JAMA. 2007;298(2):179–86. https://doi.org/10.1001/jama.298.2.179.
4. National Institute for Health and Care Excellence. Urinary tract infections in children and young people. 2013. www.nice.org.uk/guidance/qs36.
5. Stein R, Dogan HS, Hoebeke P, Kočvara R, Nijman RJ, Radmayr C, Tekgül S, European Association of Urology, European Society for Pediatric Urology. Urinary tract infections in children: EAU/ESPU guidelines. Eur Urol. 2015;67(3):546–58. https://doi.org/10.1016/j.eururo.2014.11.007.
6. Żurowska A, Wasilewska A, Jung A, Kiliś-Pstrusińska K, Pańczyk-Tomaszewska M, Sikora P, Tkaczyk M, Zagożdżon I. Zalecenia Polskiego Towarzystwa Nefrologii Dziecięcej dotyczące postępowania z dzieckiem z zakażeniem układu moczowego. Forum Medycyny Rodzinnej. 2016;10(4):159–78.
7. Subcommittee on Urinary Tract Infection. Reaffirmation of AAP clinical practice guideline: the diagnosis and management of the initial urinary tract infection in febrile infants and young children 2–24 months of age. Pediatrics. 2016;128:595–610.
8. Garin EH, Olavarria F, Garcia Nieto V, Valenciano B, Campos A, Young L. Clinical significance of primary vesicoureteral reflux and urinary antibiotic prophylaxis after acute pyelonephritis: a multicenter, randomized, controlled study. Pediatrics. 2006;117(3):626–32.
9. Amdekar S, Singh V, Singh DD. Probiotic therapy: immunomodulating approach toward urinary tract infection. Curr Microbiol. 2011;63(5):484–90. https://doi.org/10.1007/s00284-011-0006-2 **(Epub 2011 Sep 7. Review)**.
10. Lee SJ, Cha J, Lee JW. Probiotics prophylaxis in pyelonephritis infants with normal urinary tracts. World J Pediatr. 2016;12(4):425–9 **(Epub 2016 April 8)**.
11. Mohseni MJ, Aryan Z, Emamzadeh-Fard S, Paydary K, Mofid V, Joudaki H, Kajbafzadeh AM. Combination of probiotics and antibiotics in the prevention of recurrent urinary tract infection in children. Iran J Pediatr. 2013;23(4):430–8.
12. Tewary K, Narchi H. Recurrent urinary tract infections in children: preventive interventions other than prophylactic antibiotics. World J Methodol. 2015;5(2):13–9. https://doi.org/10.5662/wjm.v5.i2.13 **(eCollection 2015 Jun 26)**.
13. Lee SJ, Shim YH, Cho SJ, Lee JW. Probiotics prophylaxis in children with persistent primary vesicoureteral reflux. Pediatr Nephrol. 2007;22(9):1315–20 **(Epub 2007 May 26)**.
14. Lee SJ, Lee JW. Probiotics prophylaxis in infants with primary vesicoureteral reflux. Pediatr Nephrol. 2015;30(4):609–13. https://doi.org/10.1007/s00467-014-2988-z **(Epub 2014 Oct 30)**.
15. Reid G, Bruce AW. Probiotics to prevent urinary tract infections: the rationale and evidence. World J Urol. 2006;24(1):28–32 **(Epub 2005 Dec 31. Review)**.
16. Grin PM, Kowalewska PM, Alhazzan W, Fox-Robichaud AE. Lactobacillus for preventing recurrent urinary tract infections in women: meta-analysis. Can J Urol. 2013;20(1):6607–14.
17. Ng QX, Peters C, Venkatanarayanan N, Goh YY, Ho CYX, Yeo WS. Use of *Lactobacillus* spp. to prevent recurrent urinary tract infections in females. Med Hypotheses. 2018;114:49–54.
18. Schwenger EM, Tejani AM, Loewen PS. Probiotics for preventing urinary tract infections in adults and children. Cochrane Database Syst Rev. 2015. https://doi.org/10.1002/14651858.CD008772.pub2.
19. Hosseini M, Yousefifard M, Ataei N, Oraii A, Mirzay Razaz J, Izadi A. The efficacy of probiotics in prevention of urinary tract infection in children: a systematic review and meta-analysis. J Pediatr Urol. 2017;13(6):581–91. https://doi.org/10.1016/j.jpurol.2017.08.018 **(Epub 2017 Oct 9)**.
20. Gupta V, Nag D, Garg P. Recurrent urinary tract infections in women: How promising is the use of probiotics? Indian J Med Microbiol. 2017;35(3):347–54. https://doi.org/10.4103/ijmm.IJMM_16_292.
21. Rodríguez JM. The origin of human milk bacteria: is there a bacterial entero-mammary pathway during late pregnancy and lactation? Adv Nutr. 2014;5:779–84.
22. Bouchard DS, Seridan B, Saraoui T, Rault L, Germon P, Gonzalez-Moreno C, Nader-Macias FME, Baud D, François P, Chuat V, Chain F, Langella P, Nicoli J, Loir YL, Even S. Lactic acid bacteria isolated from bovine mammary microbiota: potential allies against bovine mastitis. PLoS ONE. 2015;10(12):e0144831. https://doi.org/10.1371/journal.pone.0144831.
23. Cerbo A, Palmieri B, Aponte M, Morales-Medina JC, Iannitti T. Mechanisms and therapeutic effectiveness of lactobacilli. J Clin Pathol. 2016;69:187–203. https://doi.org/10.1136/jclinpath-2015-202976.
24. Manzoor A, Ul-Haq I, Baig S, Qazi JI, Seratlic S. Efficacy of locally isolated lactic acid bacteria against antibiotic-resistant uropathogens. Jundishapur J Microbiol. 2016;9(1):e18952.
25. Salvetti E, O'Toole PW. The genomic basis of lactobacilli as health-promoting organisms. Microbiol Spectr. 2017. https://doi.org/10.1128/microbiolspec.BAD-0011-2016.
26. Salah RB, Trabelsi I, Hamden K, Chouayekh H, Bejar S. *Lactobacillus plantarum* TN8 exhibits protective effects on lipid, hepatic and renal profiles in obese rat. Anaerobe. 2013;23:55–61.
27. Sadeghi-bojd S, Naghshizadian R, Mazaheri M, Ghane Sharbaf F, Assadi F. Efficacy of probiotic prophylaxis after the first febrile urinary tract infection in children with normal urinary tracts. J Pediatric Infect Dis Soc. 2019. https://doi.org/10.1093/jpids/piz025.
28. Beerepoot MA, ter Riet G, Nys S, van der Wal WM, de Borgie CA, de Reijke TM, et al. Lactobacilli versus antibiotics to prevent urinary tract infections: a randomized, double-blind, noninferiority trial in postmenopausal women. Arch Intern Med. 2012;172:704–12.
29. Urinary tract infection (recurrent): antimicrobial prescribing NICE guideline. 2018. www.nice.org.uk/guidance/ng112.

7

Urethrocutaneous fistulas after voluntary medical male circumcision for HIV prevention —15 African Countries, 2015–2019

Todd Lucas[1*], Jonas Z. Hines[1], Julia Samuelson[2], Timothy Hargreave[3], Stephanie M. Davis[1], Ian Fellows[4], Amber Prainito[5], D. Heather Watts[5], Valerian Kiggundu[6], Anne G. Thomas[7], Onkemetse Conrad Ntsuape[8], Kunle Dare[9], Elijah Odoyo-June[10], Leonard Soo[11], Likabelo Toti-Mokoteli[12], Robert Manda[13], Martin Kapito[14], Wezi Msungama[15], James Odek[16], Jotamo Come[17], Marcos Canda[18], Nuno Gaspar[19], Aupokolo Mekondjo[20], Brigitte Zemburuka[21], Collen Bonnecwe[22], Peter Vranken[23], Susan Mmbando[24], Daimon Simbeye[25], Fredrick Rwegerera[26], Nafuna Wamai[27], Shelia Kyobutungi[28], James Exnobert Zulu[29], Omega Chituwo[30], Sinokuthemba Xaba[31], John Mandisarisa[32] and Carlos Toledo[1]

Abstract

Background: Voluntary medical male circumcision (VMMC) is an HIV prevention strategy recommended to partially protect men from heterosexually acquired HIV. From 2015 to 2019, the President's Emergency Plan for AIDS Relief (PEPFAR) has supported approximately 14.9 million VMMCs in 15 African countries. Urethrocutaneous fistulas, abnormal openings between the urethra and penile skin through which urine can escape, are rare, severe adverse events (AEs) that can occur with VMMC. This analysis describes fistula cases, identifies possible risks and mechanisms of injury, and offers mitigation actions.

Methods: Demographic and clinical program data were reviewed from all reported fistula cases during 2015 to 2019, descriptive analyses were performed, and an odds ratio was calculated by patient age group.

Results: In total, 41 fistula cases were reported. Median patient age for fistula cases was 11 years and 40/41 (98%) occurred in patients aged < 15 years. Fistulas were more often reported among patients < 15 compared to ≥ 15 years old (0.61 vs. 0.01 fistulas per 100,000 VMMCs, odds ratio 50.9 (95% confidence interval [CI] = 8.6–2060.0)). Median time from VMMC surgery to appearance of fistula was 20 days (interquartile range (IQR) 14–27).

Conclusions: Urethral fistulas were significantly more common in patients under age 15 years. Thinner tissue overlying the urethra in immature genitalia may predispose boys to injury. The delay between procedure and symptom onset of 2–3 weeks indicates partial thickness injury or suture violation of the urethral wall as more likely mechanisms of injury than intra-operative urethral transection. This analysis helped to inform PEPFAR's recent decision to change VMMC eligibility policy in 2020, raising the minimum age to 15 years.

Keywords: Male circumcision, Intraoperative complications, HIV, Fistula

Background

Voluntary medical male circumcision (VMMC) decreases the risk of men acquiring HIV through heterosexual sex by approximately 60% [1–4]. The use of VMMC as an HIV prevention measure is a vital component of the Joint United Nations Programme on HIV/AIDS strategy to combat the AIDS epidemic in high-prevalence areas [5]. Since 2009, the President's Emergency Plan

*Correspondence: tlucas@cdc.gov
[1] Division of Global HIV and Tuberculosis, Centers for Disease Control and Prevention, Atlanta, GA, USA
Full list of author information is available at the end of the article

for AIDS Relief (PEPFAR) has supported Ministries of Health (MoHs) and Ministries of Defense to provide over 22.8 million VMMCs in 15 southern and eastern African countries (Botswana, eSwatini, Ethiopia, Kenya, Lesotho, Malawi, Mozambique, Namibia, Rwanda, South Africa, South Sudan, Tanzania, Uganda, Zambia, Zimbabwe) [6].

Moderate and severe adverse events (AEs) occurred in approximately 1–3.5% of VMMC procedures in two of the initial African randomized controlled trials (RCTs), in Uganda and Kenya, while the third such RCT, from South Africa, which did not differentiate among mild, moderate, and severe AEs, reported a rate of 3.8% [1–3]. Rates of moderate and severe AEs from large, established VMMC programs are often reported as much lower in routine program monitoring data; for example, program data report AEs in 0.18% of VMMC procedures in Tanzania and 0.3% for surgical VMMC in Zimbabwe [7, 8]. Although these lower rates may reflect improved competence as a program matures, underreporting of AEs outside the study setting is assumed [9, 10].

A urethrocutaneous fistula (hereafter referred to as fistula) is an abnormal opening between the urethral lumen and the skin that diverts urinary flow from the meatus. In the context of male circumcision (MC), a fistula is an acquired condition resulting from the procedure. These are typically considered the result of damaging the urethral wall by cutting, crushing, or suturing, usually in the region of the frenulum where the urethra is closest to the skin [11–13]. Although post-MC fistulas are very rare, they are a known complication typically documented in case reports or series [12–18]. Case series reported outside a VMMC program setting typically involve fistulas after circumcision done for cultural or religious reasons in the neonatal period or post-neonatal infancy; this complication is often attributed to untrained personnel with poor surgical technique [13, 14, 18]. Concern about this possibility as VMMC programs scaled-up led to inclusion of warnings in the first edition of the World Health Organization's (WHO) *Manual for Male Circumcision Under Local Anaesthesia* about the risk of urethral injury, particularly when attempting to achieve hemostasis in the frenulum [19].

PEPFAR, through its notifiable adverse event reporting system (NAERS), has conducted routine passive surveillance since 2015 on severe AEs including: deaths, glans injuries, tetanus, AEs resulting in permanent disability (definite or probable), AEs resulting in permanent anatomic deformity (definite or probable), and AEs resulting in hospital admission for ≥ 3 days. Fistulas tend to be reported under one of the last two categories.

As the VMMC program expanded, isolated reports of post-VMMC fistulas began to emerge, mostly in patients under age 15 years. Once a fistula was diagnosed, the patient was referred for management by a specialist and an investigation ensued which then guided prevention activities consisting primarily of provider re-education on proper surgical technique, particularly in young adolescents. PEPFAR and WHO supported implementing partners and ministries in prevention efforts through development of educational materials on fistula prevention, identification, and management, subject matter expert contribution to investigations, and revision of the *Manual for Male Circumcision* to expand on fistula risk factors and mitigation [20–22]. Wide dissemination of these materials was accomplished through both distribution of print materials and webinars.

Despite these efforts, fistula adverse events continue as a rare but persistent complication of VMMC. The primary purpose of this analysis is to describe the collective experience with VMMC-related fistulas in PEPFAR-supported programs and assess the relation of patient age with fistula occurrence. Secondary goals include assessing completeness of the VMMC AE surveillance system to identify gaps in vital information and evaluating current management when fistulas occur. Results will be used to generate hypotheses on risks to guide further prevention efforts.

Methods

Data source and collection

All cases of VMMC-associated fistulas reported to PEPFAR through NAERS, from VMMCs performed during 2015–2019 (using U.S. government fiscal year which covers a one year period starting 1 October through 30 September), were retrospectively reviewed. Standardized forms submitted to NAERS contain information gathered during investigation into the procedure, post-operative care, the AE, and its management. A supplemental fistula investigation form, developed by WHO in 2018, was also reviewed when available. This WHO form was developed to improve and standardize data collection on clinical aspects of the case including anatomic variations such as foreskin adhesions, intraoperative events such as frenular bleeding, and provider characteristics including years of experience and number of previous procedures completed.

Data abstraction was performed from the NAERS record to aggregate information including patient demographics, site characteristics, provider and procedure details, fistula management and outcome, and completeness of fistula investigation reporting. Information used in this analysis is routinely collected data from patient charts, clinic registers, and AE investigations.

All patients provided informed written consent for the procedure; consenting for minors was obtained from parents or guardians and adhered to national standards. Data collection and analysis plans were reviewed for ethical considerations in accordance with US Centers for Disease Control and Prevention human research protection procedures.

Definitions

VMMC facilities were defined as static when routinely performed in a permanent structure, mobile when a team traveled with a consistent moveable structure (e.g. a tent or caravan), and outreach when VMMC teams traveled to on-site permanent or temporary structures and offered services as part of a limited engagement during periods of high demand. All AE types were recorded and classified as described on investigation forms without alteration. For example, if a diagnosis/description of wound infection was not stated, this AE was not assigned even if the patient was given antibiotics.

Initial management was classified as conservative if the patient was not taken urgently for fistula repair upon discovery and had either a catheter placed or at least a month of observation without a catheter between fistula onset and surgical repair. The true management intent of a referral physician was not always clear; this one month time frame was chosen as it implied a lack of urgency for surgical intervention and provided an interval over which improvement may be seen. Although some patients may not have presented immediately after noticing symptoms, the time between fistula onset and presentation was counted towards conservative management because it represented time without surgical intervention. Days from VMMC to fistula was defined as the length of time from the VMMC procedure to the day the patient first noticed symptoms consistent with a fistula (i.e. leakage of urine from a site other than the meatus) or if symptom onset was unknown, when they first presented for care of fistula symptoms. Date of referral is the first documented day the patient saw the referral provider who could offer surgical management of the fistula. Date fistula healed was the earliest date documented stating the fistula was healed.

Conventional surgical circumcisions are typically carried out by one of two methods: dorsal slit (DS) or forceps guided (FG). Due to risk of glans injuries with the FG method, particularly in patients with immature genitalia, WHO advised against use of FG method in prepubertal adolescents and in 2014, PEPFAR mandated use of the DS method in all patients aged 10 to 14 years to minimize the risk of glans injuries.

Analysis

A descriptive analysis was performed using frequencies for categorical variables and measures of central tendency for continuous variables. Age was dichotomized as < 15 and ≥ 15 years old and rates of fistula AEs were determined using total PEPFAR VMMCs performed in both age groups, in all 15 PEPFAR VMMC countries, and expressed as fistulas per 100,000 VMMCs. The relationship between age group and occurrence of a fistula AE was examined using Fisher's exact test. Missing data and differences in management led to different denominators for some variables; this is noted where it occurs.

Results

From 2015 to 2019, 41 post-VMMC fistulas, from 11 of 15 countries with PEPFAR-supported VMMC programs, were reported (Fig. 1). Complete NAE forms were available for review in 28/41 (68%) of fistula cases. Half of fistula cases (12/24) since 2018 had a WHO supplemental fistula form available. Some data, such as date of VMMC and age of patient, were reliably available and straightforward to collect. Other information, collected from narrative sections of the reporting forms, such as adequacy of provider training, whether a provider was overworked, or if diathermy was used during the procedure, were less often available.

During 2015 to 2019, approximately 14.9 million PEPFAR-supported VMMCs were performed with an overall rate of 0.28 fistulas per 100,000 procedures. Of the 41 cases, all but one of these fistulas occurred in patients under age 15 years with a median age of 11 years (interquartile range [IQR] 10–13 years old) (Table 1). The greatest number of fistula AEs occurred in patients ages 10 and 11 years (Fig. 2). Though the fistula adverse events were rare, leading to a wide confidence interval, the rate varied considerably by age. The reported rate of events for individuals under age 15 years was 0.61 per 100,000 procedures, while the rate for individuals age 15 years and above was 0.01 per 100,000 procedures. This difference was highly significant ($OR = 50.9$, [8.6, 2060.0], p value < 0.00001) (Table 2).

Fistula cases occurred in all types of facilities with slightly over half of involved facilities (21/41, 51%) identified as outreach sites (Table 1). The type of provider was reported for 16 of the 41 cases. Among the cases where type of provider was reported, both physician (5/16, 31%) and various types of non-physician providers (11/16, 69%) performed circumcisions that resulted in fistulas. Of the 12 cases where a WHO fistula investigation form was available, providers reported a wide range of both years of VMMC experience and number of previous VMMC procedures. Among the 17 fistula cases

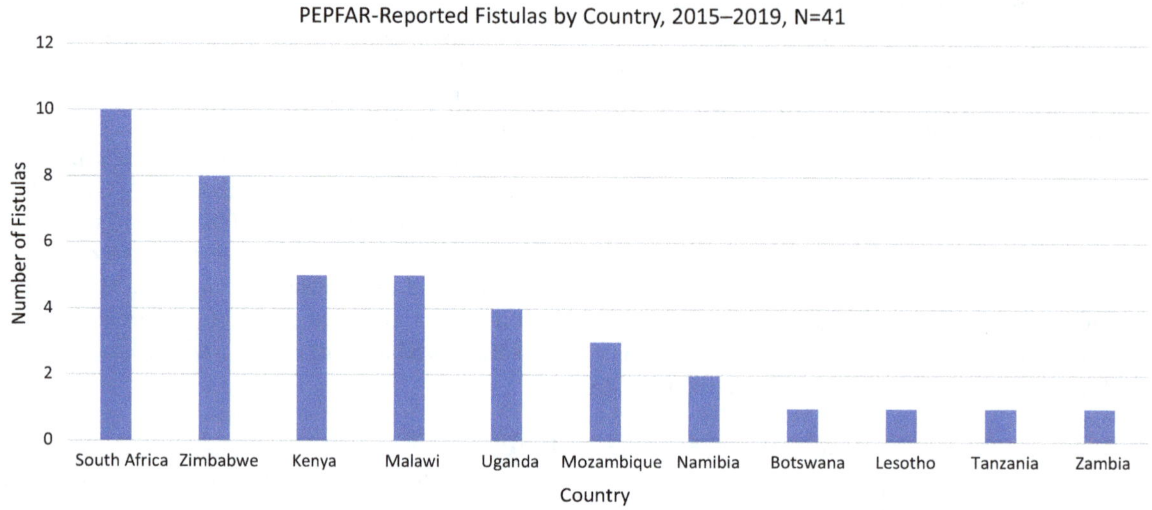

Fig. 1 Number of fistulas reported to PEPFAR by country, 2015–2019

where the records commented on diathermy use, 6 (35%) documented its use. Most cases (35/41, 85%) had their circumcision performed using the DS method and 34/41 (83%) presented for scheduled follow-up within 7 post-operative days.

The median time from VMMC to appearance of fistula symptoms was 20 days (IQR 14–27 days) (Table 3). Only 5/41 (12%) fistulas appeared within the first week after surgery. Most patients (31/41, 76%) had fistula as their initial AE diagnosis, with infection being the second most common initial diagnosis (7/41, 17%). Of the 28 cases with another type of post-VMMC AE diagnosed, 21/28 (75%) were infections. Concerning management once a fistula was diagnosed, most patients (40/41, 98%) were documented as having seen a referral specialist for fistula management where all but 2 had a documented specialty. Urologists were the most common referral specialty (29/38, 76%). Once fistula symptoms started, patients were seen by referral specialists in a median of 6 days (IQR 2–19 days) with 38/41 (93%) documenting an initial attempt at conservative management of which 4/38 (11%) had documented success, 10/38 (26%) had documented failure, and 27/38 (71%) had an unknown outcome. Nine of the total 41 patients (22%), all of whom underwent initial conservative management, had at least one attempt at surgical repair with 4/9 (44%) having documented success. Of the 9 patients with known referral and surgical dates, the median time from fistula appearance to undergoing initial surgical repair was 60 days (IQR 30–74 days). There were 40 patients with known follow-up dates who were followed for a median of 38 days after fistula onset (IQR 15–100) and in 30/41 (73%), the fistula remained unhealed on the date of last documentation.

Discussion

During 2015–2019, PEPFAR-supported programs reported 41 VMMC-related fistulas. Although these are exceedingly rare AEs, they can be very difficult to manage and often require repeated attempts at surgical repair [14]. Despite numerous attempts to prevent fistulas through provider education and training, these AEs continue to occur, and further interventions are needed.

In this analysis, age under 15 years was associated with the occurrence of a VMMC related fistula. The reported rate of fistula occurrence in <15 year olds is similar to that found for glans injuries in this same age group [23]. This finding is further supported by the biologic plausibility of a younger patient sustaining injury to less mature (smaller) genitalia during VMMC. With thinner tissue between the urethra and skin, especially at the frenulum, these patients are more prone to urethral injury with variations in surgical technique. For example, if a provider places a deep hemostatic suture in the frenulum of an adult patient, the comparatively thicker tissue may accommodate it; whereas, in an immature penis, a suture placed at the same depth could end up in the urethral lumen. Likewise, variations in contact time during application of diathermy, or method of skin suture placement, could be harmless in an adult but risk urethral injury in a young adolescent. Although other case series have noted a preponderance of post-circumcision fistulas in children, it is unclear how many adult males were being circumcised to allow comparison [13, 14, 16, 18]. Since VMMC programs for HIV prevention circumcise more older adolescents and adult males, this provides an opportunity to compare these two age groups.

Table 1 Pre- and intra-operative circumstances surrounding fistulas in PEPFAR-supported VMMC programs

	Number (%), N=41
Patient age in years	
Median (25%, 75%)	11 (10, 13)
Mean (range)	11.8 (6–25)
Modes (n=10 each)	10, 11
Facility type	
Outreach	21 (51)
Static	15 (37)
Mobile	2 (5)
Unknown	3 (7)
Cadre Type of VMMC provider	
Nurse	7 (17)
Physician	5 (12)
Clinical Officer/ Clinical Associate	3 (7)
Assistant Medical Officer	1 (2)
Unknown	25 (61)
Voluntary medical male circumcision method	
Dorsal slit	35 (85)
Forceps guided	2 (5)
Unknown	4 (10)
Use of diathermy documented	
Yes	6 (15)
No	11 (27)
Not mentioned	24 (59)
Among those completing WHO form (n=12)	
Frenular bleeding	
Yes	1 (8)
No	11 (92)
Length of MC provider experience	
6 months	3 (25)
About a year	2 (17)
About 2 years	2 (17)
3 years or more	5 (42)
Number of VMMCs done by provider	
Only a few	0
More than 10	2 (17)
More than 50	4 (33)
More than 100	6 (50)
Anatomic condition documented (e.g. adhesions, tight frenulum)	
Yes	3 (25)
No	9 (75)
Patients had at least one follow-up visit within 7 days of MC	
Yes	34 (83)
No	5 (12)
Unknown	1 (2)
Not applicable*	1 (2)

* Patient had glans injury during MC and was immediately transferred for management

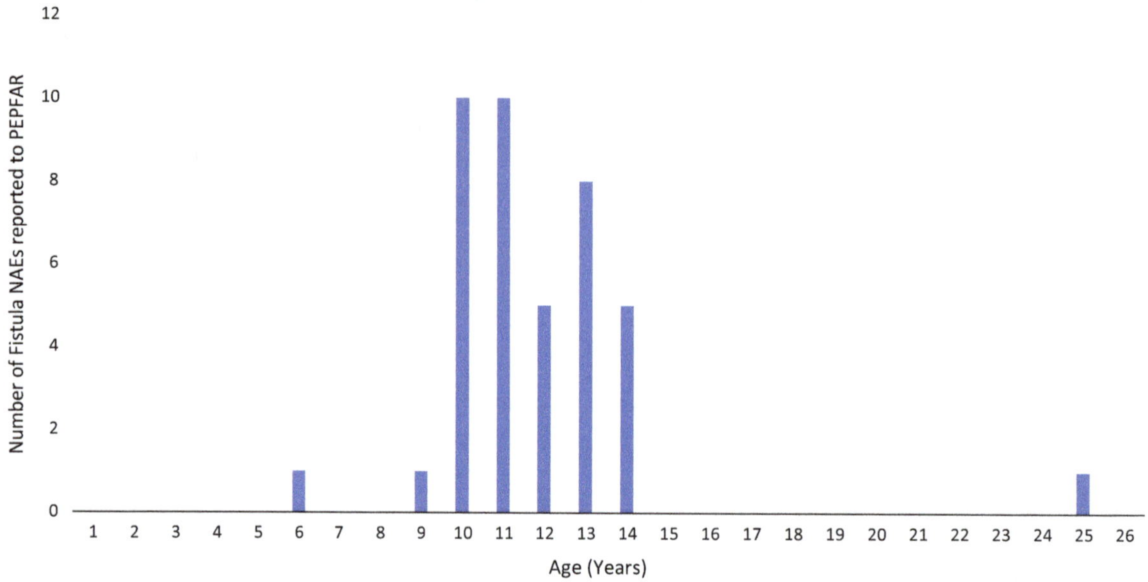

Fig. 2 Number of fistula adverse events reported to PEPFAR by age, 2015–2019, N=41

Table 2 Odds ratio of fistula occurrence in patients under age 15 years compared to those age 15 years and older in PEPFAR-supported VMMC programs, 2015–2019

	Fistula	No fistula	Odds ratio*	95% CI	Reported rate of fistula occurrence
< 15 years old	40	6,546,926	50.9	8.6–2060.0	0.61 per 100,000 VMMC
≥ 15 years old	1	8,329,144	-	–	0.01 per 100,000 VMMC

* Fisher's Exact Test, *p* value < .00001

Although the DS method of circumcision was most commonly seen in this analysis, this is likely related to this method being recommended for use in patients < 15 years of age during VMMCs due to the risk of glans injury with the alternative FG method [23]. Use of the FG method could also be under-documented due to fear of punishment for using it against policy in patients < 15 years old.

The median interval from surgery to fistula appearance of 14–27 days indicates the mechanism of injury is unlikely to be a direct cut into the urethra during the procedure since this should be evident much sooner, certainly within a day or two of surgery. However, polyglactin sutures, commonly used in VMMC programs, are typically absorbed by the body in this timeframe, and therefore if a skin or hemostatic suture is placed through the full thickness of the urethral wall, this violation may not be evident until the suture material dissolves. Ischemic injuries of the urethral wall, either from improper diathermy technique or incorporation of the wall in a suture, would also likely stay intact until tissue necrosis and sloughing takes place. All cadre types and levels of provider experience were involved with fistulas, but report forms did not collect potentially relevant information such as amount of provider experience specifically with young adolescent patients, provider workload for the day, previous fistula prevention training, adequacy of anesthesia, time of day, and adequacy of operative field lighting. Even an experienced provider could have suboptimal technique in the setting of inadequate lighting or a moving patient due to inadequate anesthesia.

Infection leading to a fistula has been reported [24]. However, most of the concurrent diagnoses of wound infection in this analysis developed after the fistula symptoms had started, which would argue against infection as an inciting event. Even in the cases where a wound infection is diagnosed first, risk factors for both, such as a large amount of ischemic tissue from excessive diathermy or hemostatic sutures, could be present as a common root cause.

Fistulas alone, although highly concerning to the patient, do not require urgent intervention. They should, however, be referred to an experienced physician who

Table 3 Post-operative circumstances surrounding fistulas in PEPFAR-supported programs

	Number (%), N = 41
Days from VMMC to fistula symptoms	
Median (25%, 75%)	20 (14, 27)
Mean (range)	30 (3–183)
Initial AE type diagnosed	
Fistula	31 (76)
Infection	7 (17)
Urinary retention	1 (2)
Glans injury	1 (2)
Wound	1 (2)
Other AE (was any other AE diagnosed in addition to fistula)	
Yes	28 (68)
Infection (% of n = 28)	21 (75)
Stricture (% of n = 28)	4 (14)
Wound/dehiscence (% of n = 28)	1 (4)
Stricture and wound (% of n = 28)	1 (4)
Glans injury (% of n = 28)	1 (4)
No	13 (32)
Referred	
Yes	40 (98)
No	0
Unknown	1 (2)
Specialty of referral provider	
Urologist	29 (71)
Pediatric Surgeon	4 (10)
Plastic Surgeon	4 (10)
Other Surgeon	1 (2)
Unknown Referral Provider Type	2 (5)
Unknown if referred	1 (2)
Days from fistula appearance to referral (if referral date known) (n = 35[†])	
Median (25%, 75%)	6 (2, 19)
Mean (range)	15 (0–75)
Antibiotic treatment	
Yes	32 (78)
No	9 (22)
Initial Management	
Conservative	38 (93)
Surgical	0
Unknown	3 (7)
Conservative management outcome (n = 38)	
Successful (% of n = 38)	4 (11)
Unsuccessful	10 (26)
Unknown	27 (71)
Ever had surgical repair	
Yes	9 (22)
No	4 (10)
Unknown	28 (68)
Days from fistula appearance to surgical repair (n = 9)	
Median (25%, 75%)	60 (30, 74)
Mean (range)	57 (16–103)

Table 3 (continued)

	Number (%), N=41
If surgery documented, what was the outcome (n=9)	
Successful (% of n=9)	4 (44)
Unsuccessful	3 (33)
Unknown	2 (22)
If surgery performed, total number of operations documented (n=9)	
One (% of n=9)	8 (89)
Two	1 (11)
Fistula healed at last documented follow up	
Yes	9 (22)
No	30 (73)
Unknown‡	2 (5)

† Outlier of 213 days excluded

‡ Two with corrective surgery performed but no follow-up results documented

is competent to perform a surgical repair. It is reassuring that patients in this analysis were seen by specialists, typically urologists, usually within a week of symptom appearance. A full discussion on appropriate management of fistulas is beyond the scope of this paper but important components of care typically involve a period of at least 3–6 months of conservative management to allow the wound time to stabilize; this may consist of time alone or may include additional measures such as placement of a urinary catheter, wound care, or antibiotics [14, 18, 25]. The median time of 60 days from fistula appearance to repair in this analysis was less than the 3–6 months recommended. Waiting longer before attempting repair represents an area for improvement in the observed fistula management. Although most final management outcomes are unknown, there were four instances of complete healing without surgery. Given the complexity of urethral reconstructions, and the increased difficulty with subsequent repairs, the first attempt should be performed by a specialist with experience in fistula repair [13, 14, 25].

Despite multiple interventions aimed at fistula prevention, primarily involving provider education and training, these rare but devastating AEs have continued to occur. Unlike glans amputations, which result from a particular surgical method that can be completely avoided, fistulas likely result from subtle variations during surgical maneuvers that cannot be avoided when performing a surgical circumcision such as sharp dissection, hemostasis, and suturing. Additional potential contributing factors such as inadequate lighting, use of diathermy in the frenulum, large needles that encourage deeper bites, surgical instruments of inappropriate size, patients who are unable to lie still, and rushing through a procedure resulting in decreased surgical precision, were identified by subject matter experts attending a recent WHO-sponsored meeting focusing on VMMC-related fistulas [25].

Strengths of this analysis include the large volume of both procedures and fistulas, standardized reporting of case investigations to allow aggregation and comparison, and wide representation of countries across the PEPFAR-supported program. This retrospective analysis includes the risk of bias due to unknown systematic errors in reporting or classification of fistulas and the risk of unknown confounding of the association of age with fistula especially given incomplete reporting forms and missing information about potential contributing risks. Some important areas where additional information would be valuable include: provider training, provider workload, adequacy of operative field lighting, use of diathermy, components of conservative management, and outcomes. Another limitation is, due to the voluntary nature of the passive reporting system, providers may have been reluctant to report fistulas due to fear of personal repercussions. While underreporting of fistulas is possible, it is unknown if systematic differences occur between age groups, or across geographic units. Given this, comparison between countries based on these data is not recommended. Furthermore, providers may underreport fistulas because the NAERS form requires them to make a judgement call about whether a fistula will result in permanent deformity or disability. Finally, aside from the increased association with age, findings from this analysis should be viewed as hypothesis-generating due to lack of comparison with controls.

Conclusions

Although improvements to any identified deficiencies at the program, facility, or provider levels can be helpful, interventions tend to be more effective the further they are from reliance on the actions of any one individual [26]. An example of this would be to avoid open surgical circumcisions in patients under age 15, the decision recently made by PEPFAR and supported by this analysis [27]. Although there is high demand among 10–14 year olds in many countries, waiting until they have matured and aged out of this high-risk group should retain the same HIV-prevention benefits while improving patient safety. The use of circumcision devices, instead of open surgical methods, in younger patients may not confer the same risk for a fistula however given the rarity of these complications, more data are needed to allow comparison. Additional recommendations including avoiding diathermy use in the frenulum, changing to a smaller needle size (19 mm instead of the typical 26 mm) [27], adequate operative field lighting, on-going monitoring and evaluation of service quality, and ensuring an adequate amount of trained staff for patient volume will likely provide improvements to safety regardless of patient age. Finally, when a fistula does occur, referral to a surgeon experienced in urethral reconstruction for all further management is needed for an optimal outcome.

Abbreviations

VMMC: Voluntary medical male circumcision; PEPFAR: President's Emergency Plan for AIDS Relief; AE: Adverse event; MoH: Ministry of Health; RCT : Randomized Controlled Trial; MC: Male circumcision; WHO: World Health Organization; NAERS: Notifiable Adverse Event Reporting System; DS: Dorsal slit; FG: Forceps-guided.

Acknowledgements

Seema Ntjabane, US Agency for International Development Lesotho for manuscript review

Authors' contributions

Conception and design: TL, JH, CT. Maintenance of surveillance database: AP, DW. Data acquisition and clinical investigation: ON, KD, EO, LS, LT, RM, MK, WM, JO, JC, MC, NG, AM, BZ, CB, PV, SM, DS, FR, NW, SK, JZ, OC, SX, JM. Drafting of manuscript: TL, JH, JS, TH, SD, IF, DH, VK, AT. Analysis and interpretation of data: TL, IF, TH, CT. Supervision: CT. All authors have read and approved the manuscript.

Competing interests

The authors declare that they have no competing interests.

Author details

[1] Division of Global HIV and Tuberculosis, Centers for Disease Control and Prevention, Atlanta, GA, USA. [2] Global HIV, Hepatitis, and STIs Programmes, World Health Organization, Geneva, Switzerland. [3] Department of Surgery, Edinburgh University, Scotland, UK. [4] Fellows Statistics, Contractor, Centers for Disease Control and Prevention, San Diego, CA, USA. [5] U.S. Office of the Global HIV/AIDS Coordinator, Washington, DC, USA. [6] Office of HIV/AIDS, U.S. Agency for International Development, Washington, DC, USA. [7] Department of Defense, Defense Health Agency, San Diego, CA, USA. [8] Ministry of Health and Wellness, Gaborone, Botswana. [9] Division of Global HIV and Tuberculosis, Centers for Disease Control and Prevention, Gaborone, Botswana. [10] Division of Global HIV and Tuberculosis, Centers for Disease Control and Prevention, Nairobi, Kenya. [11] U.S. Agency for International Development, Nairobi, Kenya. [12] Ministry of Health, Maseru, Lesotho. [13] U.S. Agency for International Development, Maseru, Lesotho. [14] Ministry of Health, Lilongwe, Malawi. [15] Division of Global HIV and Tuberculosis, Centers for Disease Control and Prevention, Lilongwe, Malawi. [16] U.S. Agency for International Development, Lilongwe, Malawi. [17] Ministry of Health, Maputo, Mozambique. [18] Division of Global HIV and Tuberculosis, Centers for Disease Control and Prevention, Maputo, Mozambique. [19] U.S. Agency for International Development, Maputo, Mozambique. [20] Ministry of Health and Social Services, Windhoek, Namibia. [21] Division of Global HIV and Tuberculosis, Centers for Disease Control and Prevention, Windhoek, Namibia. [22] National Department of Health, Pretoria, South Africa. [23] Division of Global HIV and Tuberculosis, Centers for Disease Control and Prevention, Pretoria, South Africa. [24] Ministry of Health, Dar es Salaam, Tanzania. [25] Division of Global HIV and Tuberculosis, Centers for Disease Control and Prevention, Dar es Salaam, Tanzania. [26] U.S. Agency for International Development, Dar es Salaam, Tanzania. [27] Division of Global HIV and Tuberculosis, Centers for Disease Control and Prevention, Kampala, Uganda. [28] U.S. Agency for International Development, Kampala, Uganda. [29] Ministry of Health, Lusaka, Zambia. [30] Division of Global HIV and Tuberculosis, Centers for Disease Control and Prevention, Lusaka, Zambia. [31] Ministry of Health and Child Care, Harare, Zimbabwe. [32] Division of Global HIV and Tuberculosis, Centers for Disease Control and Prevention, Harare, Zimbabwe.

References

1. Auvert B, Taljaard D, Lagarde E, Sobngwi-Tambekou J, Sitta R, Puren A. Randomized, controlled intervention trial of male circumcision for reduction of HIV infection risk: the ANRS 1265 Trial. PLoS Med. 2005;2(11):e298.
2. Bailey RC, Moses S, Parker CB, Agot K, Maclean I, Krieger JN, et al. Male circumcision for HIV prevention in young men in Kisumu, Kenya: a randomised controlled trial. Lancet (London, England). 2007;369(9562):643–56.
3. Gray RH, Kigozi G, Serwadda D, Makumbi F, Watya S, Nalugoda F, et al. Male circumcision for HIV prevention in men in Rakai, Uganda: a randomised trial. Lancet (London, England). 2007;369(9562):657–66.
4. Siegfried N, Muller M, Deeks JJ, Volmink J. Male circumcision for prevention of heterosexual acquisition of HIV in men. The Cochrane database of systematic reviews. 2009(2):Cd003362.
5. Joint United Nations Programme on HIV/AIDS (UNAIDS). On the fast-track to end AIDS. [online]. Geneva, Switzerland: UNAIDS. 2015. [cited 2020 Jan 6]. Available from URL: http://www.unaids.org/sites/default/files/media_asset/20151027_UNAIDS_PCB37_15_18_EN_rev1.pdf.
6. PEPFAR. Program Results Achieved through PEPFAR Support [online]. 2020. [cited 2020 Jan 6]. Available from URL: https://data.pepfar.gov/.
7. Hellar A, Plotkin M, Lija G, Mwanamsangu A, Mkungume S, Christensen A, et al. Adverse events in a large-scale VMMC programme in Tanzania: findings from a case series analysis. J Int AIDS Soc. 2019;22(7):e25369.
8. Bochner AF, Feldacker C, Makunike B, Holec M, Murenje V, Stepaniak A, et al. Adverse event profile of a mature voluntary medical male circumcision programme performing PrePex and surgical procedures in Zimbabwe. J Int AIDS Soc. 2017;19(1):21394.
9. Brito A, Korn A, Monteiro L, Mudender F, Maiela A, Come J, et al. Need for improved detection of voluntary medical male circumcision adverse events in Mozambique: a mixed-methods assessment. BMC Health Services Research. 2019;19(1):855.
10. Marongwe P, Gonouya P, Madoda T, Murenje V, Tshimanga M, Balachandra S, et al. Trust but verify: is there a role for active surveillance in monitoring adverse events in Zimbabwe's large-scale male circumcision program? PLoS ONE. 2019;14(6):e0218137.
11. Williams N, Kapila L. Complications of circumcision. Br J Surg . 1993;80(10):1231–6.
12. Limaye RD, Hancock RA. Penile urethral fistula as a complication of circumcision. J Pediatrics. 1968;72(1):105–6.
13. Ikuerowo SO, Bioku MJ, Omisanjo OA, Esho JO. Urethrocutaneous fistula complicating circumcision in children. Nigerian J Clin Pract. 2014;17(2):145–8.
14. Osifo OD, Odion-Obomhense H, Osagie TO. Repair-oriented categorization of circumcision urethral injury in Benin city, Nigeria. J Pediatric Urol. 2013;9(2):206–11.
15. Sancaktutar AA, Pembegul N, Bozkurt Y, Kolcu B, Tepeler A. Multiple circumferential urethrocutaneous fistulae as a rare complication of circumcision and review of literature. Urology. 2011;77(3):728–9.
16. Osifo OD, Oriaifo IA. Circumcision mishaps in Nigerian children. Ann African Med. 2009;8(4):266–70.
17. Lackey JT, Mannion RA, Kerr JE. Urethral fistula following circumcision. Jama. 1968;206(10):2318.
18. Khan I, Qureshi MA, Abbas SH, Shaukat M. Management of Post-traumatic and Iatrogenic urethrocutaneous fistula in children (a case series of seven patients). JPMA: J Pak Med Assoc. 2018;68(6):955–8.

19. World Health Organization. Manual for Male Circumcision Under Local Anesthesia. Geneva, World Health Organization, 2009. Available at: https://www.who.int/hiv/pub/malecircumcision/who_mc_local_anaesthesia.pdf?ua=1.
20. PSI, COSECSA, CDC. Adverse Event Action Guide for Voluntary Medical Male Circumcision by Surgery or Device 2nd Edition (3rd revision). 2018. Available at: https://www.malecircumcision.org/resource/adverse-event-action-guide-vmmc-surgery-or-device-2nd-edition-updated-november-2018-new. Accessed 30 June2020
21. World Health Organization. Improving Surgical Male Circumcision Practice Through Experience: Preventing Urethral Fistula, 2019. Available at: https://apps.who.int/iris/bitstream/handle/10665/311183/WHO-CDS-HIV-19.1-eng.pdf?ua=1
22. World Health Organization. Manual for Male Circumcision Under Local Anesthesia. Geneva, World Health Organization, 2018. Available at: https://apps.who.int/iris/bitstream/handle/10665/272387/9789241513593-eng.pdf?ua=1
23. Lucas TJ, Toledo C, Davis SM, Watts DH, Cavanaugh JS, Kiggundu V, et al. Case series of glans injuries during voluntary medical male circumcision for HIV prevention - eastern and southern Africa, 2015–2018. BMC Urol. 2020;20(1):45.
24. Johnson S. Persistent urethral fistula following circumcision; report of a case. US Naval Med Bull. 1949;49(1):120–2.
25. World Health Organization (2020). *WHO consultation on management of urethral fistula adverse events following voluntary medical male circumcision for HIV prevention. 1–3 October 2019, Harare, Zimbabwe* [Meeting report in preparation].
26. Centers for Disease Control and Prevention [online]. The National Institute for Occupational Safety and Health Hierarchy of Controls. [cited 30 June 2020]. Available at: https://www.cdc.gov/niosh/topics/hierarchy/default.html.
27. Office of the U.S. Global AIDS Coordinator. PEPFAR 2019 Country Operational Plan Guidance for all PEPFAR Countries. 2019. [cited 30 June 2020]. Available at: https://www.state.gov/wp-content/uploads/2020/01/COP20-Guidance.pdf.

8

Quantitative evaluation of upper urinary tract pump function in pigs with acute unilateral lower ureteral obstruction by 640-slice dynamic volume CT

Chongwen Mao[1], Cong Peng[2], Song Li[3], Liling Chen[4], Mengjing You[1], Kewei Fang[5], Shutian Xiang[1] and Yunshan Su[1*]

Abstract

Background: It is a challenging problem to differentiate obstructive hydronephrosis from noninvasive evaluation of renal pelvis and ureteral motility in patients. The purpose of this study was to explore the value of 640-slice dynamic volume CT (DVCT) in the quantitative measurement of upper urinary tract (UUT) pump function after acute unilateral lower ureteral obstruction in pigs.

Methods: In this study, a perfusion pig model was constructed by constant pressure perfusion testing of the renal pelvis and left nephrostomy. The perfusion and pressure measuring devices were connected to create a state of no obstruction and acute obstruction of the lower part of the left ureter. After successful modelling, continuous dynamic volume scanning of the bilateral renal excretion phase was performed with 640-slice DVCT, and pump functions of the renal pelvis and part of the upper ureter were calculated and analysed. No obstruction or acute obstruction of the lower part of the left ureter was observed. Pump functions of the renal pelvis and part of the upper ureter were determined.

Results: The results showed that after LUUT fistulostomy, the time difference between the average UUT volume and positive volume value increased gradually, and the calculated flow velocity decreased, which was significantly different from that of the RUUT. The volume difference of the LUUT increased significantly in mild obstruction. In the bilateral control, the volume change rate of the LUUT increased with mild obstruction and decreased with severe obstruction, and there was a significant difference between the left and right sides.

Conclusion: The continuous dynamic volume scan and measurement of 640-slice DVCT can obtain five pump function datasets of UUT in pigs with acute lower ureteral obstruction.

Keywords: Urethral obstruction, Dynamic volumetric CT, Renal pelvis constant pressure perfusion test, Upper urinary tract urodynamics, Pump function

Background

It is a challenging problem to differentiate obstructive hydronephrosis during noninvasive evaluation of the renal pelvis and ureteral motility in patients with obstructive and nonobstructive hydronephrosis [1]. At present, the evaluation of urodynamics of the upper urinary tract in clinical work mainly depends on noninvasive imaging examinations, such as ultrasound, intravenous pyelogra-

*Correspondence: wwangred@sina.cn
[1] Department of Radiology, The Fourth Affiliated Hospital of Kunming Medical University, #176 Qingnian Road, Kunming 650021, Yunnan, China
Full list of author information is available at the end of the article

phy, CT, MRI [2], radionuclide and dynamic near infrared fluorescence imaging [3], and these imaging methods can only speculate regarding the functional changes of the upper urinary tract based on morphological changes, and only some semiquantitative data have been obtained [4, 5]. The clinical quantitative evaluation of upper urinary tract urodynamics still depends on classical upper urinary tract urodynamic tests, that is, the renal pelvis constant pressure perfusion test and renal pelvis constant flow perfusion pressure test (Whitaker test) [6]. However, because the above two tests are invasive tests, they are only used in patients with nephrostomy [7].

In this experiment, a pig model of renal pelvis constant pressure perfusion (CPP) was established, and the upper urinary tract under different conditions of lower ureteral obstruction was scanned by a 640-slice dynamic volume CT scanning technique. Later, data were calculated and analysed to obtain the change rule of pump function of the upper urinary tract under different obstruction conditions to determine an imaging method for the noninvasive quantitative evaluation of upper urinary tract urodynamics instead of CPP. It is expected that this approach can replace the renal pelvis CPP test as an effective method for noninvasive quantitative imaging evaluation of UUT urodynamics.

Methods

Animals

Experimental animal modelling and grouping of healthy Diannan small-eared pigs were provided by the Experimental Animal Department of Kunming Medical University (Experimental Animal Licence No.: SYXK (Yunnan)). Ten pigs weighing 25 kg, half male and half female, were raised by the Experimental Animal Center of Kunming Medical University. The feeding conditions were as follows: room temperature 21 °C, air humidity 50% to 60%, light changes naturally with day and night, and free access to water. The kidneys of 10 pigs were divided into the left urinary tract as the experimental group and the right urinary tract as the control group. The process of this experiment was in accordance with regulations (Ministry of Science and Technology of the People's Republic of China, guidance on being kind to Experimental Animals, 2006-09-30) and was approved by the Medical Ethics Committee of Kunming Medical University.

Nephrostomy

Before anaesthesia, all experimental pigs were prevented from drinking and fasted for 12 h before the experiment, followed by intraperitoneal injection of 3% pentobarbital sodium at 10 mg/kg, establishment of an ear vein channel and maintenance of intravenous infusion after successful induction of anaesthesia, tracheal intubation and connection of the ECG monitor. An initial dose of 3% pentobarbital sodium 7.2 mg/kg (administration rate 1–2 ml/min) was given. 25–30% of the initial dose should be added at 30 min intervals according to the anesthetic condition of the animal (such as agitation and pain reaction). After successful anaesthesia, the pig was fixed in the right lying position, a left subcostal incision was made, the muscle layer and peritoneum were cut open with an electric knife, and the left kidney was exposed. Next, the left ureter on the anterior medial and inferior side was found and separated in front of the psoas major muscle, retaining the upper segment of the ureter for 3 to 4 cm, and keeping the ureter and renal hilum in a straight line, a catheter sheath was used to protect a 0.035 hard guide wire inserted retrograde into the renal pelvis from the ureteral incision and out of the kidney. The wound of the renal cortex was enlarged with the tip of the catheter sheath and then withdrawn. Then, the F8 fistulostomy tube with a length of 15 cm was inserted, the guide wire was pulled to send the fistulostomy tube into the renal pelvis, and the operator touched the tube head in the renal pelvis and fixed it. The F12 suction tube was placed on the control valve and inserted into the upper ureteral stump. The distal end of the tube was more than 3 cm from the ureteropelvic junction, the distal end was drawn out of the body and connected to the urine bag, and a catheter was inserted into the lower ureteral stump on the left to drain bladder urine. After fixing the position of the left nephrostomy tube and catheter, the kidney was moved back to original positon, the bleeding was thoroughly stopped, the abdominal cavity was closed layer by layer with sutures, and the incision was closed with a film dressing.

Perfusion

Tees were established for the left kidney CPP test to connect the manometer tube, perfusion tube and fistulostomy tube. All tubes were fully vented, and imaging was performed to ensure no bubble interference. The perfusion tube and manometer tube were suspended on the infusion rack, and the liquid level height of the manometer tube and perfusion tube was 20 cm (20 cmH_2O) above the renal pelvis plane (marked as 0 scale). The perfusion solution was a mixture of iodopropamide saline solution (10%), and a small amount of methylene blue was added for easy observation; the perfusion tube and the manometer tube were modified with the same type and length of pipeline (Fig. 1).

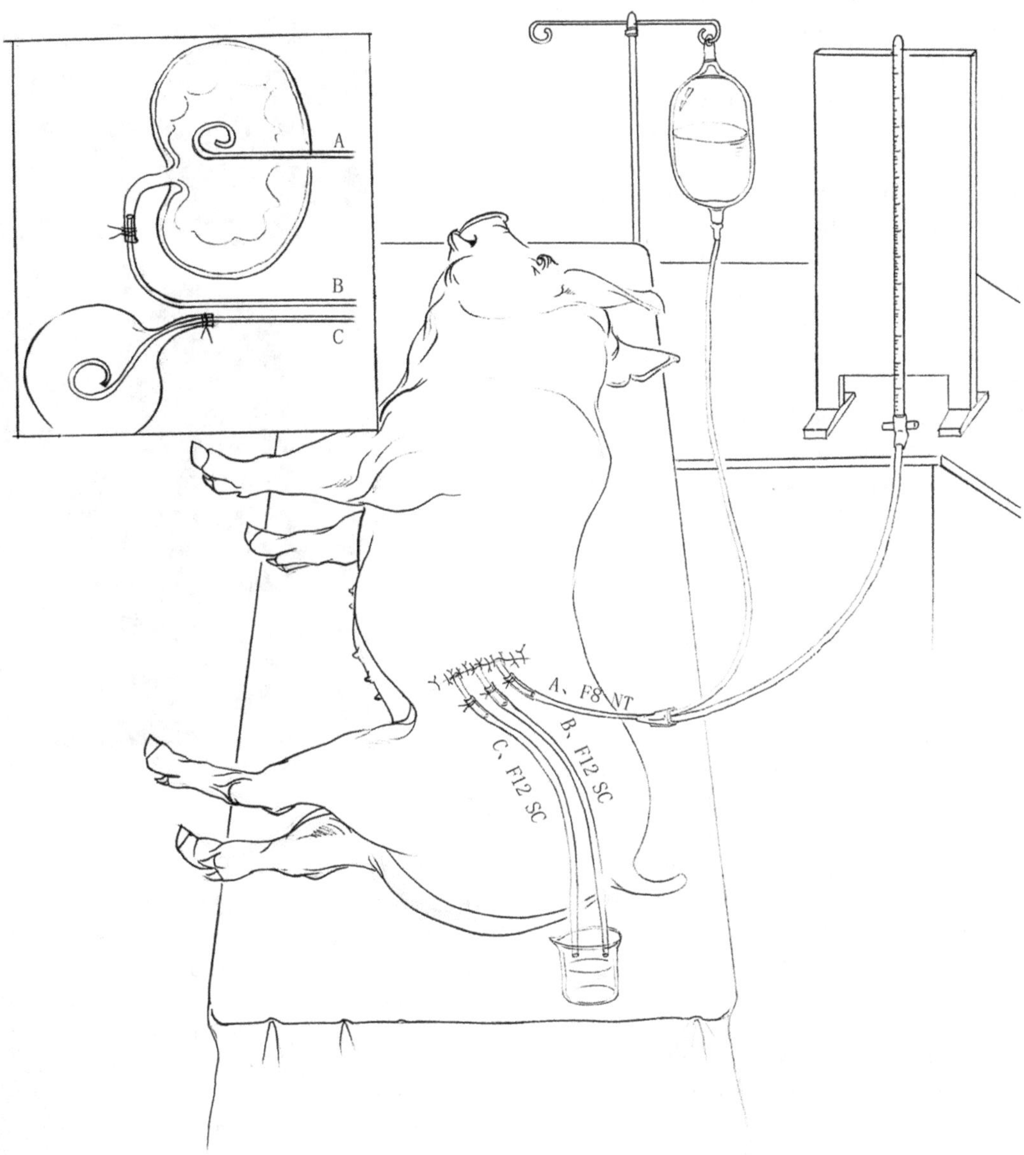

Fig. 1 Model of animals receiving perfusion

Detection

The control valve of the drainage tube at the upper end of the left ureter was set to 100, 50 and 25% open at an interval of 30 min, and the ureter was brought into a non-obstruction, mild or severe obstruction state and scanned by CT. In the experiment, the height of the perfusion solution was adjusted to control the constant perfusion pressure. The amount of liquid flowing out of 1 cm was measured when the perfusion fluid height decreased. Then, each time the liquid was removed, the perfusion bottle was raised by 1 cm to maintain a constant pressure. After the beginning of constant pressure perfusion, the perfusion velocity underwent a process of first fast, then slow, then slightly faster and finally steady, which lasted for 5 to 10 min, so the flow velocity was recorded 10 min after the beginning of perfusion, and then CT scanning was performed. The left ureteral obstruction state was set to measure the flow rate under the constant pressure perfusion of the left renal pelvis, the control valve was set to 100% open, and when the flow rate was more than 10 ml/min (0.166 ml/s), it was in a non-obstructive state; the control valve was set to a 50% open state, and the mild obstruction state was measured when the flow rate was 4–10 ml/min (average approximately 0.116 ml/s). The control valve was set to 25% open, and the flow rate was less than 4 ml/min (0.067 ml/s) for severe obstruction [8]. The bilateral kidneys and upper ureter of pigs were scanned by volume enhancement when the flow velocity was stable in the state of no obstruction, mild obstruction and severe obstruction. Scanning methods: Continuous dynamic volume scanning was performed. The auricular vein was injected with 30 ml of nonionic contrast agent iopramine (370 mgI/ml) at a speed of 3.5 ml/s with a double-barrel high-pressure syringe (OptivantageHD), and then 20 ml of saline was injected at the same flow rate. The scanning program was triggered after entering the excretion period. Scanning parameters: tube voltage 80 kV, tube current 100 mAs, rotation time 0.5 s, collimation 0.5 mm × 320 mm, scan thickness 0.5 mm, and scan interval 2 s, for a total of 10 scans. The examination bed was not moved during scanning, and 10 consecutive groups of volume images with an interval of 2 s during excretion of the double kidneys and upper ureter were obtained. The radiation dose met the required limits (DLP = 473 mGy.cm; ED = 473*k = 7.095 mSv, k = 0.015 mSv/(mGy.cm)).

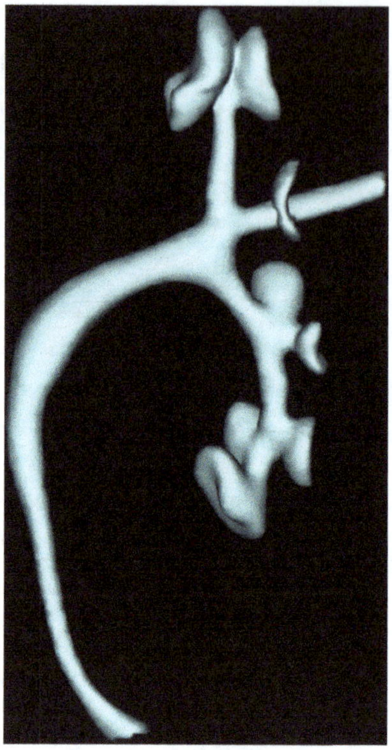

Fig. 2 Volume data of the renal pelvis and upper ureter involved in CT detection

Imaging

Image postprocessing and subjective evaluation of image quality: The original volume data of 10 groups of kidneys and upper ureters obtained by 640-slice dynamic volume CT scan were imported into the Vitreafx workstation (Vitreafx, Version 4.60) for postprocessing operation. The volume data of the renal pelvis and part of the upper ureter were obtained by setting the unified CT value of interest, as shown in Fig. 2. In the 10 groups, the development of the renal pelvis and upper ureter was good, part of the anatomical details were not clear, and there could be local artefacts, but they did not affect the volume calculation.

Data processing

All images were analysed and measured under the guidance of two experienced radiologists. The pump function values of the left and right renal pelvis and upper ureter were measured: the average volume of contrast medium (ml), volume difference (ml), time difference (s), volume change rate (%) and urine flow rate (ml/s) were calculated in all renal pelvis and renal calyx images and part of the upper ureter (above the lower pole plane) in each scanning field 3 times.

The formula is as follows:

$$\text{Volume average} = \frac{\text{Sum of continuous multi - phase volume values of ipsilateral urinary tract}}{\text{Number of periods}} \quad \text{(ml)}$$

$$\begin{aligned}&\text{Volume difference}\\&\quad = \text{The maximum value of volume data obtained by multiple collection of ipsilateral}\\&\qquad \text{urinary tract} - \text{Minimum value} \quad \text{(ml)}\end{aligned}$$

$$\begin{aligned}&\text{Time difference}\\&\quad = \text{The maximum time point in the volume data obtained by multiple collection of}\\&\qquad \text{ipsilateral urinary tract - Minimum point in time(s)}\end{aligned}$$

$$\text{Volume change rate} = \frac{\text{Ipsilateral volume difference}}{\text{Average volume of ipsilateral side}} \times 100\%$$

$$\text{Calculate the flow rate of urine} = \frac{\text{Ipsilateral volume difference}}{\text{Ipsilateral time difference}} \quad (\text{ml/s})$$

The average values measured 3 times by 2 physicians were recorded and calculated. At the same time, the urine flow velocity (ml/s) of drainage to the end of the urine bag was recorded when the left ureter formed nonobstruction and mild and severe obstruction.

Statistical analysis

All data were analysed by SPSS 23.0 statistical software. The mean and standard deviation of all values were calculated on one side. The groups were divided into two groups according to the left and right side, a paired sample t test was used for the comparison of normal distribution, a paired rank sum test was used for the comparison of skewness distribution, and the difference was statistically significant ($P < 0.05$).

Results

Among the 10 pigs, 2 pigs could not be studied because of the failure of left nephrostomy. The experimental results of 8 pigs were introduced in this paper.

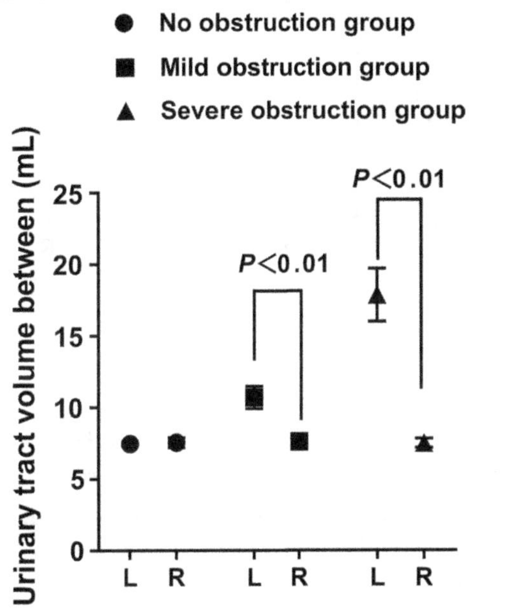

Fig. 4 Comparison of mean upper urinary tract volume between different groups

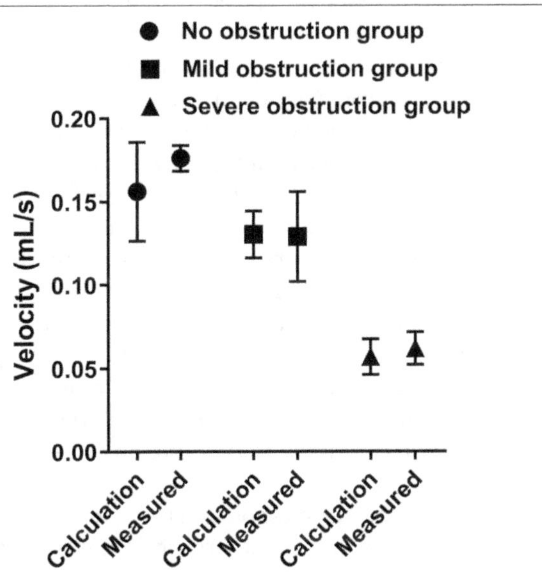

Fig. 3 Comparison of left urinary tract calculation and measured velocity

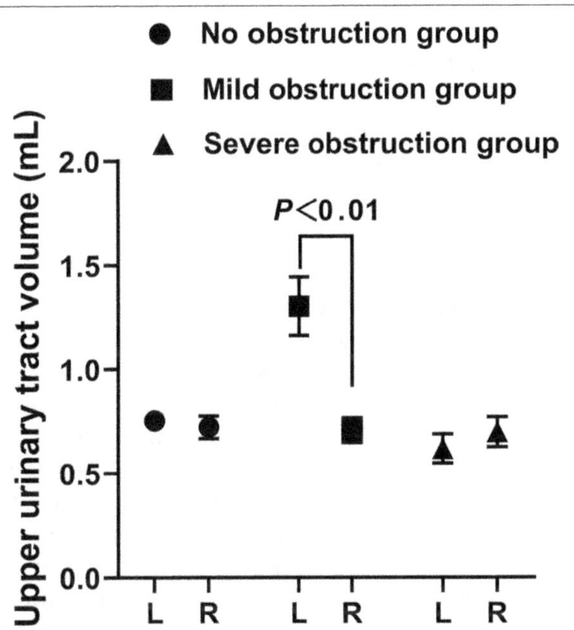

Fig. 5 Comparison of extremum differences in upper urinary tract volume between different groups

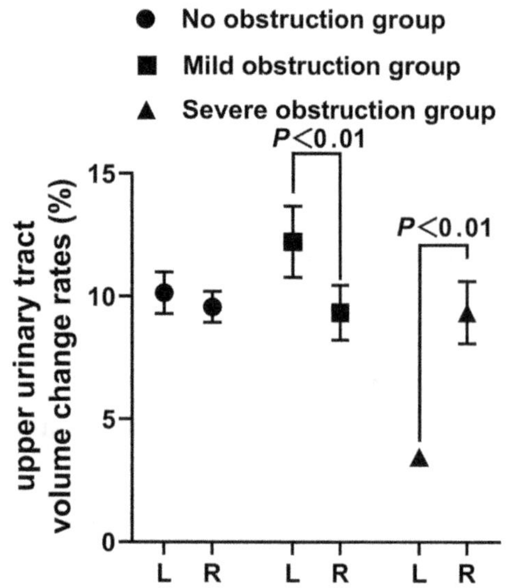

Fig. 6 Comparison of upper urinary tract volume change rates among different groups

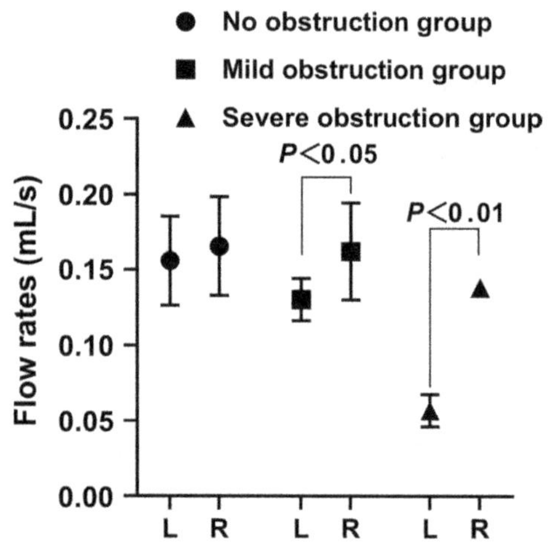

Fig. 7 Comparison of calculated flow rates in the upper urinary tract between different groups

The urine flow velocity data from the upper ureteral stump to the urine bag of 8 pigs were recorded, which showed that the urine flow velocity of the CCP test decreased linearly in normal and different obstructive states, which met the requirements of the CCP test.

Three groups of different obstructions on the left and right sides of the experimental group and the control group pump function parameters are in line with the normal distribution. Using paired T-test analysis, the statistical results are as follows: Figs. 3, 4, 5, 6, 7 and 8.

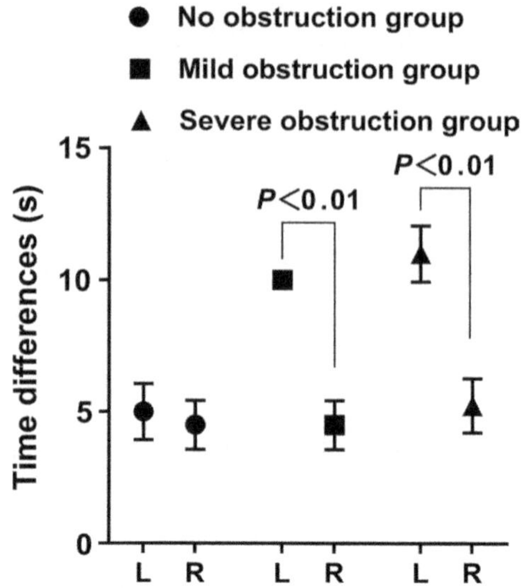

Fig. 8 Comparison of time differences between extrema of upper urinary tract volume between different groups

Discussion

Imaging examination of urodynamics of the upper urinary tract

Urinary tract dilatation does not necessarily involve obstruction, and diagnostic methods that depend on renal function may lead to misdiagnosis [7–9]. The conventional imaging method is static imaging, and functional changes are inferred according to morphological changes in the upper urinary tract [9]. For some unexplained urinary tract dilatations, it is often difficult to judge urodynamics accurately, but this is the focus of urologists. Therefore, previous urodynamic experiments of the upper urinary tract, that is, the renal pelvis constant pressure perfusion test and renal pelvis constant flow perfusion pressure measurement, were used to study and judge the urodynamics of the upper urinary tract. Among them, the renal pelvis CPP test analyses and studies the relationship between the flow rate and pressure of the upper urinary tract [7]. The perfusion fluid pressure was kept constant, and the speed of the liquid passing through the upper urinary tract was measured to determine whether there was upper urinary tract obstruction. If 20 cmH_2O pressure perfusion was used and the flow rate was less than 10 ml/min, upper urinary tract obstruction was considered. If the flow rate was always less than 4 ml/min, the obstruction was severe, while the flow velocity indicated mild obstruction at 4–10 ml/min [8].

This experimental method was implemented for a quantitative study, but the approach represents an invasive examination for patients with urinary tract dilatation without the need for nephrostomy, which is the main reason to limit the clinical application of this classical technique. Lovasz et al. verified the authenticity and accuracy of the results of upper urinary tract urodynamic diagnosis in nephrostomy patients and tried to improve the experimental method for ascertaining upper urinary tract urodynamics [10], but invasive examination has not been widely used in the clinic. Therefore, in this study, experimental animals were modelled according to the classical CPP test, and multiphase volume data were collected and calculated by 640 layers of DVCT to find a noninvasive quantitative research method to calculate the urodynamics of the upper urinary tract.

Analysis of urodynamic parameters of the upper urinary tract in this experiment

The perfusion pressure chosen to remain constant in this study was 1.96 kPa (20 cmH_2O), which was slightly higher than the human renal pelvis pressure of 0.98 kPa (10 cmH_2O). However, under this perfusion pressure, the urodynamic parameters of the upper urinary tract did not change abnormally, indicating that this pressure was within the safe pressure range of renal pelvic perfusion and was significantly lower than the clinically accepted safe pressure of renal pelvis perfusion during percutaneous nephroscopic surgery (30 mmHg) [11]. Second, because the experimental site is located in Kunming (latitude 25°02: 11\"north, longitude 102°42: 31\"east, average altitude of approximately 1891 m), the background altitude is high and the atmospheric pressure is low, so the standard pressure reference value of 1.96 kPa was adopted.

There is a certain resistance of the left nephrostomy tube itself, and the resistance of the pipe is positively correlated with the length of the tube and inversely correlated with the diameter of the tube. The resistance caused by the thin and long tube is greater. Therefore, if we want to reduce the effect on the perfusion experiment, we should choose pipes with larger diameters and shorter lengths. Before the formal implementation of this experiment, tubes with different diameters were selected for puncture fistulostomy of pig kidneys. It was found that the larger the diameter of the fistulostomy, the more serious the damage to the renal parenchyma, and the larger the diameter of the tube was, the easier it was to cause renal parenchyma rupture. For this reason, combined with the experience of Itoh [12], the catheter of F8 was finally selected to cut its length to the outside body, and a number of side holes were made at the end of the tube at the same time to reduce the resistance of the tube.

The dynamics of the upper urinary tract can be affected by the bladder filling state [13]. In the case of nondiuresis or low urine flow, the filling state of the bladder will not affect the pressure in the renal pelvis, but it will affect the peristaltic frequency of the renal pelvis and ureter and accelerate its frequency, while under high urine flow or in the constant pressure renal pelvis perfusion test, bladder filling will increase the renal pelvis pressure, resulting in a significant slowdown in the speed of urine passing through the upper urinary tract. Therefore, in this experiment, the drainage tube was placed into the bladder through the distal stump of the left ureter to drain the urine in the bladder, thus eliminating the influence of the filling state of the bladder on the experimental results.

The measured urine flow rate of the left upper ureteral stump and the calculated urine flow velocity of the left upper urinary tract decreased with the change in the state of obstruction, and there was no significant difference, indicating that the experimental fistulostomy had no definite effect on the experimental results. The follow-up data measurement are reliable.

Comparison and analysis of functional parameters of upper urinary tract pumps among groups

The function of the renal pelvis and ureter is to transport urine from the kidney to the ureter and into the bladder for storage until urination. The body works together through a series of mechanisms to achieve this goal. The basic process of regulating ureteral peristalsis is myogenic, initiated by active pacemaker cells located in the renal pelvis, and contractile impulses are transmitted from one ureteral cell to another, making the whole ureter work as a functional complex and pushing the urine into the bladder. The physiology of the urinary tract, particularly the pelvis and ureter, has been studied for nearly 100 years, including its electrical activity and contractile activity. The most important are hydrodynamic factors, such as urine flow rate, which determine the size and pattern of urine boluses, which in turn affect changes in hydrodynamic factors such as peristaltic rhythm, velocity, amplitude and baseline pressure [1]. As early as 1979, Olsen PR determined through animal experiments that renal pelvis pressure, renal pelvis volume and ureteral peristaltic frequency were important characteristics of upper urinary tract urodynamics [14]. Referring to the definition of cardiac pump function, the important characteristics of upper urinary tract urodynamics were designated "upper urinary tract pump function value" in this experiment, including the average volume value of the renal pelvis and upper ureter (ml), volume difference (ml), time difference (s) corresponding to the difference, volume change rate (%) and calculation of urinary flow velocity, which can be used to quantitatively evaluate the urodynamics of the upper urinary tract.

The results showed that the renal pelvis and ureter dilated in the early stage of upper urinary tract obstruction, and the hydronephrosis of the renal pelvis and ureter became more obvious with the deepening of the upper urinary tract obstruction. After left nephrostomy, the average volume of the non-obstruction group, mild obstruction group and severe obstruction group gradually increased, and there were significant differences between the mild and severe groups and the right upper urinary tract. The average volume shows the urine volume of the renal pelvis and upper ureter, which can quantitatively reflect the degree of dilatation of the renal pelvis and upper ureter.

Mudraya et al. [15] found that the intermittent change in the contraction frequency of the renal pelvis is related to the change in the contraction amplitude. The results of this experiment show that when the upper urinary tract is slightly obstructed, the renal pelvis and the upper part of the ureter dilate slightly and stimulate the renal pelvis and ureter to increase their contraction and peristalsis to resist the obstruction so that the contraction frequency of the renal pelvis and ureter smooth muscle is weaker than that of the normal state, but the contraction intensity is increased. Among them, the increase in contraction showed that the difference in the volume positive value was significantly larger than that on the right side, while the volume change rate was slightly higher than that on the right side. The decrease in systolic frequency is shown by the increase in the time difference, but due to the limitation of obstruction, the actual pumped urine volume accumulates in the further dilated urinary tract, which is characterized by a decrease in the urine flow rate. With the further aggravation of urinary tract obstruction, the renal pelvis and upper ureter were further dilated, resulting in overload of smooth muscle tissue, further decrease in contraction frequency and weakening of contraction strength of smooth muscle. The weakening of contraction intensity showed that there was no difference between the positive value difference of volume and that of the right side, while the volume change rate was significantly lower than that of the right side, showing ineffective contraction, resulting in a significant decrease in calculated flow velocity. The decrease in contraction frequency is shown by a further increase in the time difference. The results of this experiment proved the morphological and functional changes of the urinary tract caused by hydronephrosis after obstruction, which was consistent with the results reported by Tillig et al. [16].

In this study, porcine kidneys were scanned by 640-slice DVCT during the excretory phase, and the scanned images were segmented by a Vitreafx workstation to obtain volume images of the renal pelvis and upper ureter. Then, the volume of the upper urinary tract was measured by a workstation, and specific values were obtained; thus, the urodynamics of the upper urinary tract were evaluated accurately. Combining the CPP experiment, one of the classical experiments of upper urinary tract urodynamics, with 640 layers of DVCT, more abundant and practical data describing the renal pelvis and ureteral pump function were obtained than from the CPP experiment, which is an improvement and represents an innovation of the traditional CPP experiment.

However, there are still some limitations in our study. Because this study is a large animal experiment, the experimental tissue is difficult, so the sample size is small; at the same time, the normal state, mild obstruction state and severe obstruction state of the upper urinary tract are applied to the same sample in turn, which may lead to interference between them. Despite this, the examination methods and calculation results of the experiment were applied to patients with urinary calculi according to the approval of the ethics committee of our hospital to obtain satisfactory results.

Conclusions

In conclusion, our study showed that the continuous dynamic volume scan and measurement of 640-slice DVCT can obtain five pump function datasets of UUT in pigs with acute lower ureteral obstruction. This approach may replace the renal pelvis constant pressure perfusion test as an effective method for noninvasive quantitative imaging evaluation of UUT urodynamics.

Abbreviations

DVCT: Dynamic volume CT; UUT: Upper urinary tract; CPP: Constant pressure perfusion.

Acknowledgements

Not applicable

Declarations

The process of this experiment was in accordance with regulations (Ministry of Science and Technology of the People's Republic of China, guidance on being kind to Experimental Animals, 2006-09-30) and was approved by the Medical Ethics Committee of Kunming Medical University.

Authors' contributions

C. M conceived, designed, and performed the experiments. C. P, S. L, L. C collected the data. M. Y, K. F, S. X analysed the data. Y. S drafted or revised the manuscript. All authors approved the final version of this manuscript.

Competing interests

The authors declare no competing interests.

Author details

[1]Department of Radiology, The Fourth Affiliated Hospital of Kunming Medical University, #176 Qingnian Road, Kunming 650021, Yunnan, China. [2]Department of Radiology, The Central Hospital of Wuhan, The Tongji Medical College, Huazhong University of Science and Technology, Wuhan, Hubei, China.

[3]Department of Urology, The Fourth Affiliated Hospital of Kunming Medical University, Kunming, Yunnan, China. [4]Department of Clinical Skills Center, The Kunming Medical University, Kunming, Yunnan, China. [5]Department of Urology, The Second Affiliated Hospital of Kunming Medical University, Kunming, Yunnan, China.

References

1. Osman F, Romics I, Nyirady P, Monos E, Nadasy GL. Ureteral motility. Acta Physiol Hung. 2009;96(4):407–26.
2. Kim S, Jacob JS, Kim DC, Rivera R, Lim RP, Lee VS. Time-resolved dynamic contrast-enhanced MR urography for the evaluation of ureteral peristalsis: initial experience. J Magn Resonance Imaging: JMRI. 2008;28(5):1293–8.
3. Rowe CK, Franco FB, Barbosa JA, Minnillo BJ, Chow JS, Treves T, et al. A novel method of evaluating ureteropelvic junction obstruction: dynamic near infrared fluorescence imaging compared to standard modalities to assess urinary obstruction in a swine model. J Urol. 2012;188(5):1978–85.
4. Teodorovich OV, Vasil'ev A, Zabrodina NB, Bochkarev AB, Muchkaeva IB, Sarkhadov N, et al. Informative value of radiodiagnosis methods of pyelo-ureteral strictures in kidney anomaly. Urologiia (Moscow, Russia: 1999). 2010;2:18–21.
5. Woodbury PW, Mitchell ME, Scheidler DM, Adams MC, Rink RC, McNulty A. Constant pressure perfusion: a method to determine obstruction in the upper urinary tract. J Urol. 1989;142(2 Pt 2):632–5 (**discussion 667–638**).
6. Farrugia MK, Whitaker RH. The search for the definition, etiology, and effective diagnosis of upper urinary tract obstruction: the Whitaker test then and now. J Pediatric Urol. 2019;15(1):18–26.
7. Pegolo PT, Miranda ML, Kim S, Oliveira Filho AG, Reis LO, Silva JM. Antegrade pressure measurement of urinary tract in children with persistent hydronephrosis. Int Braz J Urol. 2012;38(4):448–55.
8. Deng X, Song L, Xie D, Fan D, Zhu L, Yao L, et al. A novel flexible ureteroscopy with intelligent control of renal pelvic pressure: an initial experience of 93 cases. J Endourol. 2016;30(10):1067–72.
9. Wolin EA, Hartman DS, Olson JR. Nephrographic and pyelographic analysis of CT urography: differential diagnosis. AJR Am J Roentgenol. 2013;200(6):1197–203.
10. Lovasz S, Lovasz L, Nyirady P, Romics I. A novel quantitative method for measuring obstruction in the upper urinary tract: the 'obstruction coefficient.' Int J Urol. 2008;15(6):499–504.
11. Zhu X, Song L, Xie D, Peng Z, Guo S, Deng X, et al. Animal experimental study to test application of intelligent pressure control device in monitoring and control of renal pelvic pressure during flexible ureteroscopy. Urology. 2016;91(242):e211-245.
12. Itoh K, Nonomura K, Matsuno T, Furudate M, Koyanagi T. Radionuclide constant pressure perfusion study on measurement of exit urine flow: experimental and preliminary clinical investigations. J Urol. 1993;150(2 Pt 1):420–6.
13. Soygur T, Burgu B, Zumrutbas A, Suer E. The need for ureteric re-implantation during augmentation cystoplasty: video-urodynamic evaluation. BJU Int. 2010;105(4):530–2.
14. Olsen PR. The renal pelvis and ureteral peristalsis. I. Pelveometry. Scand J Urol Nephrol. 1979;13(3):269–73.
15. Mudraya IS, Khodyreva LA. The role of functional urodynamic disorders in the pathogenesis of urolithiasis. Arch Ital Urol Androl. 2011;83(1):31–6.
16. Tillig B, Mutschke O, Rolle U, Gaunitz U, Asmussen G, Constantinou CE. Effects of artificial obstruction on the function of the upper urinary tract of Guinea pigs, rats and pigs. Eur J Pediatric Surg. 2004;14(5):303–15.

9

Patients with preoperative asymptomatic pyuria are not prone to develop febrile urinary tract infection after ureteroscopic lithotripsy

Kuan-Jung Lin[1,3], Eric Y. H. Huang[2,3*], I-shen Huang[2,3], Yu-Hua Fan[2,3], Chih-Chieh Lin[2,3], Tzu-Ping Lin[2,3], Hsiao-Jen Chung[2,3], Shing-Hwa Lu[2,3], Junne-Yih Kuo[2,3], Howard Hung-Hao Wu[2,3], Yen-Hwa Chang[2,3], Alex T. L. Lin[2,3] and William J. S. Huang[2,3]

Abstract

Background: This study aimed to evaluate the association of asymptomatic pyuria before ureterorenoscopic lithotripsy (URSL) with postoperative febrile urinary tract infection (UTI).

Methods: This observational case–control study identified the patients undergoing URSL for ureteral stones between May 2011 and October 2015. The included patients were classified into two groups: the asymptomatic pyuria group (6–50 white blood cells [WBCs]/high-power field [HPF]) and the non-pyuria group ($\leq$5 WBCs/HPF). All data were collected by reviewing medical records. Postoperative outcomes were collected in terms of febrile UTI, emergency visits, and stone-free rate.

Results: A total of 232 patients were included, 101 in the pyuria group, 131 in the non-pyuria group. Two (0.9%) patients developed febrile UTI after URSL and 12 (5.2%) patients visited emergency department for URSL-related symptoms. The overall stone-free rate was 90.9%. There was no significant difference between the pyuria and non-pyuria groups regarding febrile UTI, emergency visits, and stone-free rate. Multivariate analysis revealed that pyuria was neither significantly associated with postoperative febrile UTI (OR = 1.03, 95% CI = 0.06–18.10, P = 0.98), nor with emergency visits (OR = 0.48, 95% CI = 0.13–1.85, P = 0.29).

Conclusions: Compared to the patients with sterile urine prior to URSL, those with asymptomatic pyuria were not prone to develop febrile UTI after URSL.

Keywords: Pyuria, Ureteral stone, Ureterorenoscopic lithotripsy, Urinary tract infections

Background

Ureterorenoscopic lithotripsy (URSL) is a common urological management for ureteral stones. Although URSL provides satisfactory stone-free outcomes, it is also associated with an overall complication rate of 9–25% [1]. Febrile urinary tract infection (UTI) is one of the complications which is far from negligible. Asymptomatic bacteriuria is a well-documented risk factor for febrile UTI following urological procedures [2]. Both the European Association of Urology and the Infectious Diseases Society of America recommend treating asymptomatic bacteriuria before endoscopic urologic procedures [3, 4].

However, many patients with ureteral stones may present with asymptomatic pyuria instead of bacteriuria. Although current guidelines suggest the use of prophylactic antibiotics to reduce the rate of clinical UTI following

*Correspondence: yhhuang1@gmail.com
[2] Department of Urology, Taipei Veterans General Hospital, No. 201, Sec. 2, Shipai Rd., Taipei City 11217, Taiwan, ROC
Full list of author information is available at the end of the article

URSL [3, 5, 6], it lacks consensus for the management of patients with asymptomatic pyuria. Furthermore, we usually use pyuria as a surrogate for bacteriuria in real world practice. For patients with asymptomatic pyuria of less than 50 white blood cells [WBCs]/high-power field [HPF] in urinalysis, whether to eradicate pyuria prior to the operation is usually a dilemma to urologists. Therefore, this study aimed to evaluate the association of pre-URSL asymptomatic pyuria with postoperative febrile UTI. The results would provide further insight regarding the appropriate treatment of asymptomatic pyuria prior to endoscopic urologic procedures.

Methods

Study subjects

This observational case–control study was ethically approved by the Institutional Review Board of the study hospital (TPVGH-IRB 2014-11-004C). Between May 2011 and October 2015, patients who underwent URSL for ureteral stones were included. Patients were excluded for any one of the following: presence of symptoms of febrile UTI before URSL, renal staghorn stone, younger than 18 years, pregnancy, and preoperative severe pyuria (> 50 WBCs/HPF). According to preoperative midstream urine sediment which was collected one day before operation, the included patients were classified into two groups: the asymptomatic pyuria group (6–50 WBCs/HPF) and the non-pyuria group (≤ 5 WBCs/HPF). All patients received the same prophylactic antibiotics before URSL (a single dose of intravenous cefazolin 1000 mg within 30 min prior to URSL) and after URSL (oral cephalexin 500 mg every 6 h for three days).

Data collection and variables

A retrospective review of medical records was performed for the collection of patient data, including demographics (age and sex), body mass index, medical history, stone characteristics (laterality, number, size, location, and composition), operation time, double pigtail stent insertion, and pre- and intraoperative urine culture. Postoperative outcomes were collected in terms of febrile UTI, emergency visits, and stone free rate. Febrile UTI was defined as a body temperature of > 38 °C with pyuria or bacteriuria within two weeks after URSL. Bacteriuria was defined as ≥ 100,000 colony-forming units of uropathogens per mL of cultured urine. Emergency visit was recorded if the patient had visited emergency department for operation-related symptoms within two weeks after URSL, for example, fever, gross hematuria, or low abdominal pain. The status of stone free and the position of double pigtail stent were examined by plain abdominal radiography of the kidney, ureter, and bladder at postoperative day one.

Statistical analysis

Continuous variables were presented as mean (standard deviation) and categorical variables as count (percentage). Comparisons of continuous variables were performed using either Mann–Whitney U test or two-sample t test for depending on the distributional normality of the data. Either Fisher's exact test or Pearson's chi-square test was used for comparing categorical variables. Logistic regression analysis was used to determine the association of preoperative pyuria with postoperative outcomes (febrile UTI and emergency visits). Demographics, known risk factors [7], and variables with $P < 0.1$ in univariate models were taken as covariates in the multivariate models. Results of regression analyses are presented as odds ratio (OR) with 95% confidence interval (CI). A P value of < 0.05 was considered statistically significant. All statistical analyses were performed using SPSS software Version 26 (IBM Corp., Armonk, NY, USA).

Results

A total of 232 patients were included, with 101 in the pyuria group and 131 in the non-pyuria group. There was no significant difference between the pyuria and non-pyuria groups in terms of demographics, clinical data, and stone characteristics, except that the pyuria group had significantly greater mean stone size (9.0 vs. 7.5 mm, $P < 0.01$) and longer operation time (57.6 vs. 48.1 min, $P < 0.01$) than the non-pyuria group (Table 1). None of the included patients were institutionalized, immunocompromised, had renal transplants, or catheters in the urinary tract.

The most stone composition was calcium oxalate monohydrate (64.0%), followed by calcium oxalate monohydrate mixed with carbonate apatite (14.0%) and calcium oxalate dehydrate (10.0%). There was no significant difference in stone composition between the two groups ($P = 0.30$). The pyuria group had similar proportion of preoperative positive urine culture (26.1% vs. 19.1%, $P = 0.38$), preoperative bacteriuria (10.1% vs. 2.1%, $P = 0.09$), and intraoperative bacteriuria (2.6% vs, 1.2%, $P = 0.50$) to the non-pyuria group.

Regarding the postoperative outcomes, the overall stone-free rate was 90.9%. Only two (0.9%) patients experienced febrile UTI after URSL and 12 (5.2%) patients visited emergency department for URSL-related symptoms. There was no significant difference between the two groups in terms of stone-free rate, frequency of febrile UTI, and emergency visits (Table 1). The results of univariate and multivariate analysis for the association of preoperative asymptomatic pyuria with postoperative outcomes were presented in Table 2. The presence

Table 1 Demographics, clinical characteristics, and postoperative outcomes

Variables	Pyuria	Non-pyuria	*P*
Number	101	131	
Age (year)[a]	57.2 (13.7)	55.2 (12.7)	0.24
Sex			0.14
Male	65 (64.4)	96 (73.3)	
Female	36 (35.6)	35 (26.7)	
Post-menopausal women	28 (80.0)	29 (80.6)	0.95
Body mass index (kg/m^2)[a]	27.1 (5.8)	26.2 (4.2)	0.18
Diabetes	18 (17.8)	24 (18.3)	0.92
Hypertension	43 (42.6)	41 (31.3)	0.08
Chronic kidney disease	2 (2.0)	0 (0)	0.19
Laterality			0.08
Right	38 (37.6)	59 (45.0)	
Left	60 (59.4)	72 (55.0)	
Bilateral	3 (3.0)	0 (0)	
Number of stones			0.16
1	94 (93.1)	123 (93.9)	
2	7 (6.9)	4 (3.1)	
3	0 (0)	3 (2.3)	
4	0 (0)	1 (0.8)	
Mean size of stones (mm)[a]	9.0 (4.6)	7.5 (3.8)	<0.01
Size of the largest stone (mm)[a]	9.1 (4.6)	7.6 (3.8)	<0.01
Location of the largest stone			0.10
Renal pelvis	3 (3.0)	4 (3.1)	
Upper third ureter	54 (53.5)	48 (36.6)	
Middle third ureter	19 (18.8)	27 (20.6)	
Lower third ureter	16 (15.8)	35 (26.7)	
Ureterovesical junction	9 (8.9)	17 (13.0)	
Operation time (min)[a]	57.6 (23.4)	48.1 (23.0)	<0.01
Postoperative double pigtail stent insertion	98 (97.0)	122 (93.1)	0.18
Postoperative stone free	93 (92.1)	118 (90.1)	0.60
Postoperative febrile urinary tract infection	1 (1.0)	1 (0.8)	0.68
Postoperative emergency visit	3 (3.0)	9 (6.9)	0.18

[a] Data were presented as count (percentage) or mean (standard deviation)

Table 2 Logistic regression analysis for the association of preoperative pyuria with postoperative outcomes

	Odds ratio (95% confidence interval)	*P*
Febrile urinary tract infection		
Unadjusted	1.30 (0.08–21.04)	0.85
Adjusted[a]	1.03 (0.06–18.10)	0.98
Emergency visit		
Unadjusted	0.42 (0.11–1.57)	0.20
Adjusted[a]	0.48 (0.13–1.85)	0.29

[a] Covariates included age, sex, number of stones, diabetes, and positive preoperative urine culture

of preoperative pyuria was neither significantly associated with postoperative febrile UTI (OR = 1.03, 95% CI = 0.06–18.10, *P* = 0.98), nor with emergency visits (OR = 0.48, 95% CI = 0.13–1.85, *P* = 0.29).

Discussion

Currently, there is no clear consensus for the treatment of asymptomatic pyuria before endoscopic urologic procedures. In this observational study, prophylactic antibiotics with preoperative single-dose cefazolin and postoperative 3-day cephalexin was applied. The results revealed that preoperative asymptomatic pyuria before URSL was not significantly associated with postoperative febrile UTI. It suggested that prophylactic antibiotics might be sufficient for asymptomatic pyuria before URSL and the harmful consequences from overuse of antibiotics could be avoided, for example, *Clostridium difficile* infection, toxicity, and antimicrobial resistance of bacterial strains.

Risk factors of infectious complications after URSL have been evaluated in many studies [8]. However, only a few studies investigated the predictive role of preoperative asymptomatic pyuria in postoperative febrile UTI. Our results were comparable with some prior reports. The study by Morokuma et al. showed that preoperative pyuria was not a risk factor of postoperative febrile UTI in the patients undergoing URSL [9]. In a study consisting of a propensity-score matched cohort, the patients with postoperative fever after URSL had similar amount of preoperative urine leukocyte to those without postoperative fever [10]. Bai et al. also found that the proportion of preoperative pyuria did not differ between the patients complicated with and without urosepsis following URSL [11]. However, in the study by Mitsuzuka et al., the results of multivariate analysis revealed that preoperative pyuria was significantly predictive of postoperative febrile UTI (OR = 3.62, 95% CI = 1.26–8.11, *P* = 0.017) [12]. The controversial results could be explained by the heterogeneous definition of pyuria and varied incidence of postoperative febrile UTI. Among studies, pyuria was defined as a categorical variable of ≥ 5 WBCs/HPF [9], of ≥ 10 WBCs/HPF [11], of multiple levels [12], or as a continuous variable [10]. The incidence of postoperative febrile UTI also widely varied from 0.8 [11] to 18.3% [12]. These reasons may contribute to the conflict results regarding risk factors of febrile UTI after URSL, not to mention various covariates in each study. Therefore, further investigation are warranted to explore the potential role of preoperative asymptomatic pyuria in infectious complications after endoscopic urologic procedures.

There were several limitations in this study. The first came from the observational study design. Potential reporting bias and selection bias could not be avoided.

Additionally, the incidence of febrile UTI was very low, resulting in a wide 95% CI for OR. The results in the present study should be interpreted with caution. Furthermore, this was a single-institutional study, which limited the external validity of the results. Some important variables were not collected, for example, the degree of pyuria, the preoperative status of stent, and condition of glycemic control. Finally, all patients in this study received the same first-line antibiotic prophylaxis preoperatively and postoperatively and all patients were considered as low-risk of infectious complications. It deserves more research to compare different regimens of antibiotics and to focus the patients with different risk profiles.

Conclusions

In this observational case–control study, the results revealed that asymptomatic pyuria before URSL was not significantly associated with postoperative febrile UTI. It suggested that the patients with asymptomatic pyuria before URSL, compared with those with sterile urine, did not prone to develop clinically significant UTI. Intense antibiotics might not be necessary for asymptomatic pyuria before endoscopic urologic procedures and potential harms from overuse of antibiotics could be avoided.

Abbreviations

CI: Confidence interval; HPF: High-power field; OR: Odds ratio; URSL: Ureterorenoscopic lithotripsy; UTI: Urinary tract infection; WBC: White blood cell.

Acknowledgements

The authors would like to thank Miss Hui-Chen Lee for performing the statistical analysis.

Authors' contributions

KJ collected, analyzed and interpreted the patient data and was a major contributor in writing the manuscript. EYH collected, interpreted the patient data and editted the maunuscript. HK, IS, YH, CC, TP, HJ, JY, HHH, WJS, YH, and ATL contributed the patient data collection. All authors read and approved the final manuscript.

Competing interests

The authors declare that they have no competing interests.

Author details

[1]Division of Urology, Department of Surgery, Taoyuan General Hospital, Ministry of Health and Welfare, Taoyuan, Taiwan. [2]Department of Urology, Taipei Veterans General Hospital, No. 201, Sec. 2, Shipai Rd., Taipei City 11217, Taiwan, ROC. [3]Department of Urology, College of Medicine and Shu-Tien Urological Research Center, National Yang Ming Chiao Tung University, Taipei, Taiwan.

References

1. Türk C, Neisius A, Petřík A, Seitz C, Thomas K, Skolarikos A. EAU Guidelines on Urolithiasis 2020. In: European Association of Urology Guidelines 2020 Edition. Volume presented at the EAU Annual Congress Amsterdam 2020, edn. Arnhem, The Netherlands: The European Association of Urology Guidelines Office; 2020.
2. Sohn DW, Kim SW, Hong CG, Yoon BI, Ha US, Cho YH. Risk factors of infectious complication after ureteroscopic procedures of the upper urinary tract. J Infect Chemother. 2013;19(6):1102–8.
3. Bonkat G, Bartoletti R, Bruyére F, Cai T, Geerlings SE, Köves B, Schubert S, Wagenlehner F. EAU Guidelines on Urological Infections 2020. In: European Association of Urology Guidelines 2020 Edition. Volume presented at the EAU Annual Congress Amsterdam 2020, edn. Arnhem, The Netherlands: European Association of Urology Guidelines Office; 2020.
4. Nicolle LE, Gupta K, Bradley SF, Colgan R, DeMuri GP, Drekonja D, Eckert LO, Geerlings SE, Koves B, Hooton TM, et al. Clinical practice guideline for the management of asymptomatic bacteriuria: 2019 update by the infectious diseases Society of America. Clin Infect Dis. 2019;68(10):e83–110.
5. Assimos D, Krambeck A, Miller NL, Monga M, Murad MH, Nelson CP, Pace KT, Pais VM Jr, Pearle MS, Preminger GM, et al. Surgical management of stones: American Urological Association/Endourological Society Guideline, PART II. J Urol. 2016;196(4):1161–9.
6. Assimos D, Krambeck A, Miller NL, Monga M, Murad MH, Nelson CP, Pace KT, Pais VM Jr, Pearle MS, Preminger GM, et al. Surgical management of stones: American Urological Association/Endourological Society Guideline, PART I. J Urol. 2016;196(4):1153–60.
7. Bhojani N, Miller LE, Bhattacharyya S, Cutone B, Chew BH. Risk factors for urosepsis after ureteroscopy for stone disease: a systematic review with meta-analysis. J Endourol. 2021;35(7):991–1000.
8. Chugh S, Pietropaolo A, Montanari E, Sarica K, Somani BK. Predictors of urinary infections and urosepsis after ureteroscopy for stone disease: a systematic review from EAU section of urolithiasis (EULIS). Curr Urol Rep. 2020;21(4):16.
9. Morokuma F, Sadashima E, Chikamatsu S, Nakamura T, Hayakawa Y, Tokuda N. The risk factors of febrile urinary tract infection after ureterorenoscopic lithotripsy. Kobe J Med Sci. 2020;66(2):E75–81.
10. Ma YC, Jian ZY, Li H, Wang KJ. Preoperative urine nitrite versus urine culture for predicting postoperative fever following flexible ureteroscopic lithotripsy: a propensity score matching analysis. World J Urol. 2021;39(3):897–905.
11. Bai T, Yu X, Qin C, Xu T, Shen H, Wang L, Liu X. Identification of factors associated with postoperative urosepsis after ureteroscopy with holmium: yttrium-aluminum-garnet laser lithotripsy. Urol Int. 2019;103(3):311–7.
12. Mitsuzuka K, Nakano O, Takahashi N, Satoh M. Identification of factors associated with postoperative febrile urinary tract infection after ureteroscopy for urinary stones. Urolithiasis. 2016;44(3):257–62.

10

Bilateral electrical pudendal nerve stimulation as additional therapy for lower urinary tract dysfunction when stage II sacral neuromodulator fails

Shan Chen[1], Siyou Wang[2], Yunqiu Gao[3], Xiaolian Lu[1], Jiasheng Yan[3], Lihua Xuan[1] and Shenhong Wang[3*]

Abstract

Background: Sacral neuromodulation (SNM) has become an effective therapy for patients with lower urinary tract dysfunction (LUTD) who do not respond to conservative treatment. However, an effective treatment strategy for patients who fail SNM has not yet been identified. An option for LUTD is needed when the clinical response to the SNM diminishes.

Case presentation: A 51-year-old Chinese man presented to an outpatient clinic complaining of difficulty in urination for > 3 years. The patient also complained of urinary frequency and urgency, accompanied by perineal discomfort. He was diagnosed with LUTD based on his symptoms and previous examinations. The patient underwent sacral neuromodulation with a permanent implantable pulse generator (IPG) (provided free of charge by Chengnuo Medical Technology Co., Ltd.; General Stim, Hangzhou, China) in the left buttock, as he participated in the company's clinical trial to test the long-term effects of IPG. He reported loss of efficacy of the device 3 months after the implantation. We performed bilateral electrical pudendal nerve stimulation (EPNS) therapy for him. After 2 weeks of treatment, he began to report smooth voiding within 2 h after EPNS, and a moderate improvement in urinary frequency, urgency, and perineal discomfort. After 4 weeks of EPNS, the patient reported > 50% improvement in his urination, evaluated with the short form of the International Consultation on Incontinence Questionnaire for Male Lower Urinary Tract Symptoms. He reported smooth voiding, moderate improvements in urinary frequency and urgency, and the disappearance of the perineal discomfort. He also reported improved sleep and erections. The patient was discharged after 8 weeks of EPNS treatment.

Conclusion: EPNS could be an option as an additional therapy for patients with LUTD who have failed SNM.

Keywords: Sacral modulation, Lower urinary tract dysfunction, Electrical pudendal nerve stimulation, Failure, Case report

Background

Lower urinary tract dysfunction (LUTD) includes a broad spectrum of diseases ranging from failure to empty the bladder to failure to store urine [1]. Sacral neuromodulation (SNM) using InterStim is a minimally invasive therapy approved by the United States Food and Drug Administration for LUTD [2]. Over the last 20 years, SNM has become an effective therapy used in China for patients with LUTD who do not respond to conservative

*Correspondence: wsh2209@163.com
[3] Department of Urology, The First Affiliated Hospital of Zhejiang Chinese Medical University, No. 54 Youdian Road, Hangzhou 310006, Zhejiang Province, China
Full list of author information is available at the end of the article

treatment [3]. However, one-third of patients required reoperation, often due to a lack of efficacy or worsening symptoms [4]. This case report is the first to use electrical pudendal nerve stimulation (EPNS) as an additional therapy for a patient who did not respond to stage II sacral neuromodulation.

Case presentation

A 51-year-old Chinese man (height, 168 cm; weight, 59 kg) presented to an outpatient clinic complaining of difficulty urination for >3 years. He described urinary hesitancy for 2–3 min, urinary straining, and a weak urinary stream. The patient also had urinary retention 1–3 times per week for over 2 years, for which he performed intermittent self-catheterisation with around 120 mL post-void residual urine volume according to the urethral catheter output. The patient also complained of both daytime (12–14 times) and nocturnal (4–5 times) urinary frequencies and an urgency with 50–200 mL urine volume every time depending on the amount of fluid intake accompanied by perineal discomfort since he had an episode of withholding urination approximately 2 years prior. The patient also had erectile dysfunction. He had presented to multiple urology clinics over the last 3 years, undergoing multiple diagnostic examinations, including urinalysis, urinary ultrasound, urodynamic studies, cystoscope, pelvic floor muscle electromyography (PFM EMG), and magnetic resonance imaging (MRI) of the lumbar vertebrae to the sacrococcygeal vertebrae. The urinalysis result was negative. Urinary ultrasound revealed a prostate of normal size with <30 mL of post-void residual urine volume; however, prostatic calcification was noted. Urodynamics showed an underactive detrusor but no obstruction (Table 1). Cystoscopy showed lack of any anatomical obstruction and a normal bladder. PFM EMG indicated an abnormal bulbocavernosus reflex, and no abnormalities were detected on the pudendal nerve (PN) somatosensory evoked potential. No neurologic or urinary abnormalities were observed on MRI. Based on his symptoms and previous examinations, he was diagnosed with LUTD with the sub-category of overactive bladder (OAB) syndrome. The patient was prescribed tamsulosin hydrochloride (0.2 mg daily) and baclofen (10 mg daily); however, these medications were discontinued due to ineffectiveness. SNM was presented as an option to the patient more than 1 year ago. Following the first stage of SNM, the patient reported mild improvement. He then received a permanent implantable pulse generator (IPG) (Stage II) in the left buttock (Fig. 1), which was provided free of charge by Chengnuo Medical Technology Co., Ltd., (General Stim, Hangzhou, China), as he participated in the company's clinical trial to test the long-term effects of IPG. However, he reported no further improvement after the implantation with a loss of efficacy of the device 3 months later, and he also felt irritable when the IPG was turned on. The patient also complained of insomnia and depression.

The patient presented to our clinic>1 year after the IPG was implanted due to its ineffectiveness and adverse effects. We agreed with the clinical diagnosis of LUTD and OAB syndrome [5] and performed bilateral EPNS therapy for him. Four sacral points were selected (Fig. 2) [6]. The two upper points were located approximately 1 cm on either side of the sacrococcygeal joint, and the two lower points were located approximately 1 cm on either side of the tip of the coccyx. At the upper points, a needle (Suzhou Shenlong Medical Apparatus Factory, Suzhou, China) of 0.40 × 100 mm was inserted perpendicularly to a depth of 80 mm to induce a sensation referred to the urethra or anus

Table 1 Urodynamic study results

First sensation	210 mL
First desire to void	320 mL
Strong desire to void	360 mL
P detQmax	32 cm H_2O
Maximum flow rate (Qmax)	11 mL/s
Residual urine	10 mL
Rectal tone	Normal

P det pressure of the detrusor, *Qmax* the maximum flow rate

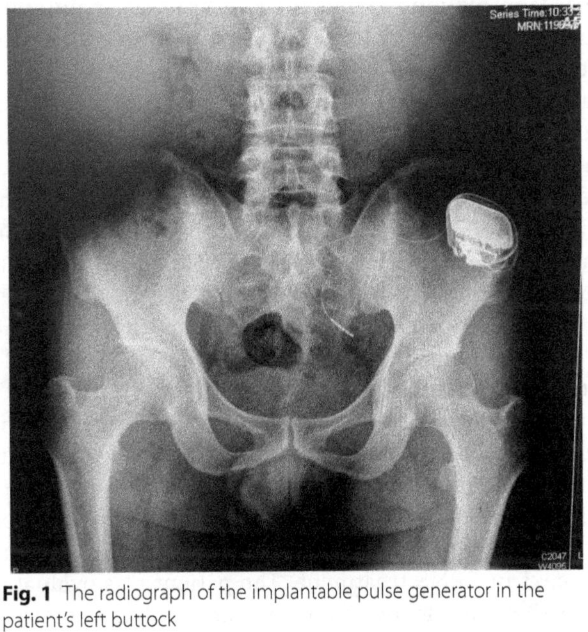

Fig. 1 The radiograph of the implantable pulse generator in the patient's left buttock

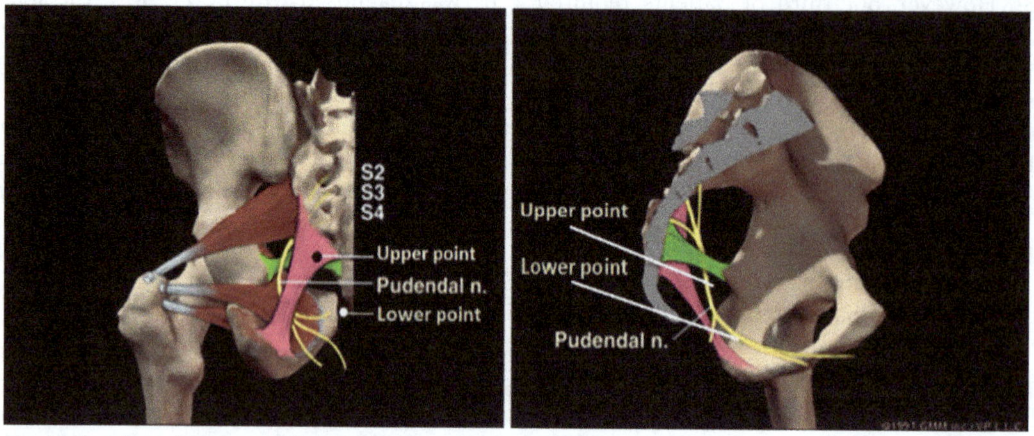

Fig. 2 The anatomical locations of the four sacral points for electrostimulation: the four points used for the electrostimulation in this patient are shown. The two upper points are located approximately 1 cm from either side of the sacrococcygeal joint, and the two lower points are located approximately 1 cm from either side of the tip of the coccyx

via stimulation of the main trunk of the PN. At the lower points, a needle of 0.40 × 100 mm was inserted obliquely toward the ischiorectal fossa to a depth of 90 mm to induce a sensation referred to the urethra via stimulation of the perineal nerve. Each pair of the ipsilaterally inserted needles were connected to two pairs of electrodes from a G6805-Aelectroacupuncture device (Shantou Medical Equipment Factory, Shantou, China), with the anode connected to the upper needle and the cathode connected to the lower needle [7, 8]. The device was set to produce electrical stimulation (biphasic 2-ms pulse) at a frequency of 2.0 Hz and a moderate intensity of 25–35 mA. Electrostimulation was performed for 60 min during each treatment. PFM contraction around the urethra was maintained during the entire electrostimulation procedure. The electrostimulation procedure was performed once daily, Monday through Friday. The patient's IPG was turned off during the procedure. During treatments, the patient was hospitalised in the acupuncture inpatient department because he lived 200 km from the clinic. After 2 weeks of treatment, he began to report smooth voiding within 2 h after EPNS and a moderate improvement in urinary frequency, urgency, and discomfort. At this time, the patient began turning off his IPG for 2–6 h instead of only during EPNS. Two weeks later, after 4 weeks of EPNS, the patient reported > 50% improvement in his urination and stopped using the IPG. He reported smooth voiding and moderate improvements of urinary frequency and urgency and a disappearance of perineal discomfort. He also reported improved sleep and erections. He was discharged after 8 weeks of EPNS treatment. The patient was evaluated with the short form of the International Consultation on Incontinence Questionnaire for Male Lower Urinary Tract Symptoms (ICIQ-MLUTS). ICIQ-MLUTS contains 13 questions on the patient's symptoms including urinary hesitancy, urinary straining, strength of urinary stream, interrupted urination, feeling of incomplete emptying, urinary urgency, urgency urinary incontinence, stress urinary incontinence, urinary incontinence for no obvious reason, enuresis, urine dribbling, urinary frequency, and nocturia. Every question was scored with 0–4 points, with a higher score indicating more severe symptoms, and the total scores ranged from 0 to 52 points. Each question had a sub-question where the patient rated the symptom's impact on quality of life from 0 to 10 points; this did not count towards the total score. The patient scored 30 points before our treatment, and scored 22, 14, and 13 points after 2, 4, and 8 weeks of EPNS therapy, respectively (Additional file 1: Table S1). He achieved > 50% improvement after 4 weeks of EPNS therapy based on the results of the ICIQ-MLUTS. The patient also indicated a reduction in the impact of the symptoms, suggesting a better quality of life.

The patient was followed up via a phone interview 1 month later, during which he reported that he experienced smooth voiding for the first 2 weeks after the EPNS was discontinued. However, in the third and fourth week, his voiding sometimes became difficult. He had no choice at home but to turn on the IPG again, which he thought might help his voiding. His voiding difficulty persisted, but to a lower degree. Other symptoms such as urinary frequency and urgency remained moderately improved. He experienced a slight discomfort around his perineum. The patient expressed interest in continuing EPNS treatment in the future. He is being followed-up via telephone at 1-month intervals.

Discussion and conclusion

SNMs have become increasingly popular in the treatment of LUTD in China in recent years [9]. However, investigations after SNM implantation regarding patients' long-term efficacy or satisfaction has received little attention [10]. A survey conducted at Toronto Western Hospital involving 71 patients who had undergone SNM implantation found that the patients' satisfaction with SNM was correlated with the need for additional medications for symptom control. Twenty-two (31%) of the patients used pain medication, intermittent self-catheterisation, intravesical Botox injections, anticholinergics, or combined mediations [11]. Additional therapy for LUTD was necessary after the clinical response to the SNM diminished.

The PN is a peripheral nerve with sympathetic fibres from the second, third, and fourth sacral nerve roots and motor and sensory functions [12]. The main trunk of the PN passes between the sacrotuberous and sacrospinous ligaments and enters Alcock's canal in the ischiorectal fossa. Within the fossa, the PN branches into the perineal nerve that innervates the PFM and the skin of the labium majus as well as the dorsal nerve of the clitoris that innervates the skin of the clitoral shaft [13]. Because SNM therapy stimulates only some of the afferent fibres of the pudendal nerve, direct neurostimulation of the PN may be more effective [14, 15]. Pudendal neurostimulation (PNM) is growing as an alternative surgical option for patients who experience a decrease in the effectiveness of SNM and in those who were never satisfied after an SNM procedure [16, 17]. The PNM procedure involves a small implantable neurostimulator device (Bion, Advanced Bionics Corporation, Valencia, CA, USA) placed directly into one side of Alcock's canal to stimulate the PN [15, 18]. The disadvantages of PNM are similar to those of SNM and include invasiveness, high cost of treatment, high surgical revision rate, device replacement when the battery runs out, and adverse events such as pain and infection [19].

In EPNS therapy, four long needles are inserted at four points near the sacrococcyx in order to stimulate the PN within the sacrococcygeal region [20]. We have previously reported that the tip of a long acupuncture needle can reach Alcock's canal where the perineal branch of the PN is located (Fig. 3) [13]. EPNS has been shown to cause PN excitation when used to treat stress urinary incontinence in women [21]. Additionally, EPNS has been used to treat female urgency-frequency syndrome and idiopathic urgency urinary incontinence [14]. A pilot study of the efficacy of EPNS on neurogenic lower urinary tract diseases compared with that of anogenital electrical stimulation found that EPNS is more effective than anogenital electrical stimulation in the short term [22].

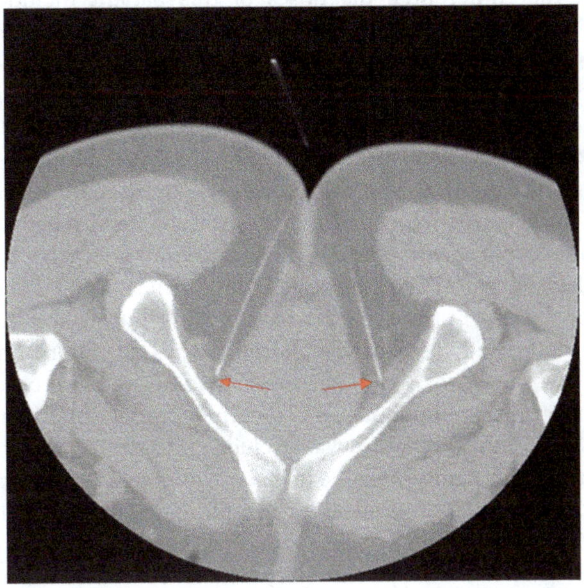

Fig. 3 Transverse computed tomography (CT) scan of the coccygeal apex: A transverse CT image of the coccygeal apex shows the tips of needles inserted at the lower sacral point in the ischiorectal fossa (adjacent to the pudendal nerve in Alcock's canal)

In this case, the patient had only mild improvement (< 50% improvement in symptoms) after Stage I. In clinical practice, clinical symptom improvement ≤ 50% was considered to indicate poor efficacy, and these patients were recommended for other treatment [3].However, the patient accepted Stage II permanent implantation as part of the company's clinical trial to test the long-term effects of IPG. Unfortunately, he failed the test, and his mood was substantially impaired because of voiding difficulty as well as urinary urgency and frequency symptoms. He described his life status as 'desperate' when he first presented to the author's clinic. This case is an example of the use of EPNS as an additional therapy for LUTD when SNM is no longer clinically effective.

However his Bladder Outlet Obstruction Index (BOOI) was 10 and Bladder Contractility Index (BCI) was 87 consistent with an underactive detrusor without any obstruction. An underactive detrusor has been defined as BCI less than 100 while obstruction has been defined as BOOI more than 40 [23]. Additionally, cystoscopy failed to demonstrate any anatomical obstruction. Therefore we diagnosed the patient with detrusor underactivity as a sub-category under LUTD.

Other differential diagnoses of this patient included benign prostatic hyperplasia, urethral stricture and bladder pain syndrome. The ultrasound revealed a prostate of normal size; thus, his lower urinary tract symptoms were not secondary to benign prostatic hyperplasia. The aetiology of urethral stricture usually involves trauma due to traffic injuries or iatrogenic causes such as late failure of surgery for hypospadia or a stricture resulting from endoscopic manipulation [24]. Urethral stricture has other signs and symptoms including urinary tract infection, epididymitis, rising post-void residual urine volume, or decreased force of ejaculation [24]. The patient had neither history of trauma, urinary surgeries, nor other symptoms including urinary tract infection or epididymitis, so urethral stricture was excluded. Diagnostic criteria for bladder pain syndrome (also known as interstitial cystitis) [25] include unpleasant symptoms associated with bladder pain (usually suprapubic) or pressure, where the pain or pressure typically increases with increased bladder volume; and other lower urinary symptoms (e.g., urinary frequency) present for at least 6 weeks and no other causes of symptoms. The patient in our case has no suprapubic pain or pressure associated with the bladder, though he had urinary frequency over 6 weeks. His perineal discomfort was not painful and stayed only at the perineum and did not increase with bladder filling. Besides, his cystoscope report was clear without finding Hunner's lesions. Since the patient did not meet the first major diagnostic criteria and cystoscope had ruled out Hunner's lesions of the bladder, he was not diagnosed with bladder pain syndrome. In summary, the diagnosis of this patient was LUTD with detrusor underactivity and OAB syndrome as sub-categories.

Regarding pharmacotherapy, the patient was prescribed 0.2 mg of tamsulosin before the EPNS treatment. Tamsulosin is a first-line treatment for male LUTD. The literature recommends 0.2 mg of tamsulosin as the initial dose for Asian men with LUTD [26]. Unfortunately, he was refractory to tamsulosin and terminated its use. Further, the main reason for his voiding difficulty was due to underactive detrusor. In our view, tamsulosin was ineffective because it helps to relax the prostatic urethra and bladder neck through alpha-adrenergic blockade. The patient was not prescribed antimuscarinics, which are used as first-line pharmacological therapy for OAB by his previous urological doctor who considered that antimuscarinics might aggravate his urinary retention through side effects of this medicine [27].

This report is not without limitations. As a case report of a single patient, the study has no statistical power. The long-term effects of EPNS was also not studied. Prospective, randomised studies with large sample sizes are required to investigate the efficacy and safety of EPNS in patients with LUTD.

In conclusion, EPNS could be an option as an additional therapy for LUTD patients who do not respond to SNM.

Abbreviations

LUTD: Lower urinary tract dysfunction; SNM: Sacral neuromodulation; EPNS: Electrical pudendal nerve stimulation; PFM EMG: Pelvic floor muscle electromyography; MRI: Magnetic resonance imaging; ICIQ-MLUTS: International Consultation on Incontinence Questionnaire for Male Lower Urinary Tract Symptoms; PN: Pudendal nerve; SEP: Somatosensory evoked potential; IPG: Implantable pulse generator; PNM: Pudendal neuromodulation; BOOI: Bladder Outlet Obstruction Index; BCI: Bladder Contractility Index; OAB: Overactive bladder.

Acknowledgements

We would like to thank Editage (www.editage.cn) for English language editing.

Authors' contributions

SC conceived and wrote the manuscript; SYW and YQG contributed to the revision of the manuscript; XLL and JSY prepared the figures and tables. LHX and SHW supervised the overall treatment of the patient. All authors have read and approved the final manuscript.

Competing interests

The authors declare that they have no competing interests.

Author details

[1] Department of Acupuncture and Moxibustion, The First Affiliated Hospital of Zhejiang Chinese Medical University, Hangzhou, China. [2] Clinical Research Section, Shanghai Research Institute of Acupuncture and Meridian, Shanghai, China. [3] Department of Urology, The First Affiliated Hospital of Zhejiang Chinese Medical University, No. 54 Youdian Road, Hangzhou 310006, Zhejiang Province, China.

References

1. Mcdonough RC, Ryan ST. Diagnosis and management of lower urinary tract dysfunction. Surg Clin N Am. 2016;96:441–52.
2. Ammirati E, Giammò A, Manassero A, Carone R. Neuromodulation in urology, state of the art. Urologia. 2019;86:177–82.
3. Zhang P, Zhang JZ, Wu LY, Zhang XD. Effects of appropriate prolonged sacral neuromodulation testing in improving implantation rate of a permanent implantable pulse generator in patients with refractory lower urinary tract dysfunctions in mainland China. Chin Med J (Engl). 2017;130:439–44.
4. Peters KM, Killinger KA, Gilleran JP, Bartley J, Wolfert C, Boura JA. Predictors of reoperation after sacral neuromodulation: a single institution evaluation of over 400 patients. Neurourol Urodyn. 2017;36:354–9.
5. Gratzke C, Bachmann A, Descazeaud A, Drake MJ, Madersbacher S, Mamoulakis C, et al. EAU guidelines on the assessment of non-neurogenic male lower urinary tract symptoms including benign prostatic obstruction. Eur Urol. 2015;67:1099–109.
6. Chen S, Wang S, Xuan Li LuH, Hu Z, Zhang C, et al. Comparison of efficacy and safety between electroacupuncture at "four sacral points" and conventional electroacupuncture for the treatment of urinary incontinence after stroke: study protocol for a randomised controlled trial. BMJ Open. 2018;8:e021783.
7. Chen S, Wang S, Xuan L, Xu F, Lu H, Lu J. Sacral electroacupuncture as a treatment for urge urinary incontinence: a prospective case series. Acupunct Med. 2020. https://doi.org/10.1177/0964528420968846.
8. Wang S, Lv J, Feng X, Lv T. Efficacy of electrical pudendal nerve stimulation versus transvaginal electrical stimulation in treating female idiopathic urgency urinary incontinence. J Urol. 2017;197:1496–501.
9. Meng L, Zhang W, Zhang Y, Wang J, Liao L, Chen G, et al. Analysis of the correlation between the clinical effect of sacral neuromodulation and

patient age: a retrospective multicentre study in China. Neuromodulation. 2020. https://doi.org/10.1111/ner.13130.

10. Cohen TN, Cohen KA, Burton CS, Kanji F, Francis SE, Patel DC. Identifying opportunities to improve patient experience with sacral neuromodulation: a human factors approach. Urology. 2020. https://doi.org/10.1016/j.urology.2020.04.092.
11. Banakhar M, Hassouna M. Patients with sacral neuromodulation: what are the factors affecting their therapy satisfaction? Urol Int. 2019;103:450–3.
12. Erdogru T, Onur R. Laparoscopic selective pudendal neuromodulation for neurogenic bladder: a review of literature. Cent Eur J Urol. 2020;73:39–41.
13. Wang S, Lv J, Feng X, Wang G, Lv T. Efficacy of electrical pudendal nerve stimulation in treating female stress incontinence. Urology. 2016;91:64–9.
14. Wang S, Zhang S, Zhao L. Long-term efficacy of electrical pudendal nerve stimulation for urgency–frequency syndrome in women. Int Urogynaecol J. 2014;25:397–402.
15. Marinkovic SP. New technologies in the management of overactive bladder: current research and future prospects. Ther Adv Urol. 2019;11:1756287219844669.
16. Li ALK, Marques R, Oliveira A, Veloso L, Girao MJBC, Lemos N. Laparoscopic implantation of electrodes for bilateral neuromodulation of the pudendal nerves and S3 nerve roots for treating pelvic pain and voiding dysfunction. Int Urogynaecol J. 2018;29:1061–4.
17. Marinkovic SP, Miller B, Hughes S, Marinkovic C, Gillen L. Successful bilateral pudendal neuromodulation to treat male detrusor areflexia following severe pubic symphysis fracture, a case report. BMC Urol. 2015;15:115.
18. Jottard K, Bonnet P, Bruyninx L, Ploteau S, De Wachter S. The ENTRAMI technique: Endoscopic transgluteal minimal invasive technique for implantation of a pudendal electrode under full visual control: a cadaver study. Neurourol Urodyn. 2019;38:130–4.
19. Lee C. Sacral neuromodulation implant infection: risk factors and prevention. Curr Urol Rep. 2017;18:16.
20. Wang S, Chen G, Li L. "Four sacral needles" therapy for female stress incontinence. J Acupunt Tuina Sci. 2006;25:15–7.
21. Wang S, Zhang S. Simultaneous perineal ultrasound and vaginal pressure measurement prove the action of electrical pudendal nerve stimulation in treating female stress incontinence. BJU Int. 2012;110:1338–43.
22. Li T, Feng X, Lv J, Cai T, Wang S. Short-term clinical efficacy of electric pudendal nerve stimulation on neurogenic lower urinary tract disease: a pilot research. Urol. 2018;112:69–73.
23. Gammie A, Kaper M, Steup A, Yoshida S, Dorrepaal C, Kos T, et al. Signs and symptoms that distinguish detrusor underactivity from mixed detrusor underactivity and bladder outlet obstruction in male patients. Neurourol Urodyn. 2018;37:1501–5.
24. Wessells H, Angermeier KW, Elliott S, Gonzalez CM, Kodama R, Peterson AC, et al. Male urethral stricture: American Urological Association guideline. J Urol. 2017;197:182–90.
25. Huffman MM, Slack A, Hoke M. Bladder pain syndrome. Prim Care. 2019;46:213–21.
26. Shim SR, Kim JH, Choi H. General effect of low-dose tamsulosin (0.2 mg) as a first-line treatment for lower urinary tract symptoms associated with benign prostatic hyperplasia: a systematic review and meta-analysis. Curr Med Res Opin. 2015;31:353–65.
27. Kelleher C, Hakimi Z, Zur R, Siddiqui E, Maman K, Aballéa S, et al. Efficacy and tolerability of mirabegron compared with antimuscarinic monotherapy or combination therapies for overactive bladder: a systematic review and network meta-analysis. Urology. 2018;74:324–33.

11

Osteochondroma of the pubic symphysis causing hematuria: A case report and literature review

Li-cheng Song[1], Qian Xu[2], Hui Li[1], Zhi-jun Li[1], Ya Li[3], Ya-fei Qin[1], Bao-long Wang[4*] and Hua-feng Zhang[1*]

Abstract

Background: Osteochondroma is the most common benign bone neoplasm and is sometimes referred to as osteocartilaginous exostosis. The symptoms caused by osteochondroma are rare, especially the urogenital complications. Therefore, this tumour is sometimes misdiagnosed.

Case presentation: This report described a 70-year-old woman with hematuria who was initially misdiagnosed with a bladder tumour in the outpatient department by a urologist. However, during cystoscopy, we found that the mass did not resemble a bladder tumor. Multidisciplinary approach with careful analysis of the imaging data suggested the diagnosis of osteochondroma. Open surgical excision of the mass was done and histology confirmed the diagnosis of benign osteochondroma. After 6 months of follow-up, the patient was still asymptomatic.

Conclusions: This case illustrates that hematuria is caused by not only urogenital disease but also osteochondroma. We present this case to draw the attention of clinicians to osteochondroma of the pubic symphysis.

Keywords: Osteochondroma, Pubic symphysis, Hematuria, Case report

Background

Osteochondroma, also called osteocartilaginous exostosis, is the most common benign bone neoplasm, accounting for 10–15% of all bone tumours and 45% of all benign bone tumours [1, 2]. However, it rarely causes complications unless the tumour is large or it is located in a crucial anatomical place [1]. Osteochondroma can present as solitary exostosis or as a part of hereditary multiple exostoses [2]. Clinical data indicate that urogenital symptoms (compression, pain, dyspareunia, haematuria, and urination difficulties) are rare. Here we report a case of osteochondroma of the pubic symphysis causing hematuria. This report intends to reinforce awareness of the disease among clinicians and to establish a clear diagnosis in the future.

Case presentation

A 70-year-old woman underwent routine physical examination 2 years ago, and the routine urine tests showed microscopic hematuria. Because of the absence of symptoms of gross hematuria and urgency, the patient did not take any further action or therapy. 3 months ago, routine urine tests still showed microscopic hematuria. Then, she went to the outpatient department for medical help from a urologist. The doctor first advised her to undergo a urinary ultrasound, and the result showed a low echogenic masses. Then, she underwent a abdominal computed tomography (CT), showed that there was a high-density mass anterior of the bladder that compressed the antetheca (Fig. 1). Combining the patient's age, imaging

*Correspondence: xiaohei67521@gmail.com; tijmuhua516@163.com
[1] Department of Orthopaedic, Tianjin Medical University General Hospital, Anshan Road No. 154, Heping District, Tianjin 300052, China
[4] Department of Urology, Tianjin Medical University General Hospital, Anshan Road No. 154, Heping District, Tianjin 300052, China
Full list of author information is available at the end of the article

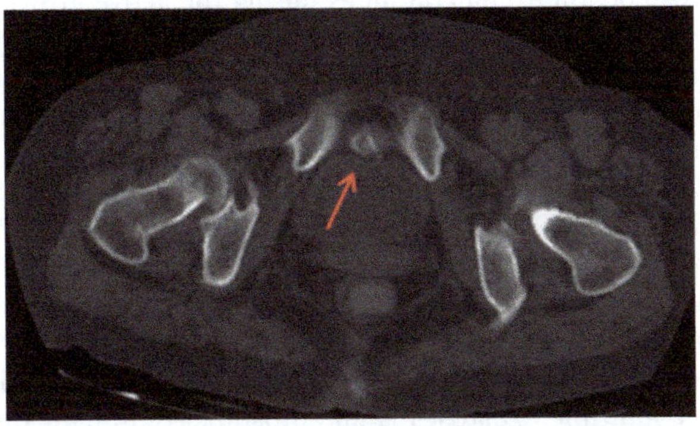

Fig. 1 Primary abdominal CT showed a high-density mass in front of the bladder that compressed the antetheca (arrow)

findings and routine urine tests, the urologist made a primary diagnosis of a bladder tumour.

On admission, the patient's physical examination was normal, without any significant pathological findings. The patient had a past medical history of hypertension. She denied smoking and drinking. Her family history was unremarkable. Routine urine showed that occult blood in the urine was 2+, the red blood cell count was 20/HPF (high-power field), the white blood cell count was 109/HPF, and the epithelial cell count was 6/HPF. Bacterial culture of the urine demonstrated no evidence of colony formation. Other laboratory data, such as routine blood tests, blood biochemistry and immune indexes, were normal.

Considering the patient's age and related high-risk factors, we arranged cystoscopy (OLYPUS) operation in the operating room. During the operation, we find that the lump was not inside but outside the bladder and that it compressed the bladder. For this situation, we immediately organized a multidisciplinary treatment (MDT). During the discussion, the orthopaedist proposed that coronary imaging and 3D reconstruction of the abdominal CT should be performed. Therefore, we performed coronary imaging and 3D reconstruction on the computer immediately (Fig. 2). According to the observation of the images, the orthopaedist made a diagnosis of osteochondroma. Our patient underwent surgery by the orthopaedist and urologist under general anaesthesia. During the operation, we found an irregular bone tumour approximately $1.5 \times 1.0 \times 0.6$ cm in size on the pubic symphysis that compressed the anterior bladder wall (Fig. 3), We resected it completely. The postoperative biopsy of the mass indicated a benign osteochondroma (Fig. 4). After resection, the microscopic hematuria disappeared. After the 6-months follow-up, the symptoms were still absent.

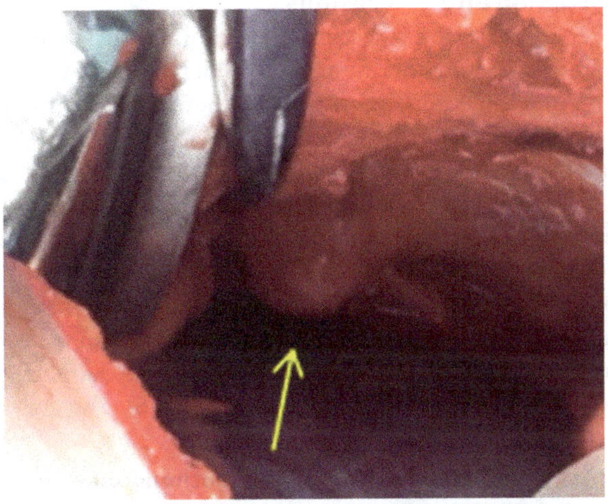

Fig. 3 Intraoperative image showed an irregularly shaped bone mass approximately 1.5 × 1.0 × 0.6 cm in size in front of the bladder (arrow)

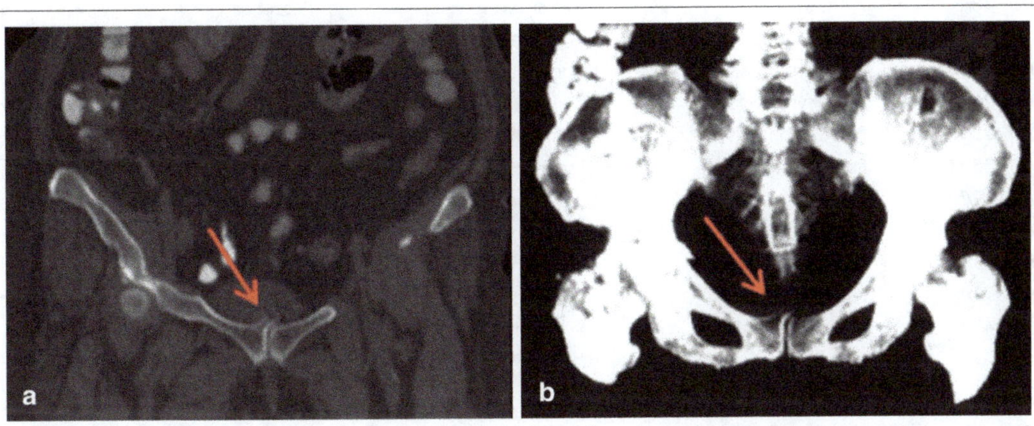

Fig. 2 **a** Coronal CT showed that a lesion arose from the superior aspect of the right pubic symphysis and grew towards the upper left region, impinging on the bladder (arrow). **b** The 3D reconstruction of the pelvis showed that the marrow and cortex of the bony mass were continuous with those of the adjacent normal bone (arrow)

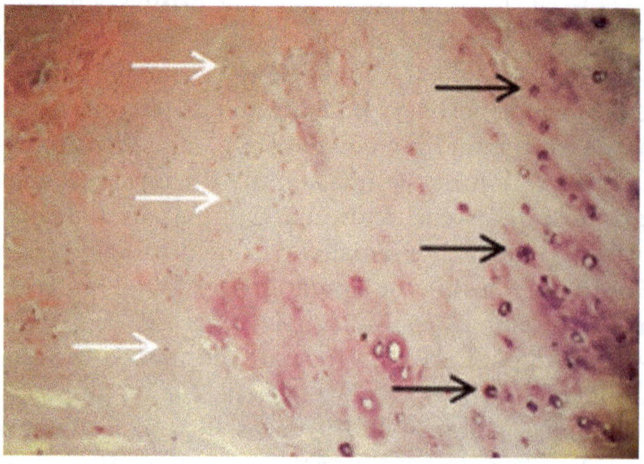

Fig. 4 Haematoxylin and eosin staining showed that the chondrocytes in the cartilage lacuna (black arrow) and osteocytes (white arrow) were diffusely distributed (magnification, × 400)

Discussion and conclusions

Osteochondroma is a benign tumour with uncertain aetiology. Osteochondroma is considered to be a developmental physeal abnormality rather than a primary bone neoplasm [3]. It is covered by a cartilaginous cap that ossifies with age to produce punctate or nodular calcification [4]. Plentiful calcification might appear on benign lesions. The marrow and cortex of osteochondroma are continuous with those of adjacent normal bone. We should be careful of the malignant transformation when the thickness of the cartilage cap exceeds 2 cm in adults and 3 cm in children [1]. The diameter of the lesion is often < 5 cm when diagnosed [5]. The growth of osteochondroma continues during the active growing period and stops in adolescence [6, 7]. Most of the symptomatic lesions are diagnosed between 10 and 20 years old due to increased skeletal growth, and the male:female ratio is approximately 2:1 [4–6].

A solitary osteochondroma usually forms at the metaphysis of a long tubular bone, particularly around the knee and at the lower femur and the upper tibia [5, 6]. Although lesions may be seen in the scapula, clavicle and ilium, their presence in the bones of the hand and foot as well as the pubic symphysis is rare [5]. Hereditary multiple exostoses is an autosomal-dominant disorder associated with the *EXT1* and *EXT2* genes [3, 5]. Only less than 1% of solitary osteochondromas transform to chondrosarcomas during later life, and the incidence of malignant changes rises to 10% in hereditary multiple exostoses (diaphyseal achalasia) [1, 4, 6, 8]. Thus, removal should be considered. It has been documented that the recurrence of osteochondroma is ~ 2% after resection [5].

The symptoms of patients usually come from mechanical irritation or compression of adjacent structures (soft tissues, bone, internal organs, peripheral nerves, spinal cord, and blood vessels), fracture, and malignant transformation [1, 9].

According to the literature, pelvic osteochondroma accounts for approximately 5% of all osteochondromas [10, 11]. Osteochondroma near the pubic symphysis is rare. We performed an extensive review of available reports about osteochondroma near the pubic symphysis from 1980 to the present (Table 1). Amis [7], Cardenas

Table 1 Available case reports of osteochondroma near the pubis symphysis

Author	Year	Age/gender	Site	Symptoms	Therapy	Follow-up	References
Kemal	2015	20/F	Pubic ramus	Groin pain, dysuria and obstructive urination	Resection	1 month	[2]
Herode	2015	18/F	Pubic ramus	Groin swelling	Resection	1 year	[3]
Phillips	1987	41/M	Pubic ramus	Hematuria	Resection	Not mentioned	[4]
Wang	2010	46/M	Pubic symphysis	Bladder outlet obstruction	Resection	> 4 years	[5]
Hoshimoto	2000	25/F	Pubic symphysis	Compression and coital pain	Resection	Not mentioned	[6]
Amis	1980	23/M	Pubic symphysis	Asymptomatic	Refused	not mentioned	[7]
Smith	1998	35/M	Pubic ramus	Dyspareunia	Resection	3 months	[8]
Mnif	2009	29/M	Pubic ramus	Dyspareunia	Resection	2 years	[11]
Cardenas	1984	27/M	Pubic symphysis	Asymptomatic	Resection	Not mentioned	[12]
Bacha	2019	35/M	Pubic symphysis	Asymptomatic	Resection	2 years	[13]
Nayak	2018	75/F	Pubic bone	Not mentioned	Not mentioned	Not mentioned	[14]
Lee W	2020	41/F	Pubic symphysis	Pelvic pain, urinary incontinence, urinary frequency, nocturia, dyspareunia	Resection	4 months	[15]
Carpintero[a]	2007	27/M; 37/M	Pubic ramus; ilio-pubic ramus	Dyspareunia; urination difficulty and dyspareunia	Resection; resection	6 years; 2 years	[16]
Peh	1999	43/M	Pubic bone	Groin swelling	Resection	2 years	[17]

[a] This article include two cases, we describe them in sequence

[12] and Bacha [13] described asymptomatic patients at the time of routine physical examination. Phillips [4] reported that exostosis arising from the superior aspect of the right pubic ramus had a close relationship with the prostate and bladder base. This is the only case report of haematuria caused by osteochondroma in the literature. Hoshimoto [6] described a 25-year-old woman with compression of the vagina and coital pain by the pubic bone. Amis [7] described a 23-year-old asymptomatic white man with a firm, enlarged and symmetrical prostate. However, this patient refused surgical intervention. Herode [3] described the reasons for resection as cosmetic, and the others opted for excision to relieve the relevant symptoms. Hence, appropriate radiographic and detailed preoperative evaluation must be carried out before any biopsy or surgical procedure to properly evaluate hard masses of the bony pelvis and to help develop a properly operative plan for management of any bone masses [5, 12].

Hematuria caused by osteochondroma of the pubic symphysis represents a rare and unusual clinical presentation. Regarding the present patient, we did not give the correct diagnosis initially due to lack of the awareness of osteochondroma. Of course, the MDT has given us great help in the diagnosis and treatment of this disease. In other words, although osteochondroma is sometimes ignored or misdiagnosed, it can be recognized by careful imaging observation and comprehensive physical examination. Surgical excision is necessary to relieve the associated complications, and the effect of surgery is obvious. We should keep this disease in mind and make a correct diagnosis in similar cases in the future.

Abbreviations

CT: Computed tomography; HPF: High-power field; MDT: Multi-disciplinary treatment.

Authors' contributions

LS, QX and YL contributed substantially to drafted the article. HZ and BW contributed to the conception and design of the article. ZL, HL and YQ conducted the literature review and extracted the data from the literature that were included. All authors read and approved the final manuscript.

Competing interests

The authors declare that they have no competing interests.

Author details

[1] Department of Orthopaedic, Tianjin Medical University General Hospital, Anshan Road No. 154, Heping District, Tianjin 300052, China. [2] School of Integrative Medicine, Tianjin University of Traditional Chinese Medicine, Tianjin 301617, China. [3] Department of the Obstetrics and Gynecology, Tianjin Medical University General Hospital, Tianjin 300052, China. [4] Department of Urology, Tianjin Medical University General Hospital, Anshan Road No. 154, Heping District, Tianjin 300052, China.

References

1. Woertler K, Lindner N, Gosheger G, Brinkschmidt C, Heindel W. Osteochondroma: MR imaging of tumor-related complications. Eur Radiol. 2000;10:832–40.
2. Gökkuş K, Atmaca H, Sağtaş E, Saylik M, Aydin AT. Osteochondromas originating from unusual locations complicating orthopedic discipline: case series. Eklem Hastalik Cerrahisi. 2015;26:100–9.
3. Herode P, Shroff A, Patel P, Aggarwal P, Mandlewala V. A rare case of pubic ramus osteochondroma. J Orthop Case Rep. 2015;5:51–3.
4. Phillips RR, Lee SH, Flannigan GM. Pelvic osteochondroma causing hematuria. Br J Urol. 1990;66:99–100.
5. Wang WY, Du LD, Lv WC, Tian Y, Shao Q, Zhang YH. Osteochondroma of the symphysis pubis: a rare cause of bladder outlet obstruction. Am Surg. 2010;76:916–8.
6. Hoshimoto K, Mitsuya K, Ohkura T. Osteochondroma of the pubic symphysis associated with sexual disturbance. Gynecol Obstet Investig. 2000;50:70–2.
7. Amis ES, Petruzzo RT. Retropubic osteochondroma simulating prostatic calcifications: a case report. J Urol. 1980;124:744–5.
8. Smith AL, Khan F. Dyspareunia due to osteochondroma of the pubic ramus. J Obstet Gynaecol. 1998;18:90.
9. Karasick D, Schweitzer ME, Eschelman DJ. Symptomatic osteochondromas: imaging features. AJR Am J Roentgenol. 1997;168:1507–12.
10. Murphey MD, Choi JJ, Kransdorf MJ, Flemming DJ, Gannon FH. Imaging of osteochondroma: variants and complications with radiologic-pathologic correlation. Radiographics. 2000;20:1407–34.
11. Mnif H, Zrig M, Koubaa M, Zammel N, Abid A. An unusual complication of pubic exostosis. Orthop Traumatol Surg Res. 2009;95:151–3.
12. Cardenas CD, Christensen AW. Osteochondroma of symphysis pubis presenting as a prostatic mass: a case report. J Urol. 1984;132:140–1.
13. Bacha D, Sassi A, Slama SB, et al. Unexpected discovery of isolated osteochondroma in the pubic symphysis. Pan Afr Med J. 2019;32:74.
14. Nayak SB, Kumar N, Sirasanagandla SR, Srinivas SP, Pamidi N, Shetty SD. Solitary osteochondroma in the body of the pubic bone: a cadaveric case report. Anat Cell Biol. 2018;51(2):136–8.
15. Lee W, Amin K, Kieras DM, Coy DL, Ruhoy SM, Lee UJ. Osteochondroma of the pubic symphysis involved with aberrantly placed minisling: a case report. Female Pelvic Med Reconstr Surg. 2020;26(1):e1-3.
16. Carpintero P, Urbano D, Segura M, de Tembleque FR, Saceda JL. Discomfort during sexual intercourse secondary to osteochondroma: a report of two cases. Joint Bone Spine. 2007;74:401–3.
17. Peh WC, Shek TW, Davies AM, Wong JW, Chien EP. Osteochondroma and secondary synovial osteochondromatosis. Skeletal Radiol. 1999;28(3):169–74.

12

The impact of *COL1A1* and *COL6A1* expression on hypospadias and penile curvature severity

Prahara Yuri[1*], Gunadi[2], Rahmadani Puji Lestari[1], Firly Putri Fardilla[1], Wiwit Ananda Wahyu Setyaningsih[3], Nur Arfian[3] and Ishandono Dachlan[4]

Abstract

Background: Hypospadias, the most frequent congenital male external genitalia abnormality, is usually associated with curvature of the ventral penis, i.e. chordee. Abnormality of darto tissue has been suggested as the pathophysiology of chordees. Collagen is one of the most abundant fibrous proteins within the extracellular matrix. In this study, we determined the expression of *collagen 1 (COL1A1)* and *COL6A1* in patients with hypospadias and associated them with the severity of penile curvature.

Methods: We included 60 children < 18 years old, consisting of 20 distal hypospadias, 20 proximal hypospadias patients, and 20 controls in our institution from 2017 – 2020. The expression of *COL1A1* and *COL6A1* in darto tissue was determined by reverse-transcriptase polymerase chain reaction (qPCR). The penile curvature severity was classified as mild (< 30 degrees), moderate (30–60 degrees), and severe (> 60 degrees).

Results: qPCR showed that *COL1A1* and *COL6A1* expression was significantly downregulated in the distal (0.88 (0.38–2.53) and 0.54 (0.16–4.35), respectively) and proximal 0.76 (0.33–2.57) and 0.57 (0.18–1.38), respectively) hypospadias groups compared to controls (1.85 (0.24–4.61) and 0.93 (0.17–4.06), respectively) with p-values of 0.024 and 0.018, respectively. Furthermore, there was a moderate correlation between *COL1A1* and *COL6A1* expression ($r = 0.458$, $p < 0.0001$). Interestingly, *COL1A1* and *COL6A1* were also significantly downregulated in the moderate and severe chordee groups compared to the mild chordee groups, with p-values of 0.003 and 0.037, respectively.

Conclusions: Aberrant *COL1A1* and *COL6A1* expression might affect abnormalities in darto tissue and penile curvature severity in hypospadias patients.

Keywords: Chordee, *COL1A1*, *COL6A1*, Expressions, Hypospadias, Penile curvature severity, qPCR

Background

Hypospadias is the most frequent congenital penile anomaly that affects male external genitalia, with an incidence of approximately 1 in 250 male newborns. It is caused by tissue underdevelopment on the ventral aspect of the penis, resulting in an abnormal location of the urethral opening on the penile underside [1]. Elastosonography found deep alteration of hypospadias penile anatomy, in which the corpus spongiosum is stiffer and less elastic with less developed cavernous corpora [2].

Hypospadias is associated with curvature of the ventral penis, called the chordee. It is caused by the insufficiency or disorganization of the complex growth (the vascular and fascial structures) of the ventral penis [3]. Resection of dartos tissue usually straightens the penis in patients with chordee and buried penis, suggesting that

*Correspondence: prahara.yuri@ugm.ac.id
[1] Division of Urology, Department of Surgery, Faculty of Medicine, Public Health and Nursing, Universitas Gadjah Mada/Dr. Sardjito Hospital, Jl. Kesehatan No.1, Yogyakarta 55281, Indonesia
Full list of author information is available at the end of the article

the pathophysiology of these anomalies is related to dartos tissue [4].

The extracellular matrix (ECM) is a noncellular macromolecular network that supports cellular processes, such as proliferation, migration, differentiation, and homeostasis [5]. One of the most abundant fibrous proteins within the ECM is collagen. It has been considered the main component of the fibrous skeleton of the corpus cavernosum penis and is ubiquitous within the erectile tissues of the human penis [6, 7].

Fibrillar collagens are widely distributed in tissues providing tensile strength. Most fibrillar collagen is type 1 collagen, which can be found throughout the tissue beneath the urethral plate [6, 7]. Type 6 collagen (COL6A1) binds to type 1 collagen (COL1A1) to form thicker collagen fibers. COL6A1 is a part of the beaded filament-forming collagens and the most studied member of its group [8]. The dartos fascia in hypospadias is an abnormal tissue, characterized by inelastic and thick tissue, but it is not the same with fibrotic tissue [9]. Therefore, we determined the expression of *collagen 1 (COL1A1)* and *COL6A1* in patients with hypospadias and associated them with the severity of penile curvature.

Methods

We included 60 children < 18 years old, consisting of 20 distal hypospadias, 20 proximal hypospadias patients, and 20 controls in our institution from 2017 – 2020. Detailed history and thorough examination of patients with hypospadias were performed by one urologist. We harvested periurethral darto tissue during urethroplasty in hypospadias patients and circumcision in normal penis samples.

Reverse-transcriptase polymerase chain reaction (qPCR) assays

Fragments of the darto tissue were kept in RNAlater (Ambion, AM7021) solution before extraction. The tissue was extracted using Genezol RNA solution (GENEzol™, Cat. No. GZR100). cDNA was synthesized using an Excel RT Reverse Transcriptase Kit (RP1300, SMOBIO, Hsinchu City, Taiwan) with PCR conditions of 25 °C for 10 min (denaturation), 42 °C for 50 min (annealing), and 85 °C for 5 min (extension).

qPCR was performed by mixing the cDNA and Taq Master Mix (GoTaq®Green Master Mix, Cat. M7122) with the following primer genes: *COL1A1* (F: 5′-TAC AGCGTCACTGTCGATGGC-3′ and R: 5′-TCAATC ACTGTCTTGCCCCAG-3′), *COL6A1* (F: 5′-GACCTC GGACCTGTTGGGTAC-3′ and R: 5′-TACCCCATC TCCCCCTTCAC-3′) [10], and *GAPDH* (F: 5′-GCACCG TCAAGGCTGAGAAC-3′ and R: 5′-TGGTGAAGACGC CAGTGGA-3′) [11]. qPCR conditions were initiated with denaturation at 94 °C for 2 min, followed by up to 40 cycles consisting of 94 °C for 10 s, annealing at 54 °C, 58 °C, 63 °C (*COL6A1, COL1A1,* and *GAPDH,* respectively) for 30 s, and 72 °C for 1 min, followed by a final extension at 72 °C for 10 min. PCR products were then separated by 2% agarose gel along with a 100-bp DNA ladder (Bioron, Germany, Cat. No. 306009) (Fig. 1). Gene expression was quantified using ImageJ software for densitometry analysis. (Fig. 2).

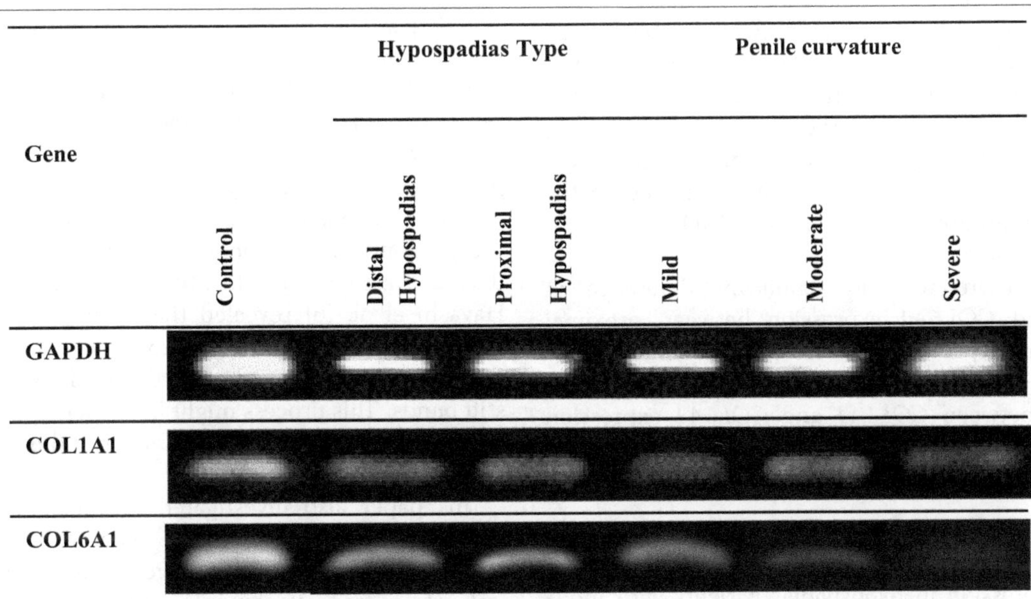

Fig. 1 Representative of qPCR products of *COL1A1* and *COL6A1*. *GAPDH* was used as reference gene

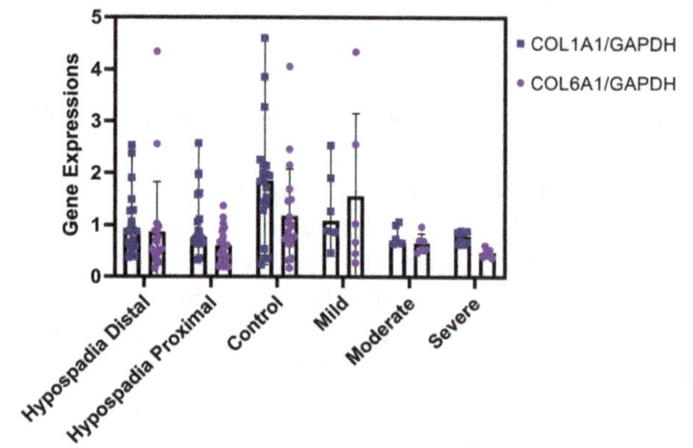

Fig. 2 The *COL1A1* and *COL6A1* gene expressions in hypospadias patients and controls and among hypospadias groups, moderate and severe penile curvature

Table 1 Characteristics of all patients in our institution

Characteristics	Mean ± SD; N (%)	*P* value
Age (years)		
Hypospadias patients	7.85 ± 3.9	0.052
Controls	5.71 ± 3.92	
Hypospadias type (n = 40)		N/A
Distal		
Glandular	1 (2.5)	
Subcoronal	5 (12.5)	
Midshaft	14 (35)	
Proximal		
Penoscrotal	13 (32.5)	
Scrotal	6 (15)	
Perineal	1 (2.5)	
Penile curvature (n = 40)		0.132
Mild (< 30 degree)	14 (35)	
Moderate (30–60degree)	12 (30)	
Severe (> 60 degree)	14 (35)	
Penoscrotal transposition		
Yes	2 (5)	0.147
No	38 (95)	
Bifid scrotum		
Yes	6 (15)	0.376
No	34 (85)	

SD standard deviation

Significant result $p < 0.05$

Statistical analysis

Data were analyzed for their normality distribution using the Kolmogorov–Smirnov test. Kruskal–Wallis and Mann–Whitney U tests were used for the data that were not normally distributed, while the normally distributed data were analyzed with one-way ANOVA tests. $p < 0.05$ was considered statistically significant.

Results

The baseline characteristics of our patients are described in Table 1. Most patients showed midshaft and penoscrotal hypospadias (67.5%) (Table 1). qPCR showed that *COL1A1* and *COL6A1* expression was significantly downregulated in the distal (0.88 (0.38–2.53) and 0.54 (0.16–4.35), respectively) and proximal (0.76 (0.33–2.57) and 0.57 (0.18–1.38), respectively) hypospadias groups compared to controls (1.85 (0.24–4.61) and 0.93 (0.17–4.06), respectively) with *p*-values of 0.024 and 0.018, respectively (Table 2). Interestingly, *COL1A1* and *COL6A1* were also significantly downregulated in the moderate and severe chordee groups compared to the mild chordee groups, with *p*-values of 0.003 and 0.037, respectively (Table 2).

Moreover, there was no significant difference in COL1A1 and COL6A1 expression between proximal and distal hypospadias or severe and moderate penile curvature (Table 3). Furthermore, there was a moderate correlation between *COL1A1* and *COL6A1* expression ($r = 0.458$, $p = 0.000$).

Discussion

Here, we are able to show downregulated *COL1A1* and *COL6A1* expression in hypospadias patients with moderate and severe penile curvature. These results are consistent with previous research, which found that the mean number of total collagen fibers in dartos tissue in hypospadias was lower but had thicker fibers compared to normal patients [9]. They also found that the hypospadias tissue anomaly consisted of a thick and inelastic tissue, although it was not always followed by an increase in collagen [9]. Another study showed no evidence of fibrous bands or dysplastic tissue in subepithelial biopsies analyzed in 17 prepubertal boys undergoing hypospadias repair [12]. Eros et al. proposed no difference in collagen intensity between normal areas and under the urethral plate of patients with hypospadias [13].

Type 1 collagen is the most abundant collagen. It is the predominant component of interstitial membranes. It is also associated with fibrosis and fibrogenesis [14]. Hayashi et al. [6] revealed that during the maturation stage of scar formation, the collagen subtype I is produced excessively, developing the fibrils with large and stiff bands. This process might be associated with the less tumescence in the penis with fibrosis of the corpus cavernosum [6].

This paper also investigated the gene expression of *COL6A1* as the most studied type of collagen in the beaded filament-forming collagen group. It plays a central role in cell attachments and connections between tissues and the surrounding matrix [15]. Type 6 collagen

Table 2 Comparison of COL1A1 and COL6A1 expressions based on hypospadias type and penile curvature severity

Hypospadias type	Distal Hypospadias	Proximal Hypospadias	Control	*P*-value
COL1A1	0.88 (0.38–2.53)	0.76 (0.33–2.57)	1.85 (0.24–4.61)	0.024*
COL6A1	0.54 (0.16–4.35)	0.57 (0.18–1.38)	0.93 (0.17–4.06)	0.018*
Penile curvature Severity	Mild (n = 14)	Moderate (n = 12)	Severe (n = 14)	*P*-value
COL1A1	1.56 (0.47–2.57)	0.69 (0.33–1.59)	0.73 (0.38–1.11)	0.003*
COL6A1	0.90 (0.16–4.35)	0.57 (0.23–1.04)	0.44 (0.18–0.89)	0.037*

* , significant result $p < 0.05$ (Kruskal Wallis test)

Table 3 Comparison of COL1A1 and COL6A1 expressions between hypospadias groups, with moderate and severe penile curvature

Gene	Hypospadias type		*p*	95% CI		Penile Curvature		*p**	95% CI	
				Lower	Upper				Lower	Upper
COL1A1	Distal	Proximal	0.957	0.963	0.972	Moderate	Severe	0.877	0.896	0.911
COL6A1	Distal	Proximal	0.570	0.570	0.596	Moderate	Severe	0.123	0.125	0.142

*Mann–Whitney test; CI, confidence interval; significant result $p < 0.05$

also regulates fibrogenesis by modulating the interactions among cells. It stimulates the activation of mesenchymal cells into myofibroblasts, resulting in extracellular matrix deposition and tissue fibrosis [15]. In lung fibrosis, type 6 collagen is increasingly expressed [15]. However, this study found decreased gene expression of COL6A1 in the hypospadias group compared to the control group. This finding might be related to the downregulation of COL1A1, which was found in this paper, suggesting that type 6 collagen is bound together to the sides of type 1 collagen to form thicker collagen fibers [7]. We found a significant positive correlation between COL1A1 and COL6A1.

The etiology of chordee in hypospadias remains unclear. Resection of dartos tissue usually can straighten the penis in patients with chordee and buried penis, suggesting that the pathophysiology of these anomalies is related to dartos tissue [4]. The composition of Dartos fibromuscular tissue determines tissue elasticity and skin mobility [4, 12].

Collagen is a part of the tissue backbone. During tissue turnover, it is formed and degraded to maintain tissue health and homeostasis. Imbalance of that process leads to fibrosis. Fibrosis is known as excessive formation of connective tissue, which damages the structure and function of its tissue [16]. Chordee occurs because of fibrosis in darto tissue, which disrupts tissue elasticity and results in penis curving [17].

We also investigated the significant difference in *COL1A1* and *COL6A1* expression among groups based on penile curvature in the hypospadias group. Mostly, severe forms of hypospadias are related to a significant chordee and a urethral meatus located proximal to the midshaft of the penis [18]. Another study proposed that the severity of chordee is generally proportional to the degree of hypospadias [19]. Many factors, such as abnormal development of the urethral plate, fibrotic mesenchymal tissue at the urethral meatus, and ventral-dorsal corporal disproportion, may be interconnected, resulting in different degrees in the final severity of curvature in each patient [20]. The Dartos tissue pattern is not influenced by age. Race and genetics may affect penis development and need further investigation [4]. Finally, for clinical implications, one of the important steps before urethroplasty is the release of fibrous tissue. The urethral plate malformation might be not associated with the most penile curvature [6]. Therefore, leaving the urethral plate is preferred by most hypospadiologists [6]. In addition, removal of the tissue under the urethral plate is still debatable [6], while excision of the inelastic dartos tissue during reconstructive surgery is recommended [9].

Conclusion

Aberrant *COL1A1* and *COL6A1* expression might affect abnormalities in darto tissue and penile curvature severity in hypospadias patients.

Abbreviation

ECM: Extracellular matrix; COL1A1: Collagen 1 subtype alpha 1; COL6A1: Collagen 6 subtype alpha 1; GAPDH: Glyceraldehyde 3-phosphate dehydrogenase; qPCR: Reverse-transcriptase polymerase chain reaction; ECM: Extracellular matrix; COL1A1: Collagen 1 subtype alpha 1; COL6A1: Collagen 6 subtype alpha 1; GAPDH: Glyceraldehyde 3-phosphate dehydrogenase; qPCR: Reverse-transcriptase polymerase chain reaction.

Acknowledgements
We thank all staff and nurses who took care of the patients.

Authors' contributions
PY collected the patient data, and PY, ID, and G analyzed and interpreted the data. PY, WAWS, NA, RPL, FPF performed PCR examination of the darto tissue. PY, ID, and G were a major contributor in writing the manuscript. All authors read and approved the final manuscript.

Competing interests
The authors declare no potential conflicts of interest with respect to the research, authorship, and/or publication of this article.

Author details
[1] Division of Urology, Department of Surgery, Faculty of Medicine, Public Health and Nursing, Universitas Gadjah Mada/Dr. Sardjito Hospital, Jl. Kesehatan No.1, Yogyakarta 55281, Indonesia. [2] Pediatric Surgery Division, Department of Surgery, Faculty of Medicine, Public Health and Nursing, Universitas Gadjah Mada/Dr. Sardjito Hospital, Yogyakarta, Indonesia. [3] Department of Anatomy, Faculty of Medicine, Public Health and Nursing, Universitas Gadjah Mada, Yogyakarta, Indonesia. [4] Division of Plastic, Aesthetic and Reconstructive Surgery, Department of Surgery, Faculty of Medicine,Public Health and Nursing, Universitas Gadjah Mada/Dr. Sardjito Hospital, Yogyakarta, Indonesia.

References

1. Marjan Waterloos PH, Spinoit A-F. Hypospadias variants Congenital anomalies of the penis. Berlin: Springer; 2017.
2. Camoglio FS, Zambaldo S, Bruno C, Zampieri N. Hypospadias anatomy: elastosonographic evaluation of the normal and hypospadic Penis. J Pediatr Urol [Internet]. 2016; Available from: http://dx.doi.org/https://doi.org/10.1016/j.jpurol.2016.02.007
3. Van Der PSCJ. Hypospadias and associated penile anomalies : a histopathological study and a reconstruction of the pathogenesis. J Plast Reconstr Aesthetic Surg. 2007;60:48–60.
4. Spinoit A, Van PC, Groen L, Van LE, Praet M, Hoebeke P. Congenital penile pathology is associated with abnormal development of the dartos muscle: a prospective study of primary penie surgery at a tertiary referra center. J Urol [Internet]. 2015;193(5):1620–4.
5. Sampaio FJB. Collagen and elastic fibers in the penis of human fetuses at 28 weeks postconception. Eur Urol. 1999;970(36):158–63.
6. Hayashi Y, Mizuno K, Kojima Y, Moritoki Y, Nishio H, Kato T, et al. Clinical investigation characterization of the urethral plate and the underlying tissue defined by expression of collagen subtypes and microarchitecture in hypospadias. Int J Urol [Internet]. 2011;18:317–22.
7. Lodish H, Berk A, Zipursky S, Al. E. Collagen: The fibrous proteins of the matrix. In: Molecular cell biology [Internet]. 4th ed. New York: W.H.Freeman; 2000. https://www.ncbi.nlm.nih.gov/books/NBK21582/
8. Theocharis AD, Skandalis SS, Gialeli C, Karamanos NK. Extracellular matrix structure. Adv Drug Deliv Rev [Internet]. 2016;97:4–27.
9. Atmoko W, Shalmont G, Situmorang GR, Wahyudi I, Tanurahardja B, Rodjani A. Abnormal dartos fascia in buried penis and hypospadias: evidence from histopathology. J Pediatr Urol [Internet]. 2018;14(6):536.e1-536.e7.
10. Schnoor M, Cullen P, Lorkowski J, Stolle K, Robenek H, Troyer D, et al. Production of type VI collagen by human macrophages: a new dimension in macrophage functional heterogeneity. J Immunol. 2008;180(8):5707–19.
11. Liu ZH, Huo JL, Wu ZG, Sun Z, Bai F, Samartzis D, et al. RASSF7 expression and its regulatory roles on apoptosis in human intervertebral disc degeneration. Int J Clin Exp Pathol. 2015;8(12):16097–103.
12. Snodgrass W, Patterson K, Plaire JC, Grady R, Mitchell ME. Histology of the urethral plate: implications for hypospadias repair. J Urol. 2000;164:988–9.
13. Erol A, Baskin L, Li Y, Liu W. Anatomical studies of the urethral plate : why preservation of the urethral plate is important in hypospadias repair. BJU Int. Nove;2000(85):728–34.
14. Henriksen K, Karsdal MA. Type I collagen. Biochemistry of collagens, laminins and elastin structure, function and biomarkers. Berlin: . Springer; 2016.
15. Sun S, Karsdal MA. Type VI collagen. Biochemistry of collagens, laminins and elastin structure, function and biomarkers. Berlin: . Springer; 2016.
16. Karsdal MA. Introduction. Biochemistry of collagens, laminins and elastin structure, function and biomarkers. Berlin: . Springer; 2016.
17. Montag S, Palmer LS. Abnormalities of penile curvature: chordee and penile torsion. Sci World J. 2011;11:1470–8.
18. Abbas TO, Mahdi E, Hasan A, AlAnsari A, Pennisi CP. Current status of tissue engineering in the management of severe hypospadias. Front Pediatr. 2018;5:283.
19. Azmy AF. Chordee (Penile Curvature). Hypospadias surgery an ilustrated guide. Berlin: . Springer; 2004. p. 117.
20. Moscardi PRM, Gosalbez R, Castellan MA. Management of High-Grade Penile Curvature Associated with Hypospadias in Children. Front Pediatr. 2017;5(189):1–8.

13

A nomogram to predict stricture-free survival in patients with ureteral stricture after balloon dilation

Jintao Hu[1,2†], Cong Lai[1,2†], Mingchao Gao[1,2†], Kaiwen Li[1,2], Wang He[1,2], Dingjun Zhu[1,2], Wenlian Xie[1,2], Haihua Wu[1], Meijuan Xu[1], Jian Huang[1,2] and Jinli Han[1,2*]

Abstract

Background: Balloon dilation is a commonly used minimally invasive endourological treatment of ureteral stricture, but the postoperative recurrence rate is relatively high. And factors contributing to recurrence after treatment are poorly understood. Herein, we sought to develop a novel clinical nomogram to predict ureteral stricture-free survival in patients suffering from ureter stricture and performed balloon dilation.

Methods: The nomogram was established based on a retrospective analysis of 321 patients who received endoscopic balloon dilation alone for ureter strictures from January 2016 to January 2020 in Sun Yat-sen Memorial Hospital using the Cox regression model. Perioperative clinical data and disease outcomes were analyzed. The primary endpoint was the onset of ureteral re-stricture after ureter balloon dilation. Discrimination of the nomogram was assessed by the concordance index (C-index) and the calibration curve. The results were internally validated using bootstrap resampling.

Results: Overall, 321 patients with a median follow-up of 590 days were enrolled in the study, among which 97 patients (30.2%) developed recurrence of ureteral stricture during follow-up. Five variables remained significant predictors of ureteral re-stricture after multivariable analyses: stricture nature ($P<0.001$), urinary nitrite ($P=0.041$), CKD ($P=0.005$), stent retention time ($P<0.001$), and balloon size ($P=0.029$). The calibration craves for the probability of 1-, 3-, and 5-years stricture-free survival (SFS) presented satisfied with the consistency of nomogram prediction and actual observation. The C-index of the model was 0.74 (95% CI 0.70–0.79).

Conclusions: Our study developed the first nomogram to effectively predict stricture-free survival in patients suffering from ureter stricture after balloon dilation. It is helpful to identify the optimal patients with ureter stricture for balloon dilation and improve treatment outcomes. However, further external validation of the nomogram is warranted.

Keywords: Nomograms, Prognosis, Recurrence, Ureteral stricture, Balloon dilation

Background

Ureteral stenosis is a well-known long-term complication that can impair kidney function, mainly caused by various factors, including benign or malignant [1]. Benign ureteral stricture occurred mainly after pelvic and abdominal surgery, ureteral injuries from lithiasis and endoscopic operation, infections, retroperitoneal fibrosis, renal transplantation, urinary diversion, endometriosis, neurogenic bladder disorder, and idiopathic causes [2–4].

*Correspondence: hanjinli@mail.sysu.edu.cn
†Jintao Hu, Cong Lai, and Mingchao Gao have contributed equally to this work
[1] Department of Urology, Sun Yat-Sen Memorial Hospital, Sun Yat-Sen University, 107 West Yanjiang Road, Guangzhou 510210, China
Full list of author information is available at the end of the article

Urothelial carcinoma, prostatic, ovarian, metastatic cervical, breast, and colorectal cancer are the primary causes of another type of ureteral stricture: malignant ureteral stenosis [5]. Open surgery is traditionally used in ureteral reconstruction surgery. With the development of minimally invasive surgery, there have been uprising cases for pure-laparoscopic and robotic-assisted surgeries for the ureteral reconstruction. But endourological procedures are often used as a first-line treatment [6, 7]. The advantageous technique is considered a safe alternative to ureteral stricture. It postpones or even potentially shuns the needs of open or laparoscopic ureteral reimplantation [8]. Besides, many documents prove that endoscopic interventions are associated with less-invasive and cost-effective [9]. Endoscopic treatments commonly used for ureteral strictures include balloon dilation and endo-ureterectomy. Balloon dilation has been applied to treat patients with ureteral stenosis for nearly 100 years. However, little is known about the long-term results of patients undergoing balloon dilation. There is still no guidelines or consensus on balloon size, dilation duration, and postoperative double-J-stent retention time and number. According to available reports, success rates of ureteral strictures with balloon dilation vary between 33 and 100% amongst all populations [10]. Many factors may affect the success rates: aetiology, stricture location, stricture length, dilation duration, stent duration, stent number, perioperative renal function, infection. In this study, we analyzed these predictive factors for the recurrence of stricture after balloon dilation and the incidence of recurrence of stricture after dilation. We aimed to build a useful and practical nomogram for predicting the stricture recurrence of patients with ureteral stricture after ureter balloon dilation.

Methods

Patient and study design

We developed the nomogram from a patient cohort from Sun Yat-sen Memorial Hospital (Guangzhou, China). We utilized a retrospective cohort study of patients diagnosed with ureteral stricture from January 2016 to January 2020.

Patients fulfilling the following eligibility criteria were enrolled for analysis: (a) individuals diagnosed with ureteral strictures confirmed by imaging and ureteroscopy. The patients received imaging checkups including ultrasound, renal scintigraphy, intravenous urography, antegrade urography, retrograde urography, computed tomography urography (CTU), or magnetic resonance urography (MRU). (b) All procedures must meet treatment with balloon dilatation alone and technical success. Technical success has defined that the ureteroscope and guidewire can pass through the ureteral stricture after balloon dilated, and then successfully indwell the double J ureteral stent. (c) Patients undergoing endoscopic balloon dilation with the postoperatively indwelling ureteral stent. Patients were excluded from analysis if they had malignant tumours that were not cured or in remission or lost follow-up.

Technique

The patient was placed in the lithotomy position or modified supine Valdivia position under local or general anaesthesia. First, retrograde ureteroscopy was used to explore the ureteral stricture, and the guidewire was inserted through the stenosis into the renal pelvis. If it failed, ultrasound-guided percutaneous nephrostomy was performed, and the guidewire was inserted into the bladder antegrade. A suitable dilatation balloon was placed into the stricture along the guidewire. Generally, according to the anatomical diameter of the ureter and clinical experience, the F24-30 balloon was selected for upper ureteral stricture, the F21-24 balloon for the middle part, and the F21 balloon for the lower segment. Under the monitoring of a ureteroscope, the balloon was filled with saline to 30 atmospheres, and the dilation time of most patients was 5 min because no better results achieved for a longer time in our preliminary trial (from 3 to 30 min) so that the stricture completely dilated without rupture of the ureter. The criteria for full dilation was that after balloon dilation, the F9.8 ureteroscope passed through the stenosis smoothly without resistance. If the first dilation didn't meet the goal, it could be dilated again or replaced with a larger balloon. After successful dilation, one or two double J stents were inserted into the ureter along the guidewire. The ureteral stent was removed after different indwelling times.

Data collection

The following demographic and clinical characteristics had extracted from medical records: age, gender, disease characteristics, dilated side, stenosis location, aetiology classification, degree of hydronephrosis, retention time and the number of stents, balloon size, dilation duration, perioperative urine leukocyte nitrite, urine culture, Scr, and so on. When processing the data, we converted part of continuous variables into categorical variables.

All participants underwent telephone follow-up and outpatient review. Follow-up data obtained from the patient's last outpatient review and contact include laboratory examinations, imaging checkups, and recorded urological symptoms available. Stricture-free had defined as a situation that the patient had a stable renal function, no urological symptoms, no evidence of worsening hydronephrosis, and no need for further treatment after the stent was removed. Patients' stricture-free survival (SFS) was from the day of withdrawing double-J-stent to the date of relapse or last contact. The overall follow-up time had defined as the interval from surgery to recurrence or the last contact. Our primary endpoint was the recurrence status of ureteral stricture and SFS time. Finally, we established a prediction model of SFS.

Statistical analysis

The primary endpoint was the onset of ureteral re-stricture after ureter balloon dilation. Log-rank test and Breslow test were used to find potentially independent prognostic variables. The missing baseline data were accounted for via multiple imputations, Cox regression analysis was used for multivariable analyses. The final model was determined by the forward LR step-down process that including all significant covariates from the univariate analysis. Statistical analysis to recognize independent prognostic factors was performed using SPSS version 25.0 for Windows (IBM Corporation, Armonk, New York, USA). On all tests, a p-value of < 0.05 demonstrated have a significant statistical difference. A nomogram was then developed based on the final model using the survival, RMS, and foreign package in R (version 4.0.2, R Foundation for Statistical Computing, Vienna, Austria) (http://www.R-project.org) [11].

The performance of the nomogram had assessed by discrimination and calibration. The bias of the nomogram had measured by the bootstrap bias-corrected estimate of concordance index (C-index) [12–14]. AUC was used to assess the specificity and sensitivity of the nomogram. And a bootstrapping-based calibration plot of the model had evaluated by comparing actual SFS probability with nomogram-predicted SFS probability [15]. We repeatedly fitted the nomogram to 2,000 bootstrap samples and assessed its performance on the original samples [16].

Results

Additional file 1: Table 1 lists the demographic and clinical characteristics. 327patients met the screening criteria of the current study. A total of 321 patients were included and analyzed due to 6 cases lost to follow-up. The ureteral stricture was most commonly secondary to ureteric lithiasis (55.96%), followed by gynaecological neoplasia surgery (11.01%) and urologic neoplasm (7.34%) (Fig. 1A). 85.02% of the ureteral stricture were benign. According to aetiology, treatment results of the obstruction have presented in Fig. 1B. During a median follow-up of 590 days, 97 of 321 patients (30.2%) developed ureteral restenosis (interquartile range (IQR) 335–1024 days). The median SFS was 406 days (IQR 93–852 days).

The overall ureteral re-stricture rate was 30.2%. Concerning etiological factors, we identified that patients who took radical cystectomy experienced the highest ureteral restenosis rate (63.1%), followed by intestinal tumours (50%). Table 1 showed the results of the univariable and multivariable Cox regression analyses used to forecast the likelihood of stricture recurrence upon dilation surgery. After applying a forward stepwise identification process, the best-simplified nomogram had developed. We found that stricture nature ($P < 0.001$), urinary nitrite ($P = 0.041$), CKD ($P = 0.005$), stent retention time ($P < 0.001$), and balloon size ($P = 0.029$) were independent risk factors for relapse of ureter stricture. Patients with malignant stricture, urinary nitrite positive, and CKD 5 were prone to ureteral restenosis, while patients with stent retention time < 3 months and dilation with F24 balloon had the highest ureteral patency rate.

The predictive nomogram that integrated all these significant predictors for 1-year, 3-year, and 5-year SFS was constructed and had depicted in Fig. 2. The nomogram had good predictive ability with a C-index of 0.74 (95% CI 0.70–0.79). Internal validation showed that the 1-, 3-, and 5-year SFS predictive accuracy of our nomogram (measured by AUC values) was 0.740, 0.768, and 0.752, respectively (Fig. 3A). Besides, a favourable consistency had shown between the predicted and actual 1-,3-, and 5-year SFS probability, which validated the accuracy of the model as demonstrated by Fig. 3B.

Discussions

To our knowledge, this study is the first to develop and validate a predictive nomogram to identify patients at increased risk of ureteral restenosis after balloon dilation. The model incorporated five items that should be evaluated with priority in clinical practice, including narrow nature, balloon size, NIT, CKD, and stent retention time.

In our study, 97 patients relapsed during follow-up, with the overall ureteral re-stricture rate was 30.2%. The results are superior to a patency rate of 41.1% reported by Campschroer et al. [8 17]. Similarly to Stehman, we observed that benign stenosis is more suitable for balloon dilation than malignant stenosis (recurrence rate:25.8%vs51.0%) [4 18]. As was shown in Fig. 1, the lowest recurrence rate had seen in stenosis secondary to both ureteral polyps (14.2%) and vascular compression (14.2%), followed by 142 secondaries to lithiasis (25.9%). All of them belonged to benign stricture. The long-term patency rate of dilation for benign stenosis was comparable to that of open surgery, which indicated that balloon dilation could replace open surgery to treat benign ureteral strictures. However, 14.6% of patients failed immediately after the stent was withdrawing, and a new stent was required to be inserting. These patients were considered not suitable for balloon dilation unless not tolerate open surgery. 41.67% of the above patients belonged

Table 1 Univariate and multivariate Cox analyses of patients with stricture recurrence after balloon dilation for stricture

Variable	Univariate Analysis			Multivariate Analysis		
	HR	95% CI	*P value*	HR	95% CI	*P value*
Nature of strictures			< 0.001			< 0.001
Benignant	1(ref)			1(ref)		
Malignant	2.558	1.617–4.046	< 0.001	3.044	2.457–3.771	< 0.001
M–S hydronephrosis			0.017			
No	1(ref)					
Yes	1.657	1.090–2.519	0.018			
Urinary nitrite (NIT)			0.020			0.041
Negative	1(ref)			1(ref)		
Positive	2.146	1.195–3.853	0.011	1.915	1.489–2.461	< 0.001
Urinary culture bacteria			0.043			
Negative	1(ref)					
Positive	1.882	1.064–3.327	0.030			
CKD			0.001			0.005
1	1(ref)		< 0.001	1(ref)		
2	1.140	0.523–2.487	0.742	1.015	0.734–1.398	0.936
3	2.055	0.953–4.432	0.066	1.460	0.966–2.206	0.006
4	2.458	0.947–6.384	0.065	1.561	1.135–2.148	0.072
5	5.021	1.975–12.764	0.001	4.120	2.806–6.049	< 0.001
Urine leukocyte			0.035			
Negative	1(ref)					
Positive	1.722	1.007–2.945	0.047			
Approach			0.028			
Retrgrade	1(ref)		0.028			
Antegrade	2.414	0.981–5.941	0.055			
Location of stenosis			0.194			
Proximal	1(ref)		0.224			
Mid	0.592	0.325–1.080	0.087			
Distal	0.854	0.535–1.363	0.508			
Balloon size			0.044			0.029
F18	1(ref)		0.035	1(ref)		
F21	0.677	0.235–1.953	0.471	0.943	0.606–1.469	0.796
F24	0.654	0.230–1.859	0.426	0.888	0.577–1.367	0.590
F30	1.273	0.448–3.613	0.650	1.814	1.164–2.827	0.008
Dilatation time			0.026			
< 5 min	1(ref)		0.034			
5–10 min	0.573	0.324–1.014	0.056			
> 10 min	1.340	0.802–2.239	0.263			
Operation side per patient			0.504			
Left	1(ref)					
Right	0.873	0.586–1.301	0.504			
Stent retention time			< 0.001			< 0.001
< 3 months	1(ref)		< 0.001	1(ref)		
3–6 months	0.996	0.584–1.700	0.989	1.13	0.902–1.416	0.289
> 6 months	3.302	2.015–5.412	< 0.001	3.043	2.455–3.772	< 0.001
Stent retention number			0.291			
1	1(ref)					
2	1.243	0.829–1.864	0.293			

M–S hydronephrosis moderate severe hydronephrosis, *CKD* chronic kidney disease, *CI* confidence intervals

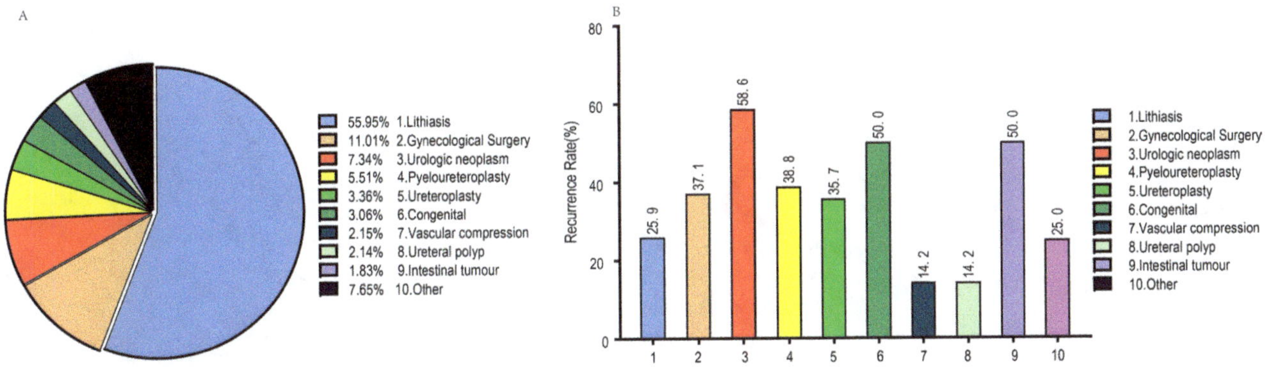

Fig. 1 **A** Etiological Classification, **B** results of dilation according to etiological

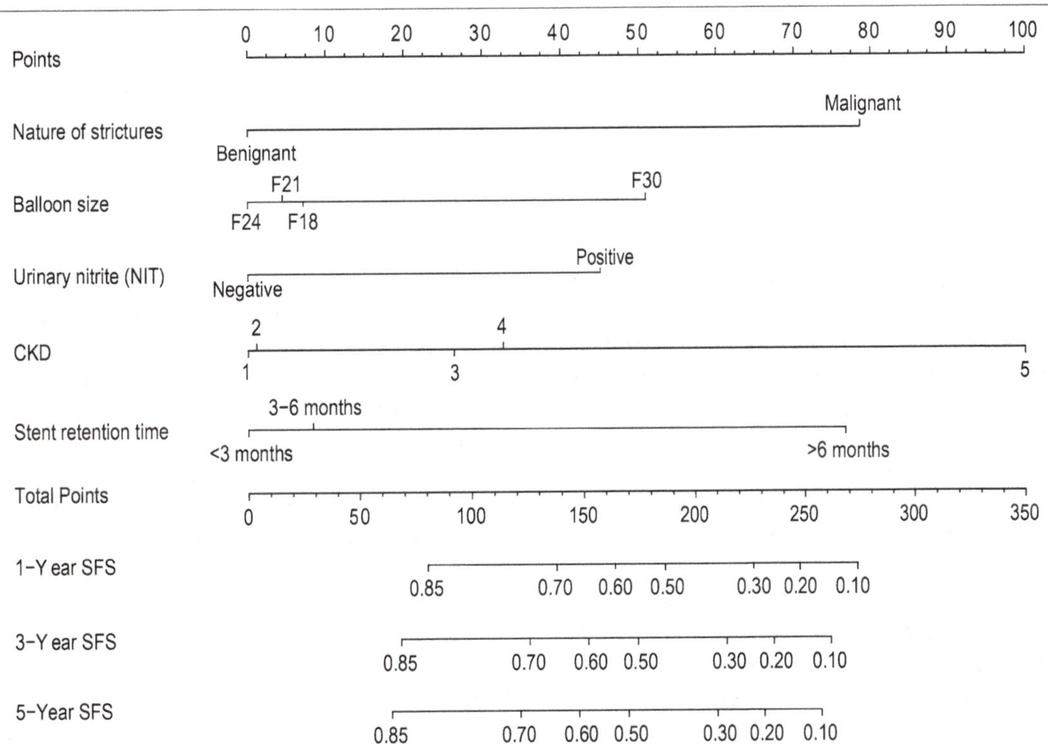

Fig. 2 Nomogram predicting 1-, 3-, and 5-year SFS for patients after balloon dilation

to malignant. Therefore, the best indication for balloon expansion is benign stenosis, such as surgery secondary to stones, ureteral polyps, vascular compression, and benign gynaecological diseases.

Some strictures (19 5.81%) were observed secondary to the laparoscopic radical cystectomy (LRC 12 3.67% recurrence rate:66.67%) or the robot-assisted radical cystectomy (RARC 7 2.14% recurrence rate:28.5%). These strictures were possibly secondary to ischemia in the context of a widespread incision [19]. It is worth noting that stenosis secondary to RARC has a lower recurrence rate after balloon dilation than other stenoses secondary to LRC.

In univariate analysis, no significant statistical difference had revealed among different stenosis sites or the number of stents retained. It is similar to previous studies that reported that there was no apparent association between stricture location (upper, mid, or distal ureter) with long-term success rate [18, 20–24]. M.J.van Son's study reported that the stricture side was an independent risk factor for stricture recurrence (P=0.009, HR 0.35, 95%CI 0.16–0.77) [8]. However, there was no significant

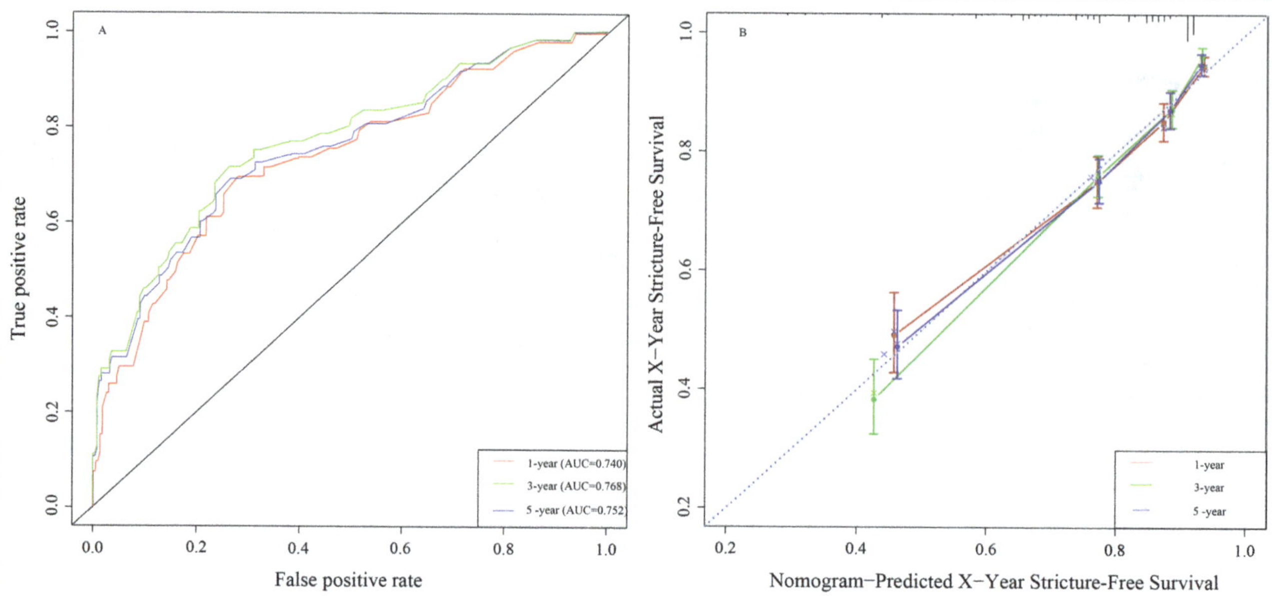

Fig. 3 **A** Receiver operating characteristic curve analysis for evaluating the accuracy of the 1-, 3-, and 5-year nomogram. **B** The calibration plots of the nomogram for predicting 1-, 3-, and 5-year stricture-free survival. Nomogram-predicted SFS is plotted on the X-axis; actual SFS is plotted on the Y-axis

difference in SFS between patients with left ureter stricture and those with the right ureter stricture in our study (P = 0.504). Interestingly, our results found no significant difference in SFS between one and two stents retention (P = 0.293). Two stents retention might cause ureteral ischemia that leads to a bad outcome.

Stavros I. reported that when indwelling stents for prolonged periods, stents may prevent tissue repair for inflammation [17]. In our study, balloon sizes were associated independently with SFS, which is consistent with several previous studies showing that appropriate size could reduce the damage to the blood supply and rupture the fibrous tissue in the stenosis [10, 25].

CKD is also considered to be an independent risk factor for patients with stenosis recurrence after balloon dilation, which is consistent with previous studies that kidney function was considered an important predictor [17, 26]. Moreover, our study showed a significant positive correlation between the five CKD stages.

Our study possesses several strengths. First, our nomogram had established through the analysis of a relatively large patients' cohort. Furthermore, the calculation method of follow-up time used more accurately reflected the recurrence of stenosis. Also, the nomogram is easily applicable in clinical practice. Therefore, it can use as an essential screening tool that allows us to improve clinical care decisions for patients with a ureteral stricture. Surgeons and patients could make better choices through this usable rating tool before surgery. However, our research also has some limitations. First, the developed nomogram was based on data obtained retrospectively from a single center. Second, due to missing data, some important factors such as the length and diameter of the stenosis and spilt renal function were not included in this study. Although this model showed good predictive ability through internal validation, it still needs external validation.

Conclusion

Our study developed the first nomogram to effectively predict stricture-free survival in patients suffering from ureter stricture after balloon dilation. It is helpful to identify the optimal patients with ureter stricture for balloon dilation and improve treatment outcomes. However, further external validation of the nomogram is warranted.

Abbreviations

US: Ureteral stricture; C-index: Concordance index; AUC: Area under the curve; SFS: Stricture-free survival; CKD: Chronic kidney disease; BMI: Body mass index; Scr: Serum creatinine; eGFR: Estimated glomerular filtration rate; SD: Standard deviation; IQR: Interquartile range.

Acknowledgements
We thank Dr. Xiaoming Rong (Department of Neurology, Sun Yat-sen Memorial Hospital, Sun Yat-sen University) her contribution to English writing and statistics of the article.

Authors' contributions
JH1, CL and MG conceived and designed the study, participated in the collection of data and data analysis, and drafted the manuscript. JH3 assisted in the design of this research and project development. KL, WH, DZ, WX, HW, MX, JH2, JH3 participated in the collection of data. All authors read and approved the final manuscript.

Competing interests
The authors declare that they have no competing interests.

Author details
[1]Department of Urology, Sun Yat-Sen Memorial Hospital, Sun Yat-Sen University, 107 West Yanjiang Road, Guangzhou 510210, China. [2]Guangdong Provincial Clinical Research Center for Urological Diseases, Guangzhou, China.

References
1. Duan H, Zhu W, Zhong W, Li X, Zeng G. Balloon dilation for failed pyeloplasty in children? Int Braz J Urol. 2019;45(3):617–20. https://doi.org/10.1590/S1677-5538.IBJU.2018.0407.
2. Netto Junior NR, Ferreira U, Lemos GC, Claro JF. Endourological management of ureteral strictures. J Urol. 1990;144(3):631–4. https://doi.org/10.1016/s0022-5347(17)39541-1.
3. Tyritzis SI, Wiklund NP. Ureteral strictures revisited trying to see the light at the end of the tunnel: a comprehensive review. J Endourol 2015;**29**(2):124–36 https://doi.org/10.1089/end.2014.0522.
4. Richter F, Irwin RJ, Watson RA, Lang EK. Endourologic management of benign ureteral strictures with and without compromised vascular supply. Urology. 2000;55(5):652–7. https://doi.org/10.1016/s0090-4295(00)00484-2.
5. Lau KO, Hia TN, Cheng C, Tay SK. Outcome of obstructive uropathy after pelvic irradiation in patients with carcinoma of the uterine cervix. Ann Acad Med Singap. 1998;27(5):631–5.
6. Varda BK, Johnson EK, Clark C, Chung BI, Nelson CP, Chang SL. National trends of perioperative outcomes and costs for open, laparoscopic and robotic pediatric pyeloplasty. J Urol. 2014;191(4):1090–5. https://doi.org/10.1016/j.juro.2013.10.077.
7. Kaouk JH, Sagalovich D, Garisto J. Robot-assisted transvesical partial prostatectomy using a purpose-built single-port robotic system. BJU Int. 2018;122(3):520–4. https://doi.org/10.1111/bju.14194.
8. van Son MJ, Lock M, Peters M, van de Putte EEF, Meijer RP. Treating benign ureteroenteric strictures: 27-year experience comparing endourological techniques with open surgical approach. World J Urol. 2019;37(6):1217–23. https://doi.org/10.1007/s00345-018-2475-4.
9. Brooks JD, Kavoussi LR, Preminger GM, Schuessler WW, Moore RG. Comparison of open and endourologic approaches to the obstructed ureteropelvic junction. Urology. 1995;46(6):791–5. https://doi.org/10.1016/s0090-4295(99)80345-8.
10. Lucas JW, Ghiraldi E, Ellis J, Friedlander JI. Endoscopic management of ureteral strictures: an update. Curr Urol Rep. 2018;19(4):24. https://doi.org/10.1007/s11934-018-0773-4.
11. Jalaeian H, Talaie R, Hunter DW, Golzarian J, Rosenberg MS. Comparison of tandem ureteral stents, cryoplasty, and cutting balloon ureteroplasty in treatment of refractory transplant ureteral strictures. Clin Transplant. 2020;34(6): e13859. https://doi.org/10.1111/ctr.13859.
12. Harrell FE Jr, Califf RM, Pryor DB, Lee KL, Rosati RA. Evaluating the yield of medical tests. JAMA. 1982;247(18):2543–6.
13. Liang W, Zhang L, Jiang G, et al. Development and validation of a nomogram for predicting survival in patients with resected non-small-cell lung cancer. J Clin Oncol. 2015;33(8):861–9. https://doi.org/10.1200/JCO.2014.56.6661.
14. Rose PG, Java J, Whitney CW, et al. Nomograms predicting progression-free survival, overall survival, and pelvic recurrence in locally advanced cervical cancer developed from an analysis of identifiable prognostic factors in patients from nrg oncology/gynecologic oncology group randomized trials of chemoradiotherapy. J Clin Oncol. 2015;33(19):2136–42. https://doi.org/10.1200/JCO.2014.57.7122.
15. Renfro LA, Goldberg RM, Grothey A, et al. Clinical calculator for early mortality in metastatic colorectal cancer: an analysis of patients from 28 clinical trials in the Aide et Recherche en Cancérologie Digestive Database. J Clin Oncol. 2017;35(17):1929–37. https://doi.org/10.1200/jco.2016.71.5771.
16. Serenari M, Han KH, Ravaioli F, et al. A nomogram based on liver stiffness predicts postoperative complications in patients with hepatocellular carcinoma. J Hepatol. 2020;73(4):855–62. https://doi.org/10.1016/j.jhep.2020.04.032.
17. Tyritzis SI, Wiklund NP. Ureteral strictures revisited…trying to see the light at the end of the tunnel: a comprehensive review. J Endourol. 2015;29(2):124–36. https://doi.org/10.1089/end.2014.0522.
18. Byun SS, Kim JH, Oh SJ, Kim HH. Simple retrograde balloon dilation for treatment of ureteral strictures: etiology-based analysis. Yonsei Med J. 2003;44(2):273–8. https://doi.org/10.3349/ymj.2003.44.2.273.
19. Tyritzis SI, Hosseini A, Collins J, et al. Oncologic, functional, and complications outcomes of robot-assisted radical cystectomy with totally intracorporeal neobladder diversion. Eur Urol. 2013;64(5):734–41. https://doi.org/10.1016/j.eururo.2013.05.050.
20. Richter F, Irwin RJ Jr, Watson RA, Lang EK. Endourologic management of malignant ureteral strictures. J Endourol. 2000;14(7):583–7. https://doi.org/10.1089/08927790050152195.
21. Lang EK, Glorioso LW 3rd. Antegrade transluminal dilatation of benign ureteral strictures: long-term results. AJR Am J Roentgenol. 1988;150(1):131–4. https://doi.org/10.2214/ajr.150.1.131.
22. Netto Júnior NR, Ferreira U, Lemos GC, Claro JF. Endourological management of ureteral strictures. J Urol. 1990;144(3):631–4. https://doi.org/10.1016/s0022-5347(17)39541-1.
23. Chang R, Marshall FF, Mitchell S. Percutaneous management of benign ureteral strictures and fistulas. J Urol. 1987;137(6):1126–31. https://doi.org/10.1016/s0022-5347(17)44426-0.
24. Lu C, Zhang W, Peng Y, et al. Endoscopic balloon dilatation in the treatment of benign ureteral strictures: a meta-analysis and systematic review. J Endourol. 2019;33(4):255–62. https://doi.org/10.1089/end.2018.0797.
25. Kaouk JH, Garisto J, Eltemamy M, Bertolo R. Robot-assisted surgery for benign distal ureteral strictures: step-by-step technique using the SP(®) surgical system. BJU Int. 2019;123(4):733–9. https://doi.org/10.1111/bju.14635.
26. Geavlete P, Niță G, Georgescu D, Mirciulescu V. Endoscopic classification and endourologic therapy in proximal incomplete ureteral duplication pathology. Eur Urol. 2001;39(3):304–7. https://doi.org/10.1159/000052458.

14

Women's barriers for contacting their general practitioner when bothered by urinary incontinence: A population-based cross-sectional study

Dorte Ejg Jarbøl*, Peter Fentz Haastrup, Sanne Rasmussen, Jens Søndergaaard and Kirubakaran Balasubramaniam

Abstract

Background: Urinary incontinence (UI) is a frequently occurring condition among women and increases with age. Effective treatments exist but many women hesitate to contact their general practitioner (GP) regarding UI. Therefore, it is important to generate knowledge regarding barriers for healthcare-seeking. Several factors such as age, duration and number of symptoms are associated with healthcare-seeking. How socioeconomic status (SES) is associated with experiencing barriers for healthcare-seeking for UI has not been explored. The objectives of this study were to: (1) analyze frequencies of barriers for healthcare-seeking, and (2) investigate associations between SES and barriers for contacting the GP, among women reporting bothersome UI.

Method: A cross-sectional web-based questionnaire study of symptoms occurrence among 51,090 randomly selected women. This study investigates reported symptoms of three types of UI (stress UI, urge UI and UI without stress or urge) and reported barriers for GP contact combined with register data on SES.

Results: A total of 4,051 (16.4%) women reported to be bothered by either stress UI (9.1%), urge UI (4.0%) or incontinence without stress or urge (2.4%) and 76.3%, 70%, and 64% respectively, had not contacted their GP regarding the symptom(s). The most frequently reported barriers were 'being too embarrassed' (19.3%) and 'being too busy' (18.4%) for stress incontinence, and 'being too embarrassed (19.0%) or 'worried about wasting the doctor's time' (16.9%) for women with bothersome urge UI or UI without stress or urge. Younger women had higher odds of reporting barriers and the barriers embarrassment and being worried about what the doctor might find were significantly associated with lower educational level.

Conclusion: Women with lower educational level have an increased risk of not seeking healthcare for UI symptoms. The GP should be aware of identifying women bothered by UI for whom effective treatment options to alleviate the symptoms are available.

Keywords: Urinary incontinence, Healthcare-seeking, Socioeconomic characteristics, Barriers

Introduction

Urinary incontinence (UI) is frequent among women worldwide [1]. UI may be classified due to the nature of the symptom, such as stress incontinence, urge incontinence and mixed incontinence [2]. The prevalence varies substantially among different study populations and is highly age dependent [3–5]. It has been estimated that

*Correspondence: djarbol@health.sdu.dk
Research Unit of General Practice, Department of Public Health, University of Southern Denmark, J.B. Winsløws Vej 9A, 2. Sal, 5000 Odense C, Denmark

substantially among different study populations and is highly age dependent [3–5]. It has been estimated that 20% of Danish women in the age group 40–60 years and 44% in the age group 80+ years report UI [6]. Not only is UI common, it has also been shown to have a negative impact on daily activity and health related quality of life [7].

There are several approaches to alleviate UI including both non-pharmacological, pharmacological and surgical treatment strategies [8]. A prerequisite for treatment is, however, that women experiencing UI seek healthcare. A review of five studies showed that less than 38% of women reporting UI contacted their general practitioner (GP) [9]. The decision of whether to contact the GP may be affected by numerous factors where some act as barriers and others as drivers for healthcare-seeking. Previous studies have found that healthcare-seeking with UI is strongly associated with age, the duration of symptoms, the number of symptoms and the symptoms being worrying or influencing the everyday life [6]. Other studies have demonstrated that embarrassment and negative attitudes towards healthcare use are negatively associated with healthcare-seeking for UI [10]. Further, healthcare-seeking for intimate symptoms varies between socioeconomic groups [11]. To facilitate diagnose and treatment for women bothered by UI but hesitating to seek healthcare it is important to generate knowledge regarding barriers for healthcare-seeking. How socioeconomic status (SES) is associated with experiencing barriers for healthcare-seeking for UI has not yet been explored.

Hence, the aim of this study was to analyze (1) frequencies of barriers for healthcare-seeking, and (2) the associations between commonly described barriers towards GP contact and SES among women bothered by UI.

Material and methods

This study is part of a nationwide cross-sectional cohort study, the Danish Symptom Cohort (DaSC). DaSC was designed as a web-based questionnaire study to which 100 000 individuals aged 20 years or above were randomly selected from the Danish Civil Registration System (CRS). The CRS contains information about date of birth, gender and a unique identification number for every Danish resident [12], which is used as the key identifier in all health and social registers. The selected individuals received a letter explaining the purpose of the study. The letter included a login for a secure web page with the questionnaire. Those without internet access were able to complete the questionnaire as a telephone interview. Individuals who did not respond within two weeks received a reminder letter, and after additional two weeks non-responders were contacted by telephone by a private marketing company. During this reminder procedure, reasons for non-participation were assessed when possible. Data were collected from June to December 2012. Details about the study sample and validity of the questionnaire are reported in Rasmussen et al. [13].

Questionnaire

The questionnaire was covering 44 predefined symptoms regarding a wide area of clinically relevant symptoms. When the respondents confirmed a symptom experience, a number of follow-up questions were asked concerning the onset of the symptom, the symptom's influence on daily activities, concerns about the symptom, whether the respondent had consulted the GP regarding the symptom and considerations about contacting the GP with the symptom in question.

The reporting of three types of UI (stress UI, urge UI and UI without stress or urge) form the basis of this paper. *The questions were phrased;* Have you within the last 4 weeks experienced any of the these? *That the urge to urinate is so strong that you cannot make it to the toilet in time (Urge UI), Involuntary urination during exertion, e.g. coughing, sneezing, lifting and exercise (Stress UI), and Involuntary urination (incontinence) without effort and urge (leakage).* To report to what extent, they were concerned about UI and to what extent UI interfered with their usual daily activities, five-point Likert scale with the options: "not at all", "slightly", "moderate", "quite a bit" and "extremely", was used. Respondents who were either moderately to extremely concerned and/or moderately to extremely influenced in their daily activities due to UI were considered bothered by UI, in the following described as bothersome UI.

This paper focuses on the women who had not contacted the GP with bothersome UI and the possible barriers for contacting the GP. Four common barriers for healthcare-seeking were included based on a literature search [14]. For each reported symptom without GP contact, the question was phrased: "You have not been in contact with your general practitioner regarding the symptom or discomfort you have experienced; did you have any of the following considerations about contacting your general practitioner?" The following options were given: "I would be too embarrassed", "I would be worried about wasting the doctor's time", "I would be worried about what the doctor might find", and "I was too busy to make time to go to the doctor" (Each of the questions could be answered with "yes" or"no"). Further, an "other" option was given, which was a free text box, where the respondents could elaborate on other options than the abovementioned. The free text box answers were not included in the present study.

The methodological framework for developing, and pilot- and field-testing the questionnaire is described in detail elsewhere [13].

Register data

For all respondents register data regarding SES (educational level, household income, cohabitation status, ethnicity and labor market affiliation) were collected from Statistics Denmark using the unique identification number in CRS enabling linkage between registers [15–17].

Statistical analyses

The study includes women reporting UI with the primary focus on women who reported bothersome UI and further reported, that they had not contacted their GP regarding the symptom(s). The term bothersome covers UI which was reported as either moderately to extremely concerning and/or moderately to extremely influencing on daily activities.

The proportions of women with bothersome UI and with no GP contact, respectively, are presented with the distribution of each covariate. The proportions of reported barriers among women with no GP contact with bothersome UI are presented for each type of UI. Logistic regression models were used to calculate unadjusted and adjusted odds ratios (ORs) for associations between each reported barrier towards GP contact among women who did not contact the GP and each of the covariates for the separate types of bothersome UI. The variables considered for analyses were age group, educational level, income, labor market affiliation, cohabitation status and ethnicity. Because of too few women reporting bothersome urge UI and UI without stress or urge we were not allowed to perform separate analyses of the associations between SES and barriers for GP contact for these respondents due to Danish data protection legislation. Hence, the two categories were merged in these analyses.

Age was categorized as 20–39, 40–59, 60–79 or 80+ years old. Education was categorized according to the highest attained educational level: low (< 10 years, i.e. primary and lower secondary school); middle (10–14 years, i.e. vocational education, upper secondary school and shorter education); or high (≥ 15 years, i.e. medium- or long-term higher education). Average disposable income was defined as the entire household income after taxation, adjusted for number of persons in the household in the year of filling in the questionnaire. Disposable income was categorized as low income (1st quartile), middle income (2nd and 3rd quartiles) or high income (4th quartile). Labor market affiliation was categorized as working, retirement pension, disability pension or out of the workforce according to the status each respondent predominantly had in the year of filling in the questionnaire. Cohabitation status at the time of participating in the survey was categorized as cohabiting/married or single. Ethnicity was categorized as people of Danish origin, immigrants, or descendants of immigrants.

All statistical tests used a significance level of $p < 0.05$. Data analyses were conducted using STATA statistical software 13.1 (StataCorp, College Station, TX, USA).

Results

A total of 51,090 Danish women were invited to participate in the survey. Among those 24,624 (48.2%) did not respond to the questionnaire or were ineligible for the study since they had either died, could not be reached due to unknown addresses, had severe illness (including dementia), had language problems, or had moved abroad. Among the 26,466 respondents 24,683 (93.3%) had complete data regarding the survey and register data.

A total of 4051 (16.4%) women reported to be bothered by either stress UI (9.1%), urge UI (4.0%) or incontinence without stress or urge (2.4%). Some 70% of those bothered by stress UI had not contacted their GP regarding the symptom. Similarly, 76.3% and 64% had not contacted their GP regarding bothersome urge UI and bothersome UI without stress or urge, respectively, Table 1.

In the analyses of associations between not contacting the GP regarding each UI subtype and SES we found that women with high educational level had higher odds of no GP contact with stress UI (OR = 1.42, 95% CI 1.05–1.93). Women on disability pension had lower odds of reporting no GP contact regarding both stress UI (OR = 0.50, 95% CI 0.35–0.72) and urge UI (OR = 0.53, 95% CI 0.34–0.81) (Table 2).

A total of 64.6% of the women with bothersome stress incontinence and no GP contact reported barriers for GP contact. The most frequent predefined barriers were 'being too embarrassed' and 'being too busy' reported by 19.3% and 18.4%, respectively (See Additional file 1: Table 1A).

Among women with bothersome urge incontinence or incontinence without stress or urge a total of 61.2% of the women with no GP contact reported at least one barrier towards GP contact. Most women reported 'being too embarrassed (19.0%) or 'worried about wasting the doctor's time' (16.9%). (See Additional file 1: Table 2A).

In total, 27% of the women with bothersome UI reported 'other' barriers for both symptom categories, indicating that the women had other barriers than the predefined barriers (See Additional file 1: Table 1A and 2A).

In the analyses of associations between age, SES and reported barriers for GP contact regarding stress UI we found that high age was associated with lower odds of

Table 1 Socioeconomic characteristics for women with bothersome* urinary incontinence (UI) and with no GP contact

	Total N	Stress UI		Urge UI		UI without stress or urge	
		N (%)	No GP contact (%)	N (%)	No GP contact (%)	N (%)	No GP contact (%)
All	24,683	2246 (9.1)	1713 (76.3)	1211 (4.9)	848 (70.0)	594 (2.4)	380 (64.0)
Age							
20–39	5554	281 (5.1)	224 (79.7)	126 (2.3)	89 (70.6)	46 (0.8)	30 (65.2)
40–59	10,680	1012 (9.5)	811 (80.1)	465 (4.4)	356 (76.6)	206 (1.9)	158 (76.7)
60–79	7732	861 (11.1)	617 (71.7)	543 (7.0)	354 (65.2)	293 (3.8)	165 (56.3)
80+	717	92 (12.8)	61 (66.3)	77 (10.7)	49 (63.6)	49 (6.8)	27 (55.1)
Marital status							
Single	6326	579 (9.2)	420 (72.5)	375 (5.9)	247 (65.9)	205 (3.2)	122 (59.5)
Married/Cohabiting	18,357	1667 (9.1)	1293 (77.6)	836 (4.6)	601 (71.9)	389 (2.1)	258 (66.3)
Educational level							
Low (< 10 years)	3069	403 (13.1)	278 (69.0)	263 (8.6)	171 (65.0)	135 (4.4)	72 (53.3)
Middle (10–14 years)	12,644	1196 (9.5)	922 (77.1)	609 (4.8)	437 (71.8)	306 (2.4)	204 (66.7)
High (>=15 years)	8970	647 (7.2)	513 (79.3)	339 (3.8)	240 (70.8)	153 (1.7)	104 (68.0)
Labor market affiliation							
Working	16,429	1263 (7.7)	1022 (80.9)	529 (3.2)	398 (75.2)	235 (1.4)	172 (73.2)
Pension	5820	682 (11.7)	480 (70.4)	470 (8.1)	307 (65.3)	267 (4.6)	148 (55.4)
Out of workforce	1360	129 (9.5)	99 (76.7)	90 (6.6)	69 (76.7)	35 (2.6)	27 (77.1)
Disability pension	1074	172 (16.0)	112 (65.1)	122 (11.4)	74 (60.7)	57 (5.3)	33 (57.9)
Equivalence weighted disposable income							
Low (1st quartile)	4189	425 (10.1)	301 (70.8)	277 (6.6)	180 (65.0)	140 (3.3)	82 (58.6)
Middle (2nd and 3rd quartile)	13,004	1217 (9.4)	928 (76.3)	649 (5.0)	455 (70.1)	320 (2.5)	201 (62.8)
High (4th quartile)	7490	604 (8.1)	484 (80.1)	285 (3.8)	213 (74.7)	134 (1.8)	97 (72.4)
Ethnicity							
Danish	23,155	2130 (9.2)	1628 (76.4)	1149 (5.0)	808 (70.3)	567 (2.4)	364 (64.2)
Immigrants/descendants of immigrants	1528	116 (7.6)	85 (73.3)	62 (4.1)	40 (64.5)	27 (1.8)	16 (59.3)

*Bothersome UI is defined by being either moderately to extremely concerned and/or moderately to extremely influenced in their daily activities due to UI

reporting all four barriers for GP contact. Further, high income and high educational level were associated with lower odds of reporting embarrassment and being worried about what the doctor might find but higher odds for choosing the "other" category as barrier. Women being outside the workforce had lower odds of being too busy to go to the GP whereas non-Danish ethnicity was associated with higher odds of being too busy (Table 3).

When analyzing the associations between age, SES and reported barriers for GP contact regarding urge UI or UI without stress or urge we found that high age was associated with lower odds of being worried about wasting the GP's time and being too busy to see the GP. Women with high educational level had lower odds of reporting being embarrassed, being worried about what the doctor might find and being worried about wasting the GP's time. Women being outside the workforce had lower odds of being too busy. Cohabiting was associated with higher odds of being worried about wasting the GP's time (Table 4).

Discussion

Main findings

We found that bothersome UI is common among women in the general population. Most women bothered by UI had not contacted their GP regarding their incontinence symptoms. Younger women had higher odds of reporting barriers and the barriers embarrassment and being worried about what the doctor might find were significantly associated with lower educational level.

Strengths and limitations

A major strength of this study is that we included a large number of randomly selected women (51,090 women) and had a relatively high response rate (54.5% among women) comparable to other studies of UI in the general population [5]. We obtained SES information from high-quality registers with a high degree of coverage and

Table 2 Associations between not contacting the GP and SES regarding women reporting bothersome urinary incontinence (UI)

	Stress UI		Urge UI		UI without stress or urge	
	Crude OR (95% CI)	Adj OR (95% CI)	Crude OR (95% CI)	Adj OR (95% CI)	Crude OR (95% CI)	Adj OR (95% CI)
Age						
20–39	1	1	1	1	1	1
40–59	1.03 (0.74–1.43)	1.06 (0.76–1.48)	1.36 (0.88–2.11)	1.35 (0.87–2.10)	1.76 (0.88–3.49)	1.77 (0.89–3.53)
60–79	0.64 (0.46–0.89)	0.72 (0.51–1.01)	0.78 (0.51–1.19)	0.81 (0.53–1.25)	0.69 (0.36–1.32)	0.77 (0.40–1.49)
80+	0.50 (0.30–0.84)	0.62 (0.36–1.07)	0.73 (0.40–1.33)	0.81 (0.44–1.50)	0.65 (0.29–1.50)	0.75 (0.32–1.76)
Marital status						
Single	1	1	1	1	1	1
Married/Cohabiting	1.31 (1.05–1.62)	1.18 (0.94–1.47)	1.33 (1.02–1.72)	1.27 (0.97–1.66)	1.34 (0.94–1.90)	1.17 (0.81–1.70)
Educational level						
Low (< 10 years)	1	1	1	1	1	1
Middle (10–14 years)	1.51 (1.18–1.94)	**1.32 (1.02–1.71)**	1.37 (1.00–1.86)	1.21 (0.88–1.66)	1.75 (1.16–2.65)	1.42 (0.92–2.18)
High (>= 15 years)	1.72 (1.30–2.29)	**1.42 (1.05–1.93)**	1.30 (0.92–1.84)	1.14 (0.80–1.63)	1.86 (1.15–3.00)	1.47 (0.89–2.42)
Labor market affiliation						
Working	1	1	1	1	1	1
Retirement pension	0.56 (0.45–0.70)	0.77 (0.54–1.09)	0.62 (0.47–0.82)	0.94 (0.62–1.43)	0.46 (0.31–0.66)	0.77 (0.43–1.38)
Out of workforce	0.78 (0.51–1.20)	0.82 (0.53–1.27)	1.08 (0.64–1.83)	1.10 (0.65–1.88)	1.24 (0.53–2.86)	1.60 (0.66–3.89)
Disability pension	0.44 (0.31–0.62)	**0.50 (0.35–0.72)**	0.51 (0.34–0.77)	**0.53 (0.34–0.81)**	0.50 (0.28–0.92)	0.57 (0.30–1.08)
Equivalence weighted disposable income						
Low (1st quartile)	1	1	1	1	1	1
Middle (2nd and 3rd quartile)	1.32 (1.03–1.69)	1.12 (0.86–1.46)	1.26 (0.94–1.70)	1.11 (0.81–1.53)	1.19 (0.80–1.79)	0.97 (0.63–1.51)
High (4th quartile)	1.66 (1.24–2.22)	1.30 (0.94–1.80)	1.59 (1.11–2.29)	1.29 (0.85–1.95)	1.85 (1.12–3.08)	1.24 (0.70–2.21)
Ethnicity						
Danish	1	1	1	1	1	1
Immigrants/ descendants of immigrants	0.85 (0.55–1.29)	0.81 (0.53–1.25)	0.77 (0.45–1.31)	0.70 (0.41–1.21)	0.81 (0.37–1.78)	0.78 (0.35–1.76)

Bold indicates a p value below 0.05

accuracy [15–17] compared to self-reported SES which may be subject to reporting bias. An overall responder analysis of the entire study cohort including both men and women showed that respondents were more often cohabiting, had higher educational level, had higher income, were of Danish origin and were more often working [18].

Our design using a web-based questionnaire is an advantage as it provides anonymity and thereby may enhance response rate from women not wishing to talk about UI. Moreover, the survey explored a range of different symptoms, and thereby trying to avoid women with UI to be more prone to answer questionnaire. The understanding and interpretation of the questions regarding UI might depend on SES, e.g. age and educational level. However, the field and pilot testing did not reveal problems in relation to this. Participants were asked to recall symptom experience during the preceding four weeks. The short recall period reduces risk of recall error. As we addressed bothersome UI i.e. which either worried or influenced daily activities, it seems reasonable to assume a correct recall within this time frame.

A minority of the respondents (2.4%) responded to the questionnaire via telephone interview. It is possible that information from the interviews are different from the information derived from the online version. The difference was sought minimised by using trained interviewers who were instructed only to read the questions out loud and ask the respondent to choose between the available answers. The interviewers were explicitly instructed not to engage in the interpretation of the questions with the respondent. The difference is explored more in depth in Rasmussen et al. [13].

The definition of bothersome UI was a constructed by two questions regarding worry related to having UI and the degree of influence on daily activity. It is possible that some respondents have answered negatively on these two questions but still feel bothered by UI.

Table 3 Associations between age, SES and reported barriers for GP contact regarding stress UI among women with no GP contact

	Being too embarrassed		Wasting the GP's time		Worried about what the GP might find	
	Crude OR (95% CI)	Adj. OR* (95% CI)	Crude OR (95% CI)	Adj. OR* (95% CI)	Crude OR (95% CI)	Adj. OR* (95% CI)
Age						
20–39	1	1	1	1	1	1
40–59	0.72 (0.51–1.01)	**0.68 (0.48 0.96)**	0.61 (0.43–0.86)	**0.58 (0.41–0.83)**	0.74 (0.46–1.19)	0.66 (0.41–1.07)
60–79	0.46 (0.32–0.67)	**0.41 (0.28–0.61)**	0.49 (0.34–0.72)	**0.48 (0.32–0.70)**	0.49 (0.29–0.82)	**0.39 (0.22–0.68)**
80+	0.34 (0.15–0.79)	**0.31 (0.13–0.73)**	0.38 (0.16–0.87)	**0.37 (0.15–0.87)**	0.98 (0.40–2.37)	**0.78 (0.31–2.00)**
Marital status						
Single	1	1	1	1	1	1
Married/Cohabiting	1.21 (0.91–1.62)	1.09 (0.81–1.47)	1.11 (0.82–1.50)	1.02 (0.75–1.38)	1.18 (0.78–1.78)	1.19 (0.77–1.84)
Educational leve						
Low (< 10 years)	1	1	1	1	1	1
Middle (10–14 years)	1.02 (0.73–1.42)	0.82 (0.57–1.16)	1.36 (0.94–1.98)	1.19 (0.81–1.76)	0.91 (0.58–1.42)	0.75 (0.47–1.21)
High (>= 15 years)	0.90 (0.62–1.30)	**0.65 (0.44–0.96)**	1.14 (0.75–1.71)	0.91 (0.59–1.40)	0.56 (0.32–0.95)	**0.42 (0.23–0.74)**
Labor market affiliation						
Working	1	1	1	1	1	1
Retirement pension	0.64 (0.48–0.86)	1.00 (0.61–1.66)	0.70 (0.52–0.95)	0.87 (0.53–1.43)	0.83 (0.55–1.26)	1.20 (0.55–2.61)
Out of workforce	1.39 (0.87–2.24)	1.33 (0.82–2.16)	1.44 (0.88–2.36)	1.42 (0.86–2.35)	1.74 (0.93–3.25)	1.60 (0.85–3.03)
Disability pension	0.58 (0.33–1.01)	0.60 (0.34–1.08)	0.81 (0.47–1.39)	0.91 (0.52–1.58)	0.96 (0.47–1.97)	0.98 (0.47–2.07)
Equivalence weighted disposable income						
Low (1st quartile)	1	1	1	1	1	1
Middle (2nd and 3rd quartile)	0.96 (0.70–1.32)	0.85 (0.61–1.20)	1.15 (0.81–1.63)	1.08 (0.75–1.58)	0.58 (0.38–0.88)	**0.53 (0.34–0.83)**
High (4th quartile)	0.65 (0.45–0.94)	**0.58 (0.38–0.88)**	0.97 (0.65–1.44)	0.96 (0.62–1.49)	0.41 (0.25–0.68)	**0.38 (0.22–0.68)**
Ethnicity						
Danish	1	1	1	1	1	1
Immigrants and descendants of immigrants	1.40 (0.84–2.33)	1.31 (0.78–2.20)	1.23 (0.71–2.14)	1.17 (0.67–2.04)	0.99 (0.45–2.20)	0.91 (0.41–2.03)

	Being too busy		Other		None	
	Crude OR (95% CI)	Adj. OR* (95% CI)	Crude OR (95% CI)	Adj. OR* (95% CI)	Crude OR (95% CI)	Adj. OR* (95% CI)
Age						
20–39	1	1	1	1	1	1
40–59	0.89 (0.63–1.26)	0.90 (0.63–1.27)	0.97 (0.70–1.34)	1.17 (0.84–1.64)	1.17 (0.84–1.63)	1.07 (0.76–1.50)
60–79	0.37 (0.25–0.54)	**0.37 (0.25–0.56)**	0.78 (0.55–1.09)	1.15 (0.80–1.65)	2.35 (1.67–3.29)	**1.91 (1.35–2.71)**
80+	0.38 (0.17–0.89)	**0.38 (0.16–0.91)**	0.41 (0.19–0.89)	0.69 (0.31–1.54)	3.85 (2.14–6.94)	**2.83 (1.53–5.23)**
Marital status						
Single	1	1	1	1	1	1
Married/Cohabiting	1.05 (0.79–1.40)	0.87 (0.65–1.18)	1.17 (0.91–1.51)	1.03 (0.79–1.35)	0.74 (0.59–0.93)	0.90 (0.71–1.14)
Educational leve						
Low (< 10 years)	1	1	1	1	1	1
Middle (10–14 years)	1.61 (1.09–2.37)	1.24 (0.83–1.85)	2.12 (1.44–3.12)	**2.08 (1.41–3.09)**	0.55 (0.42–0.72)	**0.68 (0.51–0.90)**
High (>= 15 years)	1.71 (1.14–2.59)	1.20 (0.78–1.86)	4.77 (3.21–7.09)	**4.73 (3.14–7.13)**	0.36 (0.26–0.48)	**0.47 (0.34–0.65)**
Labor market affiliation						
Working	1	1	1	1	1	1
Retirement pension	0.27 (0.19–0.39)	**0.32 (0.19–0.54)**	0.61 (0.47–0.79)	0.78 (0.52–1.18)	2.64 (2.11–3.31)	**1.77 (1.23–2.56)**
Out of workforce	0.52 (0.29–0.94)	**0.50 (0.28–0.90)**	0.58 (0.35–0.97)	0.70 (0.42–1.18)	1.30 (0.84–2.02)	1.17 (0.75–1.83)

Table 3 (continued)

	Being too busy		Other		None	
	Crude OR (95% CI)	Adj. OR* (95% CI)	Crude OR (95% CI)	Adj. OR* (95% CI)	Crude OR (95% CI)	Adj. OR* (95% CI)
Disability pension	0.20 (0.09–0.44)	**0.20 (0.09–0.44)**	0.80 (0.52–1.25)	1.05 (0.66–1.69)	1.88 (1.26–2.80)	**1.54 (1.01–2.33)**
Equivalence weighted disposable income						
Low (1st quartile)	1	1	1	1	1	1
Middle (2nd and 3rd quartile)	1.03 (0.73–1.46)	0.90 (0.62–1.32)	1.39 (1.01–1.91)	1.03 (0.73–1.44)	0.84 (0.64–1.10)	1.14 (0.85–1.52)
High (4th quartile)	1.40 (0.96–2.03)	1.25 (0.82–1.90)	1.89 (1.35–2.65)	1.19 (0.82–1.75)	0.63 (0.47–0.86)	0.96 (0.68–1.34)
Ethnicity						
Danish	1	1	1	1	1	1
Immigrants and descendants of immigrants	1.81 (1.11–2.95)	**1.68 (1.02–2.77)**	0.77 (0.46–1.31)	0.74 (0.43–1.26)	0.80 (0.50–1.28)	0.85 (0.53–1.38)

*Adjustments were made for all other covariates

Bold indicates a p value below 0.05

Including stratified analyses based on gravity of bothersome UI could have added to the results but was not a specific aim of this study.

We included three different types of UI for the survey. UI without stress or urge may include different kinds of UI, e.g. postural incontinence, continuous incontinence, insensible incontinence, and coital incontinence, but the study does not provide any details about this. We did not ask specific about mixed incontinence, rather we explored urge and stress UI separately, but it was possible to report more than one of the symptoms and considerable overlap may have been reported.

In addition to the predefined barriers, the questionnaire comprised an "other" category with the possibility to express other barriers. In total, 27% of the women with bothersome UI reported 'other' barriers for healthcare-seeking. Qualitatively exploring the statements in the "other" category is however beyond the scope of this study, but the relative high degree of answers in this category indicates that other barriers than those predefined should be explored in future studies.

Comparison with existing literature

A Danish study specifically about UI in the general population reached a slightly higher response rate (66.6%) and found a much higher prevalence of 46.4% [3] compared to the total prevalence of 16.4% in the present study. However, the study by Schreiber Pedersen et al. measured UI in general and not only bothersome UI which may explain the substantial difference. Further, it has been shown that the prevalence of UI varies greatly between studies depending on definitions and designs [4]. Therefore, it is recommended to assess the bothersomeness of UI and to use non-UI focused surveys to assess the prevalence of UI in the general population as symptomatic women may be more prone to answer questionnaires leading to an overestimation of the prevalence [4].

Regarding the associations between SES and healthcare-seeking one study found that ethnicity and education were not significantly associated with seeking treatment for UI [19]. However, this study focused only on women during the menopausal transition and consequently only a minor part of the general population of women. In contrast, we included adult women of all ages in our study, which may explain why we found SES to be associated with healthcare-seeking with UI.

Conclusion

Bothersome UI is common, often not presented to the GP, and younger women are more likely to report barriers for GP contact with UI. Women with lower educational level are more likely to be worried about what the doctor might find and be too embarrassed to contact their GP when being bothered by UI. This knowledge underlines the importance of the GP being aware of identifying women bothered by UI for whom effective treatment options to alleviate the symptoms are available. A special focus should be on women with lower educational level who might be at increased risk of hesitating to contact the GP and on practice organization and structure which may play a role in the way patients and GPs meet in general practice.

Table 4 Associations between age, SES and reported barriers for GP contact regarding urge UI or UI without stress or urge among women with no GP contact

	Being too embarrassed		Wasting the GP's time		Worried about what the GP might find	
	Crude OR (95% CI)	Adj. OR* (95% CI)	Crude OR (95% CI)	Adj. OR* (95% CI)	Crude OR (95% CI)	Adj. OR* (95% CI)
Age						
20–39	1	1	1	1	1	1
40–59	1.20 (0.73–2.00)	1.16 (0.70–1.93)	0.62 (0.38–1.02)	**0.58 (0.35–0.97)**	0.74 (0.40–1.39)	0.70 (0.38–1.32)
60–79	0.66 (0.39–1.11)	0.59 (0.35–1.02)	0.57 (0.35–0.95)	**0.52 (0.31–0.87)**	0.69 (0.37–1.29)	0.59 (0.31–1.12)
80+	0.56 (0.23–1.33)	0.54 (0.22–1.31)	0.59 (0.26–1.31)	0.59 (0.26–1.34)	0.43 (0.14–1.37)	0.38 (0.12–1.23)
Marital status						
Single	1	1	1	1	1	1
Married/Cohabiting	1.40 (0.99–2.00)	1.32 (0.92–1.88)	1.47 (1.01–2.13)	**1.48 (1.01–2.17)**	1.11 (0.71–1.73)	1.09 (0.69–1.70)
Educational level						
Low (< 10 years)	1	1	1	1	1	1
Middle (10–14 years)	0.84 (0.57–1.25)	0.69 (0.46–1.04)	0.93 (0.62–1.40)	0.85 (0.56–1.29)	0.75 (0.46–1.21)	0.68 (0.41–1.12)
High (>=15 years)	0.74 (0.48–1.16)	**0.60 (0.37–0.95)**	0.60 (0.37–0.97)	**0.53 (0.32–0.87)**	0.50 (0.28–0.90)	**0.44 (0.24–0.81)**
Labor market affiliation						
Working	1	1	1	1	1	1
Retirement pension	0.63 (0.44–0.89)	1.06 (0.57–1.97)	0.90 (0.63–1.28)	1.06 (0.58–1.93)	0.91 (0.57–1.45)	0.87 (0.42–1.78)
Out of workforce	1.05 (0.60–1.84)	1.00 (0.56–1.78)	1.10 (0.60–2.01)	1.02 (0.55–1.90)	2.20 (1.17–4.15)	2.00 (1.04–3.83)
Disability pension	1.02 (0.59–1.74)	0.99 (0.56–1.73)	1.17 (0.67–2.06)	1.21 (0.68–2.18)	1.59 (0.83–3.08)	1.47 (0.74–2.90)
Equivalence weighted disposable income						
Low (1st quartile)	1	1	1	1	1	1
Middle (2nd and 3rd quartile)	0.90 (0.61–1.33)	0.82 (0.54–1.24)	1.10 (0.74–1.65)	1.08 (0.70–1.66)	0.74 (0.46–1.17)	0.74 (0.45–1.21)
High (4th quartile)	0.89 (0.57–1.38)	0.76 (0.46–1.25)	0.70 (0.42–1.14)	0.70 (0.40–1.22)	0.44 (0.24–0.81)	**0.45 (0.23–0.89)**
Ethnicity						
Danish	1	1	1	1	1	1
Immigrants and descendants of immigrants	1.44 (0.75–2.75)	1.32 (0.68–2.55)	1.51 (0.77–2.93)	1.49 (0.76–2.94)	1.65 (0.76–3.60)	1.60 (0.72–3.53)

	Being too busy		Other		None	
	Crude OR (95% CI)	Adj. OR* (95% CI)	Crude OR (95% CI)	Adj. OR* (95% CI)	Crude OR (95% CI)	Adj. OR* (95% CI)
Age						
20–39	1	1	1	1	1	1
40–59	0.74 (0.45–1.22)	0.76 (0.46–1.24)	1.47 (0.92–2.37)	1.62 (1.00–2.63)	0.94 (0.60–1.47)	0.90 (0.57–1.42)
60–79	0.35 (0.21–0.60)	**0.36 (0.21–0.63)**	1.01 (0.62–1.64)	1.24 (0.75–2.04)	2.13 (1.36–3.32)	**1.97 (1.25–3.09)**
80+	0.39(0.16–0.95)	**0.39 (0.16–0.96)**	0.81 (0.38–1.71)	0.90 (0.42–1.94)	2.49 (1.32–4.72)	**2.35 (1.23–4.50)**
Marital status						
Single	1	1	1	1	1	1
Married/Cohabiting	0.96 (0.67–1.38)	0.87 (0.60–1.25)	0.87 (0.65–1.16)	0.79 (0.58–1.07)	0.91 (0.70–1.19)	1.03 (0.78–1.37)
Educational level						
Low (< 10 years)	1	1	1	1	1	1
Middle (10–14 years)	1.41 (0.87–2.29)	1.15 (0.70–1.89)	1.73 (1.14–2.62)	**1.67 (1.09–2.55)**	0.73 (0.53–1.01)	0.89 (0.64–1.25)
High (>=15 years)	1.65 (0.98–2.77)	1.29 (0.76–2.21)	3.55 (2.29–5.50)	**3.48 (2.22–5.44)**	0.48 (0.33–0.70)	**0.60 (0.41–0.88)**
Labor market affiliation						
Working	1	1	1	1	1	1
Retirement pension	0.23 (0.14–0.35)	**0.17 (0.09–0.33)**	0.59 (0.43–0.80)	0.62 (0.38–1.00)	2.52 (1.91–3.32)	1.75 (1.12–2.73)
Out of workforce	0.34 (0.16–0.73)	**0.31 (0.14–0.67)**	0.84 (0.50–1.42)	0.96 (0.56–1.64)	0.98 (0.59–1.64)	0.96 (0.57–1.62)

Table 4 (continued)

	Being too busy		Other		None	
	Crude OR (95% CI)	Adj. OR* (95% CI)	Crude OR (95% CI)	Adj. OR* (95% CI)	Crude OR (95% CI)	Adj. OR* (95% CI)
Disability pension	0.26 (0.12–0.57)	**0.25 (0.11–0.55)**	0.75 (0.46–1.24)	0.86 (0.51–1.44)	1.57 (0.99–2.48)	1.43 (0.89–2.29)
Equivalence weighted disposable income						
Low (1st quartile)	1	1	1	1	1	1
Middle (2nd and 3rd quartile)	1.10 (0.71–1.71)	1.05 (0.65–1.69)	1.46 (1.00–2.13)	1.29 (0.87–1.93)	0.81 (0.60–1.11)	0.94 (0.67–1.32)
High (4th quartile)	1.39 (0.85–2.26)	1.33 (0.76–2.32)	2.39 (1.58–3.60)	**1.89 (1.19–3.00)**	0.65 (0.45–0.93)	0.84 (0.56–1.27)
Ethnicity						
Danish	1	1	1	1	1	1
Immigrants and descendants of immigrants	1.68 (0.86–3.28)	1.54 (0.78–3.03)	0.97 (0.52–1.82)	0.89 (0.46–1.69)	0.69 (0.38–1.26)	0.80 (0.43–1.47)

*Adjustments were made for all other covariates

Bold indicates a p value below 0.05

Abbreviations

UI: Urinary incontinence; GP: General practitioner; SES: Socioeconomic status; OR: Odds ratio; CI: Confidence interval.

Acknowledgements

The initial survey was conducted in collaboration between the Research Unit of General Practice, University of Southern Denmark and the Research Centre for Cancer Diagnosis in Primary Care, Aarhus University.

Authors' contributions

KB, PH, DEJ, JS, and SR participated in the design of the study, development of the questionnaire, the logistics concerning the survey, analyses, and the drafting of the manuscript. DEJ drafted the first version of the manuscript. All authors read and approved the final manuscript.

Competing interests

The authors declare no competing interests.

References

1. Hagan KA, Erekson E, Austin A, Minassian VA, Townsend MK, Bynum JPW, et al. A prospective study of the natural history of urinary incontinence in women. Am J Obstet Gynecol. 2018;218(5):502.e1–.e8.
2. Minassian VA, Hagan KA, Erekson E, Austin AM, Carmichael D, Bynum JPW, et al. The natural history of urinary incontinence subtypes in the Nurses' Health Studies. Am J Obstet Gynecol. 2020 Feb;222(2):163.e1-163.e8.
3. Schreiber Pedersen L, Lose G, Høybye MT, Elsner S, Waldmann A, Rudnicki M. Prevalence of urinary incontinence among women and analysis of potential risk factors in Germany and Denmark. Acta Obstet Gynecol Scand. 2017;96(8):939–48.
4. Bedretdinova D, Fritel X, Panjo H, Ringa V. Prevalence of female urinary incontinence in the general population according to different definitions and study designs. Eur Urol. 2016;69(2):256–64.
5. O'Donnell M, Lose G, Sykes D, Voss S, Hunskaar S. Help-seeking behaviour and associated factors among women with urinary incontinence in France, Germany, Spain and the United Kingdom. Eur Urol. 2005;47(3):385–92; discussion 92.
6. Raasthoj I, Elnegaard S, Rosendal M, Jarbol DE. Urinary incontinence among women-which personal and professional relations are involved? A population-based study. Int Urogynecol J. 2019;30(9):1565–74.
7. Hagglund D, Walker-Engstrom ML, Larsson G, Leppert J. Quality of life and seeking help in women with urinary incontinence. Acta Obstet Gynecol Scand. 2001;80(11):1051–5.
8. Lukacz ES, Santiago-Lastra Y, Albo ME, Brubaker L. Urinary incontinence in women: a review. JAMA. 2017;318(16):1592–604.
9. Koch LH. Help-seeking behaviors of women with urinary incontinence: an integrative literature review. J Midwifery Womens Health. 2006;51(6):e39-44.
10. Kinchen KS, Burgio K, Diokno AC, Fultz NH, Bump R, Obenchain R. Factors associated with women's decisions to seek treatment for urinary incontinence. J Women's Health. 2003;12(7):687–98.
11. Balasubramaniam K, Elnegaard S, Rasmussen S, Haastrup PF, Christensen RD, Sondergaard J, et al. Lifestyle, socioeconomic status and healthcare seeking among women with gynaecological cancer alarm symptoms: a combined questionnaire-based and register-based population study. BMJ Open. 2018;8(7):e021815.
12. Pedersen CB. The Danish civil registration system. Scand J Public Health. 2011;39(7 Suppl):22–5.
13. Rasmussen S, Sondergaard J, Larsen PV, Balasubramaniam K, Elnegaard S, Svendsen RP, et al. The Danish Symptom Cohort: Questionnaire and Feasibility in the Nationwide Study on Symptom Experience and Healthcare-Seeking among 100 000 Individuals. Int J Fam Med. 2014;2014:187280.
14. Simon AE, Forbes LJ, Boniface D, Warburton F, Brain KE, Dessaix A, et al. An international measure of awareness and beliefs about cancer: development and testing of the ABC. BMJ Open. 2012;2(6):e001758.
15. Jensen VM, Rasmussen AW. Danish education registers. Scand J Public Health. 2011;39(7 Suppl):91–4.
16. Baadsgaard M, Quitzau J. Danish registers on personal income and transfer payments. Scand J Public Health. 2011;39(7 Suppl):103–5.
17. Petersson F, Baadsgaard M, Thygesen LC. Danish registers on personal labour market affiliation. Scand J Public Health. 2011;39(7 Suppl):95–8.
18. Elnegaard S, Andersen RS, Pedersen AF, Larsen PV, Sondergaard J, Rasmussen S, et al. Self-reported symptoms and healthcare seeking in the general population–exploring "The Symptom Iceberg." BMC Public Health. 2015;15:685.
19. Waetjen LE, Xing G, Johnson WO, Melnikow J, Gold EB. Study of Women's Health Across the N Factors associated with seeking treatment for urinary incontinence during the menopausal transition. Obstet Gynecol. 2015;125(5):1071–9.

15

Cross-organ sensitization between the prostate and bladder in an experimental rat model of lipopolysaccharide (LPS)-induced chronic pelvic pain syndrome

Ozgu Aydogdu[1], Pinar Uyar Gocun[2], Patrik Aronsson[1], Thomas Carlsson[1] and Michael Winder[1*]

Abstract

Background: The aim of the current study was to investigate the effects of chronic prostatitis/chronic pelvic pain syndrome (CP/CPPS) on bladder function via prostate-to-bladder cross-sensitization in a rat model of lipopolysaccharide (LPS)-induced prostate inflammation.

Methods: Male rats were intraprostatically injected with LPS or saline, serving as control. Micturition parameters were examined in a metabolic cage 10 or 14 days later. Subsequently, to evaluate bladder function, cystometry was performed. Micturition cycles were induced by saline infusion and cholinergic and purinergic contractile responses were measured by intravenous injection with methacholine and ATP, respectively. Thereafter, the prostate and bladder were excised and assessed histopathologically for possible inflammatory changes.

Results: Metabolic cage experiments showed increased urinary frequency in rats with LPS-induced CP/CPPS. Cystometry showed a significant increase in the number of non-voiding contractions, longer voiding time and lower compliance in CP/CPPS animals compared to controls. Induction of CP/CPPS led to significantly reduced cholinergic and purinergic bladder contractile responses. Histopathological analysis demonstrated prostatic inflammation in CP/CPPS animals. There were no significant differences between the groups regarding the extent or the grade of bladder inflammation. Prostate weight was not significantly different between the groups.

Conclusions: The present study shows that prostate-to-bladder cross-sensitization can be triggered by an infectious focus in the prostate, giving rise to bladder overactivity and alterations in both afferent and efferent signalling. Future studies are required to fully understand the underlying mechanisms.

Keywords: Lipopolysaccharide (LPS), CPPS, Prostate, Bladder, LUTS, Overactive bladder

*Correspondence: michael.winder@pharm.gu.se

[1] Department of Pharmacology, Institute of Neuroscience and Physiology, The Sahlgrenska Academy, University of Gothenburg, Gothenburg, Sweden

Full list of author information is available at the end of the article

Introduction

Chronic prostatitis/chronic pelvic pain syndrome (CP/CPPS) constitutes an important part of urology visits [1]. Despite rare association between bacterial foci in the prostate and CP/CPPS, infection has for long been speculated to be a potential factor that can trigger inflammatory pathways in the pelvic region [1, 2]. Some studies have demonstrated the presence of bacterial DNA in prostate tissues from men with CP/CPPS [1, 3, 4] and it has been suggested that an initial intraprostatic bacterial colonization could provoke chronic inflammation that possibly entails insistent structural changes in the prostate [5].

A large number of male patients diagnosed with CP/CPPS suffer from lower urinary tract symptoms (LUTS), including urgency and frequency, similar to patients with overactive bladder (OAB) [6, 7]. The potential mechanisms by which chronic prostatic inflammation contributes to LUTS has recently been highlighted [6, 8–10]. Cross-organ sensitization between the urinary bladder and prostate has been speculated as a potential mechanism to explain the possible negative effects of chronic prostate inflammation on bladder function [10–12]. A recent study on zymosan-induced CP/CPPS in rats supports this notion [13].

Interstitial cystitis/bladder pain syndrome (IC/BPS) is often referred to as a disease that more commonly affects women [14]. Nevertheless, studies have suggested that the true prevalence of IC/BPS in men is higher than thought, which may be due to an underdiagnosis of this pathology in male patients [15, 16]. I.e., that many men diagnosed with CP/CPPS may also have concomitant IC/BPS. It is noteworthy that male patients suffering from CP/CPPS frequently experience inadequate treatment [17]. Besides a lack of effective medication, possible negative effects of chronic prostate inflammation on urinary bladder function and urothelial pathophysiology may explain the unsatisfactory management of men with CP/CPPS. Considering the relatively large number of patients who do not respond positively to treatment for CP/CPPS, more effort is required to find an explanation for the potential cross-organ sensitization between prostate and bladder. For this, it is necessary to understand possible underlying mechanisms for inflammatory processes in the pelvic region. This will potentially lead to the discovery of new and more effective pharmacological targets for the treatment of male patients with CP/CPPS.

In the present study, it was hypothesized that an intraprostatic infectious focus could be an inducing factor for CP/CPPS which subsequently leads to pelvic cross-sensitization. For this, prostatic inflammation was induced in male rats by intraprostatic injection with lipopolysaccharide (LPS), a component of the outer layer of the cell wall of gram-negative bacteria. LPS can activate the immune system and cause chronic inflammation, which in turn can cause release of various pro-inflammatory cytokines including interleukin-1 (IL-1), interleukin-6 (IL-6) and tumor necrosis factor alpha (TNF-α) [2]. Micturition parameters were studied in a metabolic cage at 10 and 14 days after LPS injection. Subsequently, urodynamic properties were examined during cystometry by repeated bladder filling. Further, methacholine (MeCh) and adenosine-5′-triphosphate (ATP) were used to examine cholinergic and purinergic responses, respectively. Lastly, inflammatory changes in the prostate and urinary bladder were studied immunohistochemically.

Materials and methods

The current study aimed to investigate if bacterially induced chronic prostate inflammation leads to symptoms of bladder overactivity. Further, the study aimed to examine the potential underlying mechanisms causing these alterations. Eighteen adult male Sprague–Dawley rats (300–450 g; Charles River Laboratories, Calco, Italy) were used in the current study which was approved by the local ethics committee at the University of Gothenburg, Sweden (permit number: 1794/2018). All experiments were designed to minimize the suffering of the animals during and after the surgical and experimental procedures. The number of animals were chosen based on previous studies and to ensure obtainment of objective and reliable results, i.e. avoid underpowering, but at the same time minimize the number of animals used, i.e. avoid overpowering. All drugs were purchased from Sigma-Aldrich, St Louis, USA unless otherwise stated.

Study design

The animals were randomly divided into three groups ($n=6$ in each group; Fig. 1). In group 1 and 2, LPS (100 μL; 100 $\mu g*kg^{-1}$) was injected into the dorsal and ventral lobes of the prostate (50 μL in each lobe). In group 3, the rats were similarly injected with vehicle (100 μL saline, serving as control). During intraprostatic injections, the needle tip was tunnelled 2–3 mm subcapsularly and the needle was held in injection site for approximately 20 s as a standard procedure to avoid a possible leakage from the prostate. All intraprostatic injections were performed with laparotomy under deep anaesthesia with 3% isoflurane on a thermo-regulated heating pad. Following the injection procedure, abdominal muscle and skin were closed with separate surgical sutures. A single dose of subcutaneous buprenorphine (0.1 $mg*kg^{-1}$) was used as postoperative analgesia.

Metabolic cage

Ten or 14 days after intraprostatic LPS injection (termed as group L10 and L14, respectively) or 10 days after

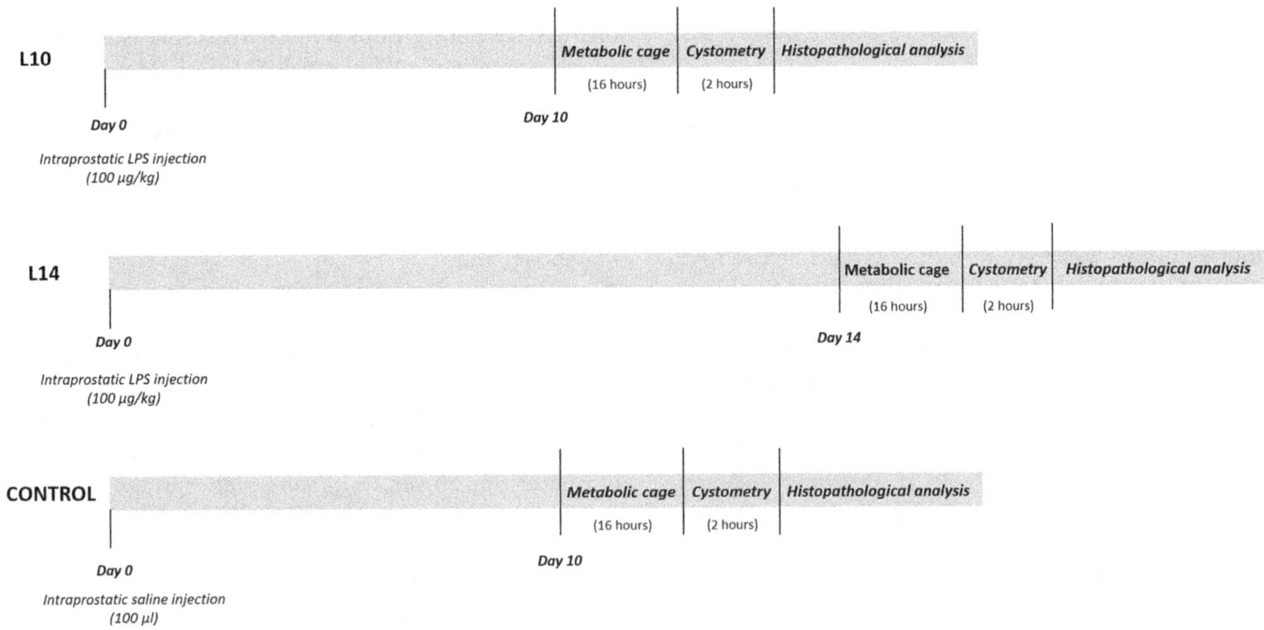

Fig. 1 Study flowcharts. Timelines for the experimental procedures in each treatment group. Male rats were injected intraprostatically with either lipopolysaccharide (LPS; (L10 and L14; 100 $\mu g * kg^{-1}$) or saline (Control; 100 µL). After 10 (L10, Control) or 14 (L14) days the rats were placed in a metabolic cage for 16 h. Subsequently, cystometry was performed. This was followed by histopathological analysis of bladder and prostate tissues

intraprostatic saline injection (control), metabolic cage experiments were carried out. The time intervals were chosen based on previous observations of inflammatory responses in the prostate [2, 13]. These previous studies demonstrate possible differences at 10 and 14 days after intraprostatic LPS injection, respectively. Further, they indicate that 7 days may be too short of an interval for observations of prostatitis after a single injection and that differences that are seen after 14 days are not significantly increased at later time points (i.e. after 21 days). Similar to previous studies, the animals were currently placed in a metabolic cage with free access to water and the voided urine was collected continuously for 16 h, typically from 4 PM to 8 AM. [18, 19]. The total water intake and total amount of expelled urine were measured. For registration of the number of micturitions, a laser Doppler (WFL30-40B416; SICK, Richmond Hill, Canada) that registered each drop of voided urine was used. This allowed for micturition frequency and voided volume per micturition to be calculated. A MP150WSW data acquisition system and the AcqKnowledge 3.8.1 software (BioPac Systems, Goleta, USA) were used to record the metabolic cage data.

Cystometry

Immediately following each metabolic cage experiment, cystometry was performed. Deep anaesthesia was induced with 3% isoflurane and maintained during the entirety of the cystometry investigations. The surgical procedure followed previous similar studies [20]. Briefly, the urinary bladder was exposed by laparotomy and the femoral artery and vein were catheterized to monitor blood pressure and administer drugs (MeCh and ATP), respectively. After the catheterization of the femoral blood vessels, a pressure sensing catheter and a cannula were placed in the urinary bladder via a midline incision in the bladder dome and subsequently fixed with a ligature. Saline was infused via the cannula to induce simulated micturition cycles. The bladder was emptied before each infusion and was filled until the rat voided (approx. 30–40 s). The change in intravesical pressure that occurred during bladder filling (ΔP), volume change in the bladder (ΔV), voiding time and non-voiding contractions (NVCs), defined as increases in intravesical pressure more than 10 mmHg over baseline pressure without any voiding, were noted during the experiments. For standardization purposes, NVCs were counted during a two hour period, from the beginning of the first induced micturition cycle and onwards. Bladder compliance was calculated by dividing ΔV by ΔP. Simulated micturition cycles were performed five times before and after concentration–response series of the cholinergic agonist MeCh (1, 2 and 5 $\mu g * kg^{-1}$ i.v.) and the purinergic agonist ATP (5, 10 and 100 $\mu g * kg^{-1}$ i.v.). Each concentration–response series was performed two times. Calculations were performed on the average responses during the induced micturition cycles and the concentration–response series.

Histopathology

After the cystometry experiments, the dorsal and ventral prostate lobes as well as the urinary bladder were excised and the rats were euthanized. Total prostate weight was noted and paraformaldehyde (4% in 0.1 M phosphate-buffer solution) was used to fix the tissues before histopathological analysis. After fixation (48–72 h), the tissues were embedded in paraffin and sectioned into 8 μm thin tissue sections (Histolab Products AB, Gothenburg, Sweden). Haematoxylin–eosin staining was performed and the histopathological analysis followed the same procedure as previous studies [13, 21], including the use of a similar grading scale (see Table 1). Prostatic inflammation was scored based on the magnitude or density of lymphocytes (grade) and the extent or distribution of lymphocyte infiltration (extent). The grade of inflammation was scored from 0 to 3 where 0 represented no inflammation and 3 represented severe inflammation while the extent of inflammation was scored as focal (1), multifocal (2) or diffuse (3), respectively (Fig. 2).

Statistics

Statistical measurements were performed using GraphPad Prism version 8.2.1 (GraphPad Software Inc., San Diego, USA). One-way ANOVA or two-way ANOVA followed by Tukey`s correction for multiple comparisons was used for statistical comparisons of metabolic cage and cystometry findings, as these data were assumed to be normally distributed. Histopathological findings were statistically compared using the non-parametric Kruskal–Wallis test followed by Dunn`s test for multiple comparisons, to compare the mean ranks between each of the treatment groups and controls. Statistical significance was regarded for p-values < 0.05. Metabolic cage and cystometry data are presented as mean ± SEM while histopathological data are presented as median with range.

Results

Metabolic cage

There were no significant differences between the groups regarding total water intake ($p = 0.299$) or total amount of voided urine ($p = 0.735$) during the metabolic cage experiments (Table 2). The number of micturitions per hour were significantly higher in the L14 group as compared to controls ($p = 0.035$). Similarly, the total number of micturitions (over 16 h) were higher in the L14 group as compared to controls ($p = 0.035$, Table 2). No significant differences were seen between the L10 and L14 groups regarding the number of micturitions per hour or the total number of micturitions. The volume/micturition was significantly lower in both L10 and L14 as compared to controls (L10 vs control, $p = 0.016$; L14 vs control, $p = 0.018$). Again, there was no significant difference between the L10 and L14 group (Table 2).

Cystometry

Baseline urinary bladder pressures were similar in all groups, both before and after the administration of agonist (MeCh and ATP). However, there were significantly more NVCs in the CP/CPPS groups as compared to controls (Fig. 3; control vs L10: 2.67 ± 0.76 vs 33.00 ± 7.67, $p = 0.014$; control vs L14: 2.67 ± 0.76 vs 34.83 ± 8.43, $p = 0.009$). No significant difference was seen in regard to NVCs between the CP/CPPS groups. Similarly, lower bladder compliance ($\Delta V/\Delta P$) was observed in the CP/

Table 1 Immunohistochemical grading scales

Grade (Inflammatory cell density, cells/mm²)	
0	No inflammation
1, mild	Individual inflammatory cells (< 100 cells/mm²)
2. moderate	Confluent sheets of inflammatory cells without tissue destruction or lymphoid follicle formation (100–500 cells/mm²)
3, severe	Confluent sheets of inflammatory cells with tissue destruction or lymphoid follicle formation (> 500 cells/mm²)
Extent (Tissue area involved by inflammatory cell infiltrates)	
1, focal	< 10%
2, multifocal	10–50%
3, diffuse	> 50%

Grading scales used to score inflammatory changes in prostate and urinary bladder. The procedure for determination of grade and extent of inflammation was adapted from Inamura et al. [21]

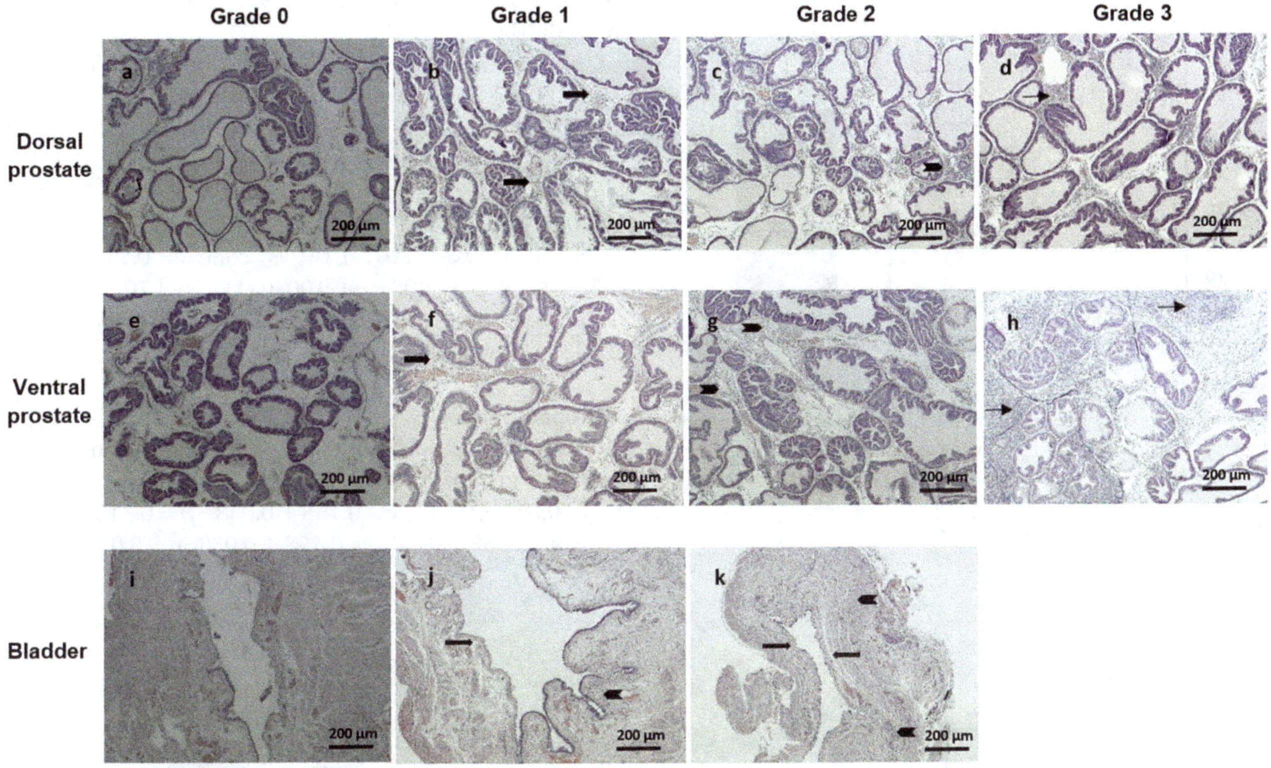

Fig. 2 Examples of inflammation scoring (grade). All tissues were stained with haematoxylin–eosin and examined at 10X (a-j) or 4X (k) magnification. **a** No signs of inflammatory cells. **b** Individual inflammatory cells (arrows) separated by distinct intervening spaces are seen around the glands (< 100 cells/mm^2). **c** Confluent sheets of inflammatory cells (arrowhead) around the glands without tissue destruction or lymphoid nodule/follicle formation (100–500 cells/mm^2). **d** Confluent sheets of inflammatory cells with lymphoid nodule formation (arrow) lie within stroma around the glands (> 500 cells/mm^2). **e** No signs of inflammatory cells. **f** Few inflammatory cells (arrow) seen around the glands (< 100 cells/mm^2). **g** Confluent sheets of inflammatory cells (arrowheads) around the glands without tissue destruction or lymphoid nodule/follicle formation (100–500 cells/mm^2). **h** Confluent sheets of inflammatory cells with lymphoid nodule formation (arrows) lie within stroma around the glands (> 500 cells/mm^2). **i.** No signs of inflammation. **j** Urinary bladder surface epithelium is partially diminished (arrow) and few inflammatory cells (arrowhead) are seen under urothelium in the lamina propria (< 100 cells/mm^2). **k** Urinary bladder surface epithelium is totally diminished (arrows), and there is lymphoid cell infiltration in the lamina propria and through the bladder wall (arrowheads) without tissue destruction or lymphoid nodule/follicle formation (100–500 cells/mm^2). The scale bar in each image indicates 200 μm

Table 2 Metabolic cage results

	Control	L10	L14
Total water intake (mL)	7.50 ± 1.12	9.83 ± 2.40	11.83 ± 1.94
Total urine output (mL)	11.92 ± 1.34	11.67 ± 1.09	13.50 ± 2.28
Total number of micturitions	6.50 ± 0.43	13.50 ± 1.41	16.50 ± 4.15*
Micturitions/hour	0.41 ± 0.03	0.84 ± 0.09	1.03 ± 0.26*
Volume/micturition (mL)	1.62 ± 0.23	0.90 ± 0.10*	0.91 ± 0.13*

Comparisons between data from saline-treated controls and 10 (L10) and 14 (L14) days after intraprostatic injection with lipopolysaccharide (LPS)

*Denotes significant difference ($p < 0.05$) between control and treatment group; n = 6 per group. No significant differences were noted between the L10 and L14 groups

CPPS groups as compared to controls (control vs L10: 0.041 ± 0.002 vs 0.025 ± 0.001, $p < 0.0001$; control vs L14: 0.041 ± 0.002 vs 0.024 ± 0.001, $p < 0.0001$; Fig. 4a). Rats in the CP/CPPS groups had significantly longer voiding times compared to controls (L10 vs control, 133.70 s ± 2.99 vs 44.61 s ± 0.81, $p < 0.0001$; L14 vs control, 141.2 s ± 3.19 vs 44.61 s ± 0.81, $p < 0.0001$; Fig. 4b). There were no significant differences between the CP/CPPS groups in regard to voiding time or compliance.

Significantly decreased contractile responses (intravesical pressure change, ΔP) to MeCh were seen in the L14 group as compared to controls (at 1 $\mu g * kg^{-1}$: L14 vs control, 0.69 ± 0.14 vs 2.98 ± 0.79, $p = 0.013$; at 2 $\mu g * kg^{-1}$: L14 vs control, 1.27 ± 0.35 vs 3.93 ± 0.72, $p = 0.004$). However, there were no significant differences between the L10 group and controls in regards to ΔP at the same doses. At a dose of 5 $\mu g * kg^{-1}$ MeCh, a significantly decreased response was seen in both the L10 and L14 groups, as compared to controls (Fig. 5a; L10 vs control, 3.26 ± 0.48 vs 7.47 ± 1.01,

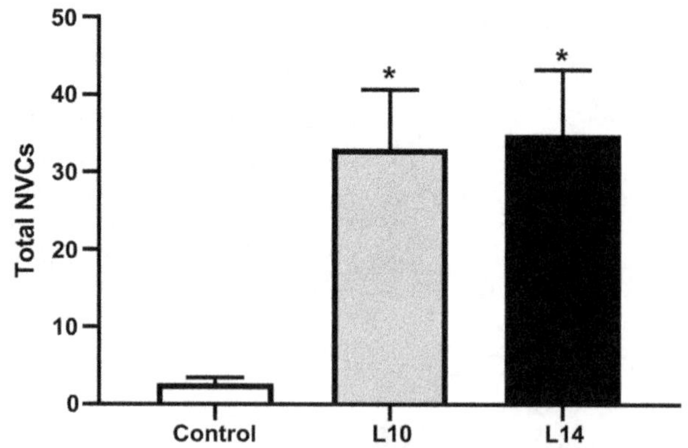

Fig. 3 Total number of non-voiding contractions (NVCs) during cystometry. The observed number of NVCs were low in saline-treated controls. Following intraprostatic injection with LPS, the number of NVCs were significantly increased after 10 (L10) and 14 (L14) days. * denotes significant difference ($p < 0.05$) between control and treatment group; n = 6 per group

$p < 0.0001$; L14 vs control, 1.82 ± 0.43 vs 7.47 ± 1.01, $p < 0.0001$).

The contractile responses to all doses of ATP (5, 10 and 100 μg*kg^{-1}) were significantly decreased in both the L10 and L14 groups as compared to controls (Fig. 5b; at 5 μg*kg^{-1}: L10 vs control, 0.12 ± 0.04 vs 1.01 ± 0.24, $p = 0.002$; L14 vs control, 0.08 ± 0.03 vs 1.01 ± 0.24, $p = 0.001$; at 10 μg*kg^{-1}: L10 vs control, 0.24 ± 0.09 vs 1.58 ± 0.23, $p < 0.0001$; L14 vs control, 0.13 ± 0.05 vs 1.58 ± 0.23, $p < 0.0001$; at 100 μg*kg^{-1}: L10 vs control, 1.52 ± 0.41 vs 3.30 ± 0.60, $p < 0.0001$; L14 vs control, 0.80 ± 0.20 vs 3.30 ± 0.60, $p < 0.0001$).

Histopathology

Prostate weight was not significantly altered in the L10 and L14 groups, as compared to controls (L10 vs control, 0.864 ± 0.037 vs 0.758 ± 0.038, $p = 0.113$; L14 vs control, 0.888 ± 0.042 vs 0.758 ± 0.038, $p = 0.063$). Grade

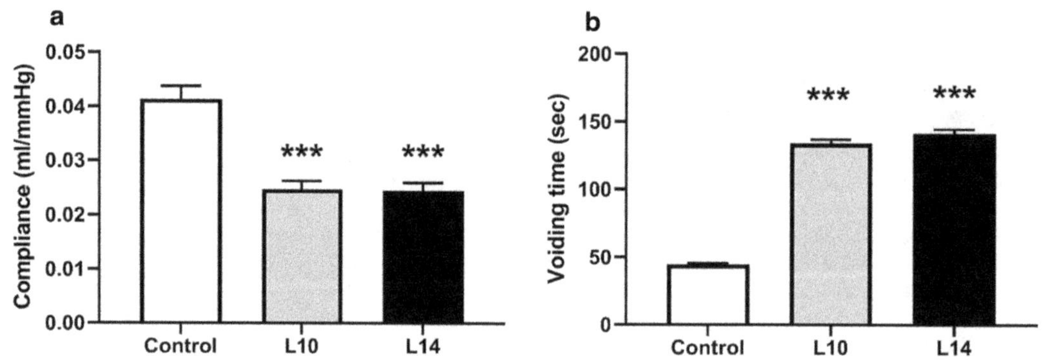

Fig. 4 Bladder compliance (ΔV/ΔP) and voiding times during cystometry. To calculate compliance, the bladder was infused with saline while continuously monitoring intravesical pressure. **a** Bladder compliance was significantly decreased at 10 (L10) and at 14 (L14) days after intraprostatic injection with LPS. **b** Voiding times were significantly increased 10 (L10) and 14 (L14) days after intraprostatic injection with LPS. *** denotes significant difference ($p < 0.001$) between control and treatment groups; n = 6 per group

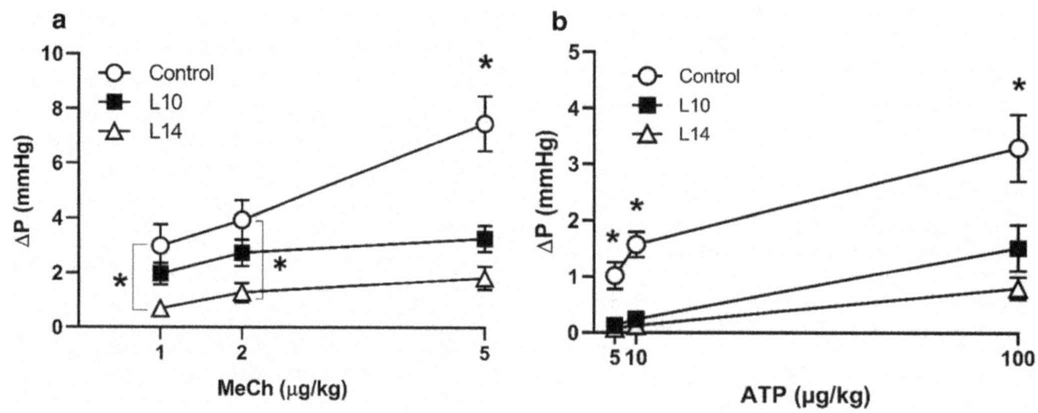

Fig. 5 Intravesical pressure changes (ΔP) upon agonist stimulation. Bladder contraction as a response to **a** methacholine (MeCh;1, 2 and 5 μg*kg^{-1} i.v.) and **b** ATP (5, 10 and 100 μg*kg^{-1} i.v.) in saline-treated controls (O) and 10 (L10; ■) and 14 (L14; Δ) days post intraprostatic injection with LPS. * denotes significant difference ($p < 0.05$) between control and treatment groups; n = 6 per group

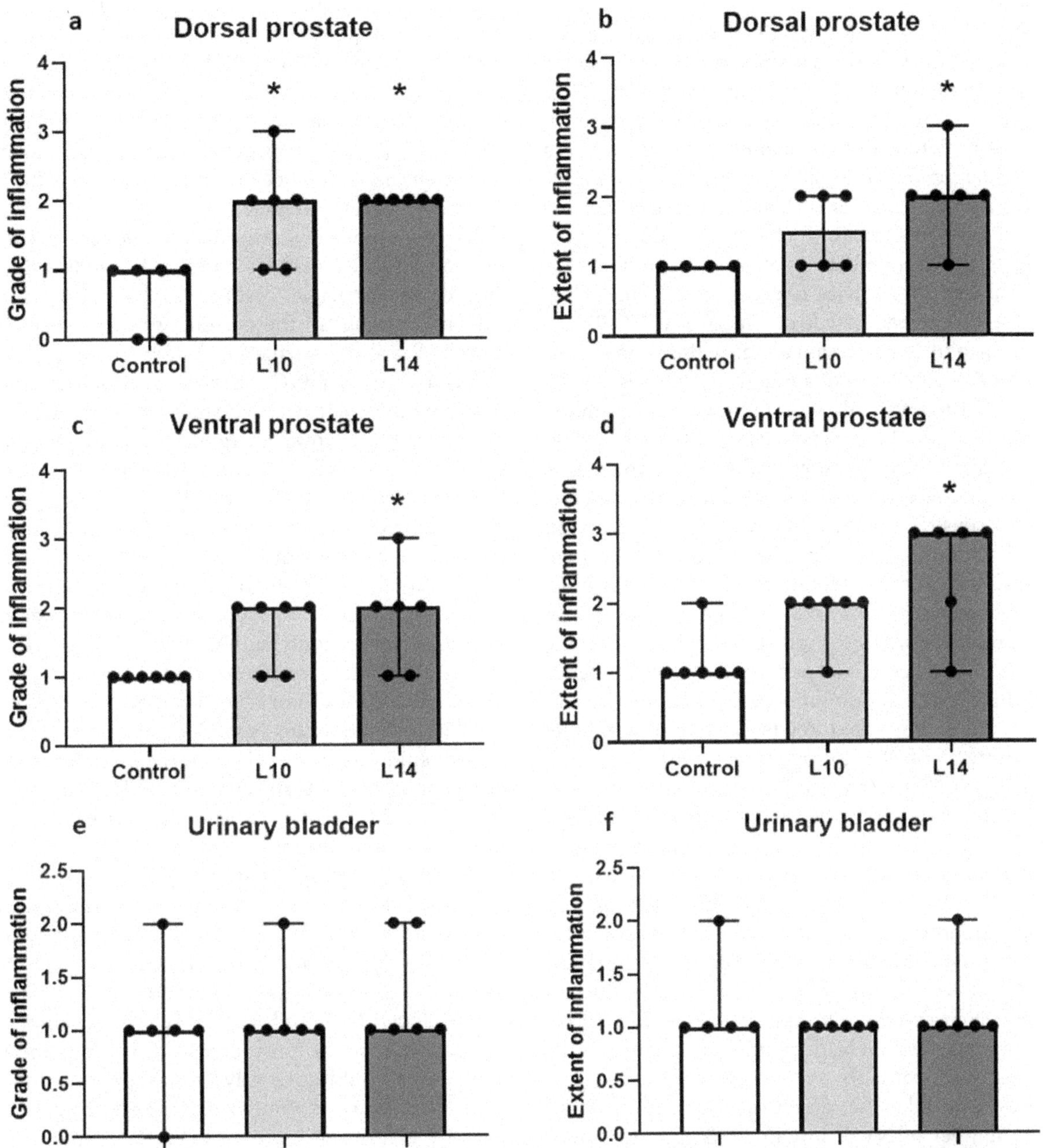

Fig. 6 Histopathological analysis of prostate and bladder inflammation. Scatter plots with bars indicate the grade of inflammation (**a**, **c**, **e**) and the extent of inflammation (**b**, **d**, **f**) in discrete individual values in controls and 10 (L10) or 14 (L14) days after intraprostatic injection with LPS. Analysis was performed on tissue slices from dorsal prostate (**a-b**), ventral prostate (**c–d**) and urinary bladder (**e–f**). Extent of inflammation was graded for all tissues that display a grade of inflammation > 0. * denotes significant difference ($p < 0.05$) between the treatment groups and controls in terms of mean rank values (Dunn`s test); n = 6 per group

of inflammation in the dorsal prostate was significantly higher in the L10 and L14 groups as compared to controls (Fig. 6a). The extent of inflammation in the dorsal prostate was higher in the L14 group as compared to controls (Fig. 6b). Both grade (Fig. 6c) and extent (Fig. 6d) of prostatic inflammation in the ventral prostate were significantly higher in the L14 group as compared to controls. Regarding the bladder, the grade (Fig. 6e) and extent (Fig. 6f) of inflammation were similar between all groups.

Discussion

In the present in vivo study it was investigated if a primary intraprostatic infectious focus could be an inducing factor for an inflammatory state mimicking CP/CPPS. Further, the potential effects of CP/CPPS were examined on both afferent (NVCs, compliance) and efferent (voiding time, cholinergic and purinergic contractile responses) nervous control of bladder function as well as on possible inflammatory changes in the bladder. Metabolic cage experiments confirmed experimentally induced bladder overactivity and cystometry investigations showed significant negative effects of CP/CPPS on both afferent and efferent signalling, without any demonstration of significant inflammatory changes in the bladder. Taken together, these data show that an initial infectious focus in the prostate can provoke prostate-to-bladder cross-organ sensory pathways in the pelvic region. These observations may be of clinical relevance as cross-organ sensitization in the pelvic region is believed to be a contributing cause for the frequently observed unsatisfactory treatment of men with CP/CPPS. Previous studies advocated that CP/CPPS could be associated with bacterial colonization in the prostate, at least in some patients [1, 4]. Rudick et al. speculated that characteristics of the pathogen and immunogenetic background of the host could be important key features in determining the development of chronic pelvic pain after an initial infectious focus in the prostate [1]. The outcomes of the present study support the idea that a primary infectious focus in the prostate could be a more imperative cause of CP/CPPS than previously assumed.

The current findings confirm that induction of CP/CPPS by intraprostatic injection with LPS was a valid choice of method. Metabolic cage experiments showed increased urinary frequency in rats with LPS-induced CP/CPPS, which could be interpreted as CP/CPPS having a sensitizing effect on bladder afferent signalling. This finding was in concordance with the outcomes of a previous study [13]. Likewise, cystometry data revealed an increased number of NVCs in CP/CPPS groups, as well as decreased compliance, which is in line with the findings in previous studies that investigated the effect of chemically induced prostate inflammation on bladder function [10, 13]. Although no significant differences between the groups regarding prostate weight could be observed, histopathological examination of the prostate tissues revealed chronic inflammation following LPS injection.

Voiding times were significantly longer in both LPS-injected groups, as compared to controls. This is interpreted as a demonstration of the effect of CP/CPPS on efferent signalling. However, the increase in voiding times in CP/CPPS groups could also be due to bladder outlet obstruction, potentially due to an increase in innate urethral contractile activity or BPH. Some previous studies have shown a correlation between chronic prostate inflammation and BPH [2]. Chronic inflammation in the prostate is also related with a higher risk for disease progression and acute urinary retention in men with BPH [2, 22]. However, as previously mentioned, no significant differences were seen between the groups regarding prostate weight.

Previous studies have shown reduced muscarinic receptor-induced bladder contractility following induction of hemorrhagic cystitis [23, 24]. This is in line with the findings in the present study. Further, the current ATP-evoked purinergic bladder contractions were reduced in both CP/CPPS groups, which is consistent with the findings in a recent study on chemically induced prostatitis [13]. However, reduced purinergic responses are not in line with previous studies that investigated bladder activity during cystitis [25–27]. This discrepancy could be explained by the simple fact that the current study is not a cystitis model. On the contrary, the current histopathological data highlight the absence of significant changes between the groups regarding bladder inflammation. Another contributing factor could be alterations in the cholinergic component of ATP-evoked bladder contractility [24]. The reduced muscarinic and purinergic bladder contractile responses that are observed in the present study, despite likely simultaneous afferent sensitization, indicate that prostate-to-bladder cross-sensitization can lead to local changes in the detrusor, urothelium and/or on efferent nerves.

The histopathological analysis showed higher scores for both the grade and extent of inflammation in the ventral as well as the dorsal prostate following LPS injection. This finding is in line with a recent study in which zymosan was used to create a model of chemically induced CP/CPPS [13]. However, dissimilar from the previous study, no increase in bladder inflammation scores could currently be observed. Much of the recent literature is controversial regarding the existence of bladder inflammation after induced prostatitis in animal models [6, 10, 13]. This dissimilarity between different studies is likely due to the different substances being used to induce prostatitis and the variety of inflammation evaluation methods. Regarding this, it is important to point out that the present study has some potential limitations. First, no pain evaluation was performed. Such an evaluation could have been beneficial to support the conclusion of induced CP/CPPS. Second, cystometry was performed under deep anaesthesia with isoflurane, which likely influenced nerve transmission. However, cystometry, including induction and maintenance of anaesthesia, was performed similarly in all groups, thus allowing valid comparisons between the groups. Third, there is a small risk that the surgical procedure that is required for the intraprostatic injection could cause minor injury to the pelvic floor, possibly affecting the bladder. Nevertheless, the same surgical procedure was performed in all groups. In addition, the prostate and bladder are in close proximity anatomically. However, the histopathological analysis did not reveal any significant inflammatory changes in the bladder which indicates that this potential pitfall was avoided.

In order to manage patients with inflammatory pain syndromes adequately it is crucial to understand the potential mechanisms underlying cross-sensitization between adjacent organs in the pelvic and abdomen region. Grundy et al. showed in a mouse model that colitis induced neuroplasticity in sensory pathways innervating the colon and bladder, resulting in bladder dysfunction [28]. It was further shown that the changes in bladder function were not due to bladder inflammation. Similar to this, the present study demonstrates induced changes in bladder function that do not correlate with inflammatory changes in the bladder. Instead, alterations in both afferent and efferent signalling are indicated. Despite not performing retrograde labelling or measuring nerve activity per se, this sheds a light on the possible mechanisms of cross-sensitization between the prostate and urinary bladder. However, the exact underlying mechanisms of prostate-to-bladder cross-organ sensitization are yet to be fully elucidated and require further investigation.

Conclusions

The model of LPS-induced chronic prostatitis used in the current study was shown to be valid for examining prostate-to-bladder cross-organ sensitization. It was shown that prostate-to-bladder sensitization could be triggered by an initial bacterial focus in the prostate, which upon development of chronic prostatitis gave rise to overactive bladder and alterations in both afferent and efferent signalling. Further clinical and intervention studies are needed to elucidate the underlying mechanisms of prostate-to-bladder cross-organ sensitization and improve the unsatisfactory management of men with CP/CPPS.

Abbreviations

ATP: Adenosine-5′-triphosphate; CP/CPPS: Chronic prostatitis/chronic pelvic pain syndrome; IC/BPS: Interstitial cystitis/bladder pain syndrome; IL-1: Interleukin-1; IL-6: Interleukin-6; LPS: Lipopolysaccharide; LUTS: Lower urinary tract symptoms; MeCh: Methacholine; NVCs: Non-voiding contractions; TNF-α: Tumor necrosis factor alpha.

Authors' contributions

OA conducted all in vivo experiments, analyzed and interpreted data and helped prepare the manuscript. PUG performed the immunohistochemical analysis and interpreted data. PA analyzed and interpreted data. TC analyzed and interpreted data. MW designed the study, analyzed and interpreted data and helped prepare the manuscript. All authors read and approved the final manuscript.

Competing interests

The authors declare that they have no competing interests.

Author details

[1]Department of Pharmacology, Institute of Neuroscience and Physiology, The Sahlgrenska Academy, University of Gothenburg, Gothenburg, Sweden. [2]Department of Pathology, School of Medicine, Gazi University, Ankara, Turkey.

References

1. Rudick CN, Berry RE, Johnson JR, Johnston B, Klumpp DJ, Schaeffer AJ, et al. Uropathogenic *Escherichia coli* induces chronic pelvic pain. Infect Immun. 2011;79(2):628–35.
2. Dos Santos Gomes FO, Oliveira AC, Ribeiro EL, da Silva BS, Dos Santos LAM, de Lima IT, et al. Intraurethral injection with LPS: an effective experimental model of prostatic inflammation. Inflamm Res. 2018;67(1):43–55.
3. Leskinen MJ, Rantakokko-Jalava K, Manninen R, Leppilahti M, Marttila T, Kylmälä T, et al. Negative bacterial polymerase chain reaction (PCR) findings in prostate tissue from patients with symptoms of chronic pelvic pain syndrome (CPPS) and localized prostate cancer. Prostate. 2003;55(2):105–10.
4. Nickel JC, Alexander RB, Schaeffer AJ, Landis JR, Knauss JS, Propert KJ. Leukocytes and bacteria in men with chronic prostatitis/chronic pelvic pain syndrome compared to asymptomatic controls. J Urol. 2003;170(3):818–22.
5. Funahashi Y, Wang Z, O'Malley KJ, Tyagi P, DeFranco DB, Gingrich JR, et al. Influence of *E. coli*-induced prostatic inflammation on expression of androgen-responsive genes and transforming growth factor beta 1 cascade genes in rats. Prostate. 2015;75(4):381–9.
6. Funahashi Y, Takahashi R, Mizoguchi S, Suzuki T, Takaoka E, Ni J, et al. Bladder overactivity and afferent hyperexcitability induced by prostate-to-bladder cross-sensitization in rats with prostatic inflammation. J Physiol. 2019;597(7):2063–78.
7. Kim HJ, Park JW, Cho YS, Cho CH, Kim JS, Shin HW, et al. Pathogenic role of HIF-1alpha in prostate hyperplasia in the presence of chronic inflammation. Biochim Biophys Acta. 2013;1832(1):183–94.
8. Wong L, Hutson PR, Bushman W. Prostatic inflammation induces fibrosis in a mouse model of chronic bacterial infection. PLoS ONE. 2014;9(6):e100770.
9. Song B, Jiang C, Wang Y, Lu Y, Li L. Newly found prostate-bladder neural reflex in rats–possible mechanism for voiding dysfunction associated with prostatitis/pelvic pain. Urology. 2009;74(6):1365–9.
10. Schwartz ES, La JH, Young EE, Feng B, Joyce S, Gebhart GF. Chronic prostatitis induces bladder hypersensitivity and sensitizes bladder afferents in the mouse. J Urol. 2016;196(3):892–901.
11. Lee S, Yang G, Xiang W, Bushman W. Retrograde double-labeling demonstrates convergent afferent innervation of the prostate and bladder. Prostate. 2016;76(8):767–75.
12. Chen Y, Wu X, Liu J, Tang W, Zhao T, Zhang J. Distribution of convergent afferents innervating bladder and prostate at dorsal root Ganglia in rats. Urology. 2010;76(3):764.e1-6.
13. Aydogdu O, Gocun PU, Aronsson P, Carlsson T, Winder M. Prostate-to-bladder cross-sensitization in a model of zymosan-induced chronic pelvic pain syndrome in rats. Prostate. 2021;81(4):252–60.
14. Patnaik SS, Lagana AS, Vitale SG, Buttice S, Noventa M, Gizzo S, et al. Etiology, pathophysiology and biomarkers of interstitial cystitis/painful bladder syndrome. Arch Gynecol Obstet. 2017;295(6):1341–59.
15. Arora HC, Shoskes DA. The enigma of men with interstitial cystitis/bladder pain syndrome. Transl Androl Urol. 2015;4(6):668–76.
16. Forrest JB, Nickel JC, Moldwin RM. Chronic prostatitis/chronic pelvic pain syndrome and male interstitial cystitis: enigmas and opportunities. Urology. 2007;69(4 Suppl):60–3.
17. Zhang J, Liang C, Shang X, Li H. Chronic prostatitis/chronic pelvic pain syndrome: a disease or symptom? Current perspectives on diagnosis, treatment, and prognosis. Am J Mens Health. 2020;14(1):1557988320903200.

18. Andersson M, Aronsson P, Giglio D, Wilhelmson A, Jerabek P, Tobin G. Pharmacological modulation of the micturition pattern in normal and cyclophosphamide pre-treated conscious rats. Auton Neurosci. 2011;159(1–2):77–83.
19. Patel B, Perez F, Aronsson P, Alothmani R, Carlsson T, Winder M. Combination drug therapy against OAB normalizes micturition parameters and increases the release of nitric oxide during chemically induced cystitis. Pharmacol Res Perspect. 2020;8(1):e00564.
20. Andersson MC, Tobin G, Giglio D. Cholinergic nitric oxide release from the urinary bladder mucosa in cyclophosphamide-induced cystitis of the anaesthetized rat. Br J Pharmacol. 2008;153(7):1438–44.
21. Inamura S, Ito H, Shinagawa T, Tsutsumiuchi M, Taga M, Kobayashi M, et al. Prostatic stromal inflammation is associated with bladder outlet obstruction in patients with benign prostatic hyperplasia. Prostate. 2018;78(10):743–52.
22. Sciarra A, Di Silverio F, Salciccia S, Autran Gomez AM, Gentilucci A, Gentile V. Inflammation and chronic prostatic diseases: evidence for a link? Eur Urol. 2007;52(4):964–72.
23. Barut EN, Engin S, Barut B, Kaya C, Kerimoglu G, Ozel A, et al. Uroprotective effect of ambroxol in cyclophosphamide-induced cystitis in mice. Int Urol Nephrol. 2019;51(5):803–10.
24. Stenqvist J, Winder M, Carlsson T, Aronsson P, Tobin G. Urothelial acetylcholine involvement in ATP-induced contractile responses of the rat urinary bladder. Eur J Pharmacol. 2017;809:253–60.
25. Burnstock G. Purinergic signalling in the urinary tract in health and disease. Purinergic Signal. 2014;10(1):103–55.
26. Kumar V, Chapple CR, Surprenant AM, Chess-Williams R. Enhanced adenosine triphosphate release from the urothelium of patients with painful bladder syndrome: a possible pathophysiological explanation. J Urol. 2007;178(4 Pt 1):1533–6.
27. Sun Y, Chai TC. Augmented extracellular ATP signaling in bladder urothelial cells from patients with interstitial cystitis. Am J Physiol Cell Physiol. 2006;290(1):C27-34.
28. Grundy L, Harrington AM, Castro J, Garcia-Caraballo S, Deiteren A, Maddern J, et al. Chronic linaclotide treatment reduces colitis-induced neuroplasticity and reverses persistent bladder dysfunction. JCI Insight. 2018;3(19).

16

Splenogonadal fusion: A case report and review of the literature

Guangjie Chen, Xiaohao Wang, Yijun Zhao, Linfeng Zhu and Daxing Tang*

Abstract

Background: Splenogondal fusion (SGF) is a rare congenital anomaly characterized by abnormal association between the splenic tissue and the gonads or mesonephric remnants. SGF that requires separate two-stage laparoscopic staged Fowler-Stephen orchiopexy on both the left and right sides is extremely rare. SGF could be misdiagnosed as testicular malignancy and leads to unnecessary orchiectomy.

Case presentation: This is a case of an 8-month old male infant presented with bilateral cryptorchidism, B-mode ultrasound visualized the left and right testes in the lower abdominal cavity and the upper margin of the left testicle as a hypoechoic mass extending to the spleen, indicating an undescended right testis and possible SGF on the left side. Single-site laparoscopic examination confirmed the diagnosis of SGF on the left side and an undescended right testis. As both testes were high and the right spermatic vessel was poorly developed and short, a routine single stage orchiopexy would be difficult and risky, therefore, separate two-stage laparoscopic staged Fowler-Stephen orchiopexies for both sides were implemented. Stage 1 of the staged Fowler-Stephen orchiopexy for the right side was performed first without treating the left side, Stage 2 for the right side, separation of the left testis from the spleen as well as Stage 1 for the left side were performed 7 months later, and Stage 2 for the left side was performed 7 months after that. Follow-up ultrasound 1 year after the surgery revealed no obvious abnormalities in the shapes of the testes or their blood supply. This treatment strategy prevented unnecessary orchiectomy.

Conclusions: We reported a rare case of SGF that needed separate two-stage laparoscopic staged Fowler-Stephen orchiopexies for both sides, and a review of the recent literature. SGF is a rare congenital anomaly often diagnosed incidentally during exploration/surgery for scrotal swelling/mass, cryptorchidism or inguinal hernia in young patients. Surgeons, especially pediatric surgeons should be aware of this rare condition to avoid unnecessary, life-altering radical orchiectomy. When routine single stage orchiopexy is not feasible or risky for either side, separate two-stage laparoscopic staged Fowler-Stephen orchiopexies could be performed on both the left and right sides to avoid unnecessary orchiectomy.

Keywords: Splenogondal fusion (SGF), Orchiopexy, Pediatric, Case report

Background

Splenogonadal fusion (SGF) is a rare benign congenital malformation characterized by an abnormal association between the splenic tissue and the gonads or mesonephric remnants [1–3]. It was first reported by Bostroem in 1883 and the first detailed review of 30 SGF cases was published by Putschar and Manion in 1956 wherein a SGF classification system was established [1–4]. In 1990, Carragher did a comprehensive review of 123 reported SGF cases, of which about 70% were pediatric cases [3]. Subsequently, Malik et al. in 2013 published a review of 61 additional SGF cases [5]. Since then, 40 new SGF cases have been reported

*Correspondence: Tangdx0206@zju.edu.cn
Department of Urology, The Children's Hospital, Zhejiang University, School of Medicine, National Clinical Research Center for Child Health, 57 Zhugan Xiang, Hangzhou 310053, China

in English [2, 6–41]. SGF is a condition that usually presents as inguinal hernia, cryptorchidism, or scrotal swelling/mass, and it could be misdiagnosed as testicular malignancy and leads to unnecessary, life-altering orchiectomy [2, 7, 12, 13]. Lack of awareness of this condition is a major reason for its misdiagnosis [2, 7, 12, 13]. SGF cases that present as cryptorchidism are often treated with single stage laparoscopic Fowler-Stephen orchiopexy [11, 30, 32]. In the current study, we report 1 unique SGF case that presented as bilateral cryptorchidism that required separate two-stage laparoscopic staged Fowler-Stephen orchiopexies on both the left and right sides, because performing routine single stage laparoscopic Fowler-Stephen orchiopexy was very difficult and risk. This strategy prevented unnecessary orchiectomy in this patient. A literature review of the 40 newly reported SGF cases [2, 6–41] was also provided. This study was approved by the ethics committee of the Children's Hospital, Zhejiang University, School of Medicine, National Clinical Research Center for Child Health, and written informed consent was obtained from the patient's caregiver for the study and the publication of this manuscript and any accompanying images. We present the following case in accordance with the CARE Guideline [42].

Case presentation

An 8-month old male infant presented with bilateral cryptorchidism since birth was referred to our hospital and hospitalized. His mother had tocolytic treatment prior to his birth. The patient's medical and family history revealed nothing unusual. The patient had received no prior treatment for the bilateral cryptorchidism. Physical examination showed that the patient was 68.5 cm high, weighed 9.5 kg, had a head circumference of 42.4 cm and was in good general health except for the bilateral cryptorchidism. Examination of the patient's four limbs and chest, palpation of the spine and musculoskeletal examination revealed no abnormality, and the patient had normal vision and hearing. An X-ray revealed no obvious pulmonary abnormality. The patient had bilateral flat and empty scrotum with no split and there was no obvious inguinal mass on either side (Fig. 1a, b). The patient had a properly developed corpus cavernosum and normal urinary meatus. B-mode ultrasound indicated bilateral cryptorchidism and visualized a left testis of 1.4 × 0.8 cm and

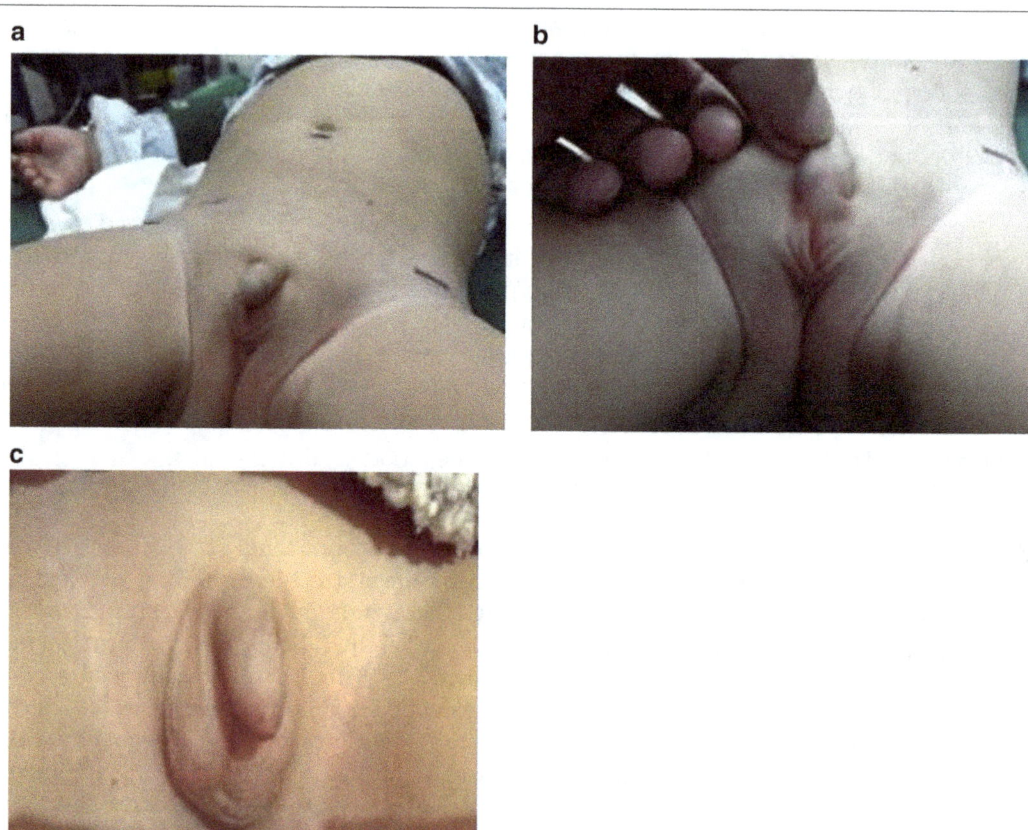

Fig. 1 The appearance of an 8-month old male infant's external genitalia. **a, b** Before the surgery; **c** after the surgery

a right testis of 1.2 × 0.6 cm in the lower abdominal cavity. In addition, the ultrasound also visualized the upper margin of the left testicle as a hypoechoic mass extending to the spleen. The ultrasound findings suggested an undescended right testis and a possible SGF on the left side (Fig. 2a). The ultrasound did not reveal any abnormality in the patient's heart, liver or spleen. Magnetic resonance imaging (MRI) visualized no obvious testis on either side and no obvious abnormality in the patient's heart, spleen or liver. In addition, MRI showed no obvious uterus, ovary or fallopian tube-like structures. As to the patient's kidneys, both the ultrasound and MRI visualized kidneys with normal sizes and shapes at normal positions, intact renal capsule, and renal pelvis and ureter that were not dilated, In addition, per our routine practice, we assessed the patient's External Masculinization Score (EMS) to summarize clinical features representing his genitalia and to determine the degree of masculinization of this male infant, he had an EMS score of 10 out of 12 [43]. Overall, our physical examination of the patient ruled out other obvious congenital disorders.

We also screened for genetic variant(s) related to disorder of sex development with panel based next generation sequencing (NGS) test using multiple ligation-dependent probe amplification (MLPA). The NGS test did not reveal any known SGF related genetic variant, although the test did indicate that the patient carries a missense mutation in the gene encoding SET binding protein 1 (SETBP1) (c.2608G>A [p.Gly870Ser]), a causative variation for Schinzel-Giedion syndrome (OMIM #269150) [44], a frameshift or nonsense mutation in SETBP1 known to cause autosomal dominant mental retardation-29 (OMIM #616078) [45], and a mutation in the oligophrenin-1 gene (OPHN1) known to cause X-linked mental retardation with cerebellar hypoplasia (OMIM #300486) [46].

The first laparoscopic surgery was performed on January 11, 2018, single-site laparoscopy revealed closed internal rings on both sides, right testis in the in the iliac fossa, positioned approximately 2 cm above the right internal ring, at about the same height as the junction between the iliac vessel and the ureter (Fig. 2b, c). It also showed that the left testis was about 3.5 cm above the left internal ring and 1.5 cm above the junction between the iliac vessel and the ureter, and that the left testis was fused to the spleen with a clear demarcation (Fig. 2d). In addition, the left and right vas deferens were also visualized. No obvious uterus, ovary or fallopian tube-like structure was visible. The laparoscopic examination further revealed that the patient's right spermatic vessel was poorly developed and short (Fig. 2b, c). A diagnosis of undescended right testis and continuous SGF on the left side was made. The patent's Internal Masculinization Score (IMS) was also assessed during the examination as part of our routine practice to summarize clinical features of his internal sex organ and to determine the degree of masculinization of the male infant, and he had an IMS score of 9 out of 10 [43].

As the European Association of Urology (EAU) guideline for paediatric urology recommends that "If a testis has not concluded its descent at the age of six months (corrected for gestational age), and since spontaneous testicular descent is unlikely to occur after that age, surgery should be performed within the subsequent year, and by age eighteen months at the latest" [47], we decided to perform the orchiopexy immediately. Considering the fact that the positions of the patient's testes were high and in the abdominal cavity, and that the right spermatic vessel was poorly developed and short, it would be very difficult and risky to complete their descent into the scrotum through the internal rings and inguina or through the straight hernia triangle with single-stage Fowler-Stephen orchiopexy. It has been reported that although the risk of postoperative testicular atrophy was comparable between single-stage and 2-stage Fowler-Stephen orchiopexy, 2-stage Fowler-Stephen orchiopexy could lead to a more favorable testicular position in the scrotum [48]. As the patient's mother had history of multiple miscarriages and received tocolytic treatment prior to the patient's birth, the patient's parents wanted the procedure to be as safe and effective as possible. Therefore, we decided to perform separate 2-stage laparoscopic staged Fowler-Stephen orchiopexies for both the left and the right sides. In order to reduce the risk of bilateral testicular atrophy, we decided against performing Stage 1 for both the left and the right sides simultaneously. Rather, we decided that Stage 1 for the right side should be performed first, if it was successful, Stage 2 for the right side and Stage 1 for the left side should then be performed months later, and if this was also successful, Stage 2 for the left side should be performed months after that. We completed stage 1 of laparoscopic staged Fowler-Stephen orchiopexy for the right testis without treating the SGF on the left side during the same single-site laparoscopic examination. Ultrasound monitoring immediately after the surgery revealed that the right testis had normal shape and good blood supply. B-mode ultrasound taken four months later (May 2, 2018) visualized a right testis of 1.2 × 0.6 × 0.6 cm with a normal shape and good blood supply and a testis-shaped hypoechoic mass of 1.5 cm × 0.8 cm extending to the spleen with good blood supply.

7 month later, on August 20, 2018, stage 2 of laparoscopic staged Fowler-Stephen orchiopexy for the right testis (descent of the right testis into the scrotum), separation of the left testis from the spleen as well as stage 1 of laparoscopic staged Fowler-Stephen orchiopexy for the

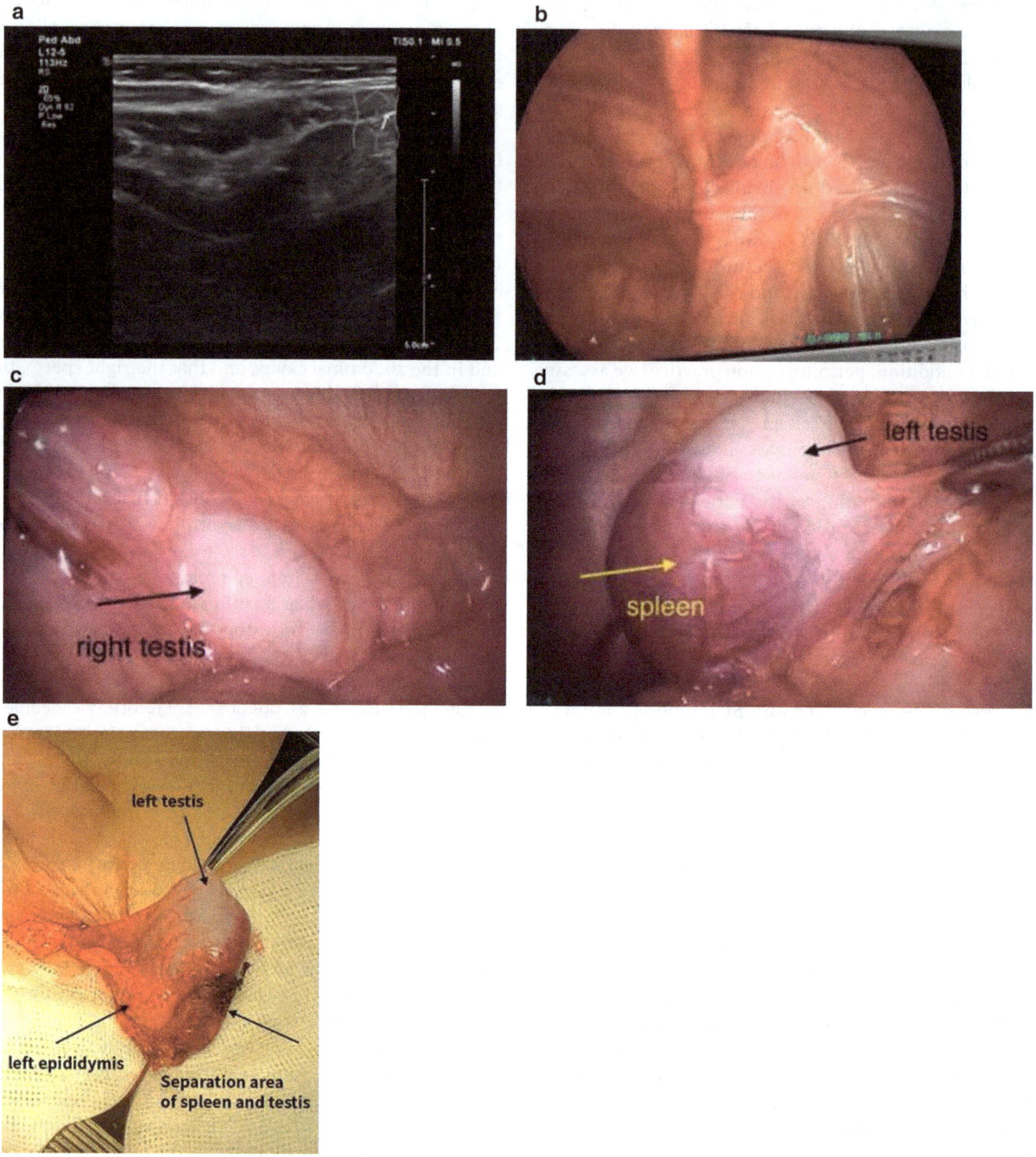

Fig. 2 Continuous splenogonadal fusion on the left side and undescended right testis in an 8-month old male infant. **a** Pre-operative B-mode ultrasound revealed possible fusion of the left testis and the kidney; **b** single site laparoscopic examination revealed closed right internal ring and the right testis in the iliac fossa, at about the same height as the junction between the iliac vessel and the right vas deferens; **c** single-site laparoscopic examination visualized the right testis located in the right iliac fossa, approximately 2 cm above the right internal ring, with poorly developed right spermatic vessel; **d** complete fusion of the spleen and the left testis in the left iliac fossa visualized by the single-site laparoscopic examination; **e** the left testis descended into the scrotum after being separated from the spleen

left testis were performed. Ultrasound monitoring immediately after surgery revealed that both testes had normal shapes and good blood supply. B-mode ultrasound taken 4 months later (December 12, 2018) showed a right testis of $1.0 \times 0.6 \times 0.6$ cm and a left testis of $1.1 \times 0.5 \times 0.4$ cm, both with adequate blood supply.

Stage 2 of laparoscopic staged Fowler-Stephen orchiopexy for the left testis was performed 7 months later (March 12, 2019), the left testis descended into the scrotum. The residual spleen tissue was cut from the left testis (Fig. 2e) and post-operative biopsy confirmed that it was accessory spleen tissue. Ultrasound monitoring immediately after surgery revealed that both testis had normal shapes and good blood supply, it also visualized smooth tunica vaginalis and multiple hyperechoic spots without acoustic shadows indicating possible testicular microlithiasis (Fig. 3a–d). B-mode ultrasound taken 1 month later (April 20, 2019) revealed that both testes were in the scrotum and that the left and right testes had a size of $1.3 \times 0.7 \times 0.6$ cm and $1.3 \times 0.8 \times 0.7$ cm, respectively. Both testes had healthy blood supply and the spleen had a normal shape. The patient had an uneventful recovery and suffered no adverse or unanticipated events. Follow-up ultrasound 1 year after the surgery revealed no obvious abnormalities in the shapes of the testes or their blood supply (Fig. 3e, f) and the patient's penis and scrotum had normal appearance (Fig. 1c).

Discussion and conclusions

SGF is a very rare congenital anomaly, and only about 220 cases have been reported in literature [2, 5–41]. Carragher published a review of 123 cases in 1990 [3] and Malik et al. published a review of an additional 61 cases in 2013 [5]; We have examined 40 cases published in English after *Malik* et al. and summarized their data [2, 6–41] along with our present case (total 41 cases) in this study (Table 1). Detailed characteristics and treatments of each included case cannot be included in this article. Interested readers can find them in a Supplementary appendix online (Additional file 1: Table S1).

SGF is a condition of male predominance (male/female ratio 14.3:1) [5], the reported male dominance is most likely due to underestimation of SGF occurrence in females as females' gonads are inside the body and therefore less accessible for examination than the male gonads, in addition, there are fewer complications associated with female gonads than with male gonads [3, 5, 12]. Consistent with previous findings, 40 of the 41 cases (97.56%) in our review occurred in males, and the remaining 1 case occurred in a newborn who is phenotypical female (a 46, XY genotype despite a female phenotype) [8]. Also consistent with previous teaching that about 70% of SGF cases were pediatric cases [3, 5], 26 of the 41 cases (63.41%) in our study were reported in patients ≤ 19 years old (Table 1). The youngest patient was a newborn with a 46, XY genotype despite a female phenotype (phenotypical sex reversal) as well as a hypoplastic left heart, and this is the first reported SGF case associated with sex reversal [8].

SGF occurs between the 5th and 8th weeks of gestation. During the 5th and 6th weeks of gestation, the spleen develops from the splenic anlage in the left dorsal mesogastrium. At about the same time, the gonadal ridge is formed between the mesonephros and dorsal mesentery. As the embryonic gut rotates during week 5 of gestation, the dorsal mesogastrium rotates to the left, placing the splenic anlage into close proximity with the left urogenital fold which contains the gonadal mesoderm. Such close proximity remains until descent of the gonads and mesonephric involution during the 8th week of gestation [1, 3, 5]. Several mechanisms have been proposed to explain the actual abnormal fusion between the splenic and gonadal tissues [5, 11]. The close proximity between the left gonad and spleen during embryogenesis explains the fact that SGF almost always occurs on the left side [1, 3, 5]. All of the 41 cases included in our study occurred on the left side as well (Table 1).

SGF can be classified into continuous and discontinuous SGF [3, 5]. Continuous SGF (55% of cases) is characterized by the presence of a cord of splenic or fibrous tissue connecting the spleen and gonad, and occasionally beads of splenic tissue could be found along the cord (splenic rosary bead), while in discontinuous SGF (45% of cases), there is no such connection. Rather, in discontinuous SGF, ectopic splenic tissue or accessory spleen is directly attached to the gonad without connecting to the native spleen [2, 3, 5, 7, 10]. During embryonic development, the descent of the testis could sometimes draw out the developing spleen fused to the testis into a long band (Continuous SGF) or to carry a portion of the splenic primordium down with the descending testis (Discontinuous SGF) [7]. 19 (46.34%) of the 41 cases in our study were continuous, and 23 (53.65%) cases were discontinuous (Table 1).

The most common malformations associated with SGF are cryptorchidism and inguinal hernia [1, 5, 12]. It has been reported that 31% of SGF patients had cryptorchidism or inguinal hernia [12], while Malik et al. found that 36% of SGF patients had cryptorchidism [5]. Other common anomalies include limb defects as well as craniofacial abnormalities such as micrognathia, most likely because active development of the limb bud and mandible occurs during 5th and 8th weeks of gestation, the same time as SGF [5]. Less common associations include cleft palate, Moebius syndrome, hypospadias, osteogenesis imperfecta, persistent mullerian duct syndrome, Potter

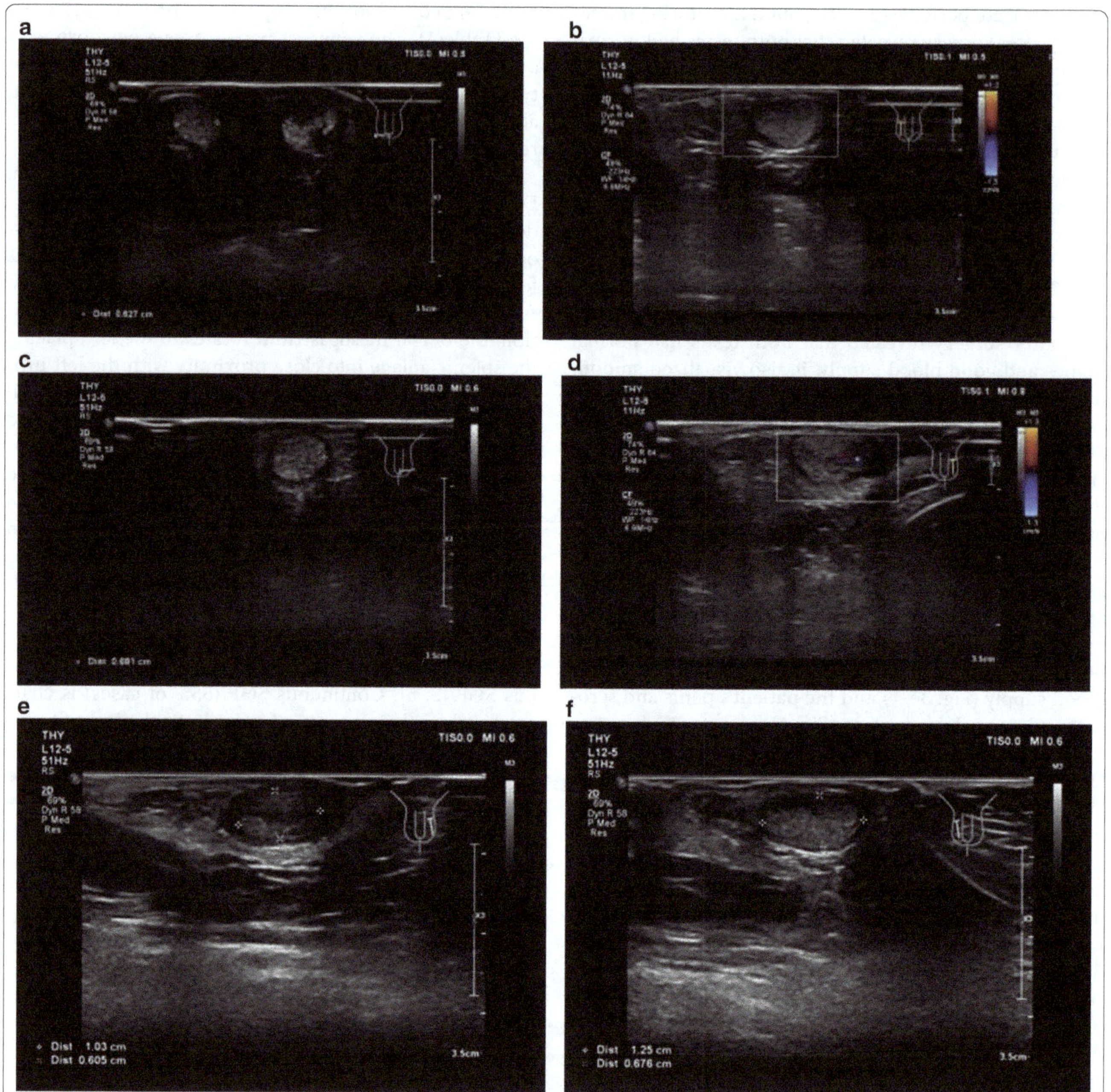

Fig. 3 Post-operative ultrasound of the testes. **a** The right testis; **b** post-operative Doppler image of blood supply for the right testis; **c** left testis; **d** post-operative Doppler image of blood supply for the left testis; **e** and **f** follow-up ultrasound 1 year after the surgery showed that the left and right testes had a size of 1.0 × 0.6 × 0.6 cm and 1.3 × 0.7 × 0.7 cm, respectively, both with a homogeneous echogenic appearance and normal blood supply

syndrome, gastrointestinal malrotation, anal stenosis, and transverse testicular ectopia [5]. In our study, 20 of the 41 SGF cases (48.78%) were associated with other congenital anomalies, the most common being cryptorchidism (12 [29.27%]) and inguinal hernia (5 [12.20%]). Other less common associations included limb and facial defects, male infertility and/or azoospermia, hypospadias, left hip dysplasia, a hypoplastic left heart and phenotypical sex reversal (Table 1).

Our present case of left SGF in a male infant presented with bilateral cryptorchidism was not unusual for known SGF cases (Table 1) [3, 5, 12]. We used ultrasound to reach a preliminary diagnosis that was further confirmed by laparoscopy, this diagnostic process was also used in

Table 1 Summary of characteristics and treatments of splenogonadal fusion (SGF) cases

	Number (N = 41)
Age at diagnosis (years), n (%)	
0–9	20 (48.78%)
10–19	6 (14.63%)
20–29	5 (12.20%)
30–39	6 (14.63%)
40–49	1 (2.44%)
50–59	2 (4.88%)
60–69	0 (0%)
70–79	1 (2.44%)
Gender, n (%)	
Male	40 (97.56%)
Phenotypical female (phenotypical sex reversal)	1 (2.44%)
Side, n (%)	
Left	41 (100%)
Right	0 (0%)
Classification, n (%)	
Continuous	19 (46.34%)
Discontinuous	22 (53.65%)
Clinical presentation	
Painful or painless inguinal / scrotal /testicular swelling/mass	28 (68.29%)
Cryptorchidism	11 (26.83%)[a]
Primary infertility	2 (4.88%) [a]
A hypoplastic left heart and phenotypical sex reversal	1 (2.44%)
Congenital anomalies associated with SGF, n (%)	
Cryptorchidism	12 (29.27%)[b,c,d]
Inguinal hernia	5 (12.20%)
Limb and /or facial defects	2 (4.88%)[c]
Male infertility and/or azoospermia	2 (4.88%)[b]
Hypospadias	2 (4.88%)[d]
Left hip dysplasia	1 (2.44%)[c]
A hypoplastic left heart and phenotypical sex reversal	1 (2.44%)
None	21 (51.22%)
Testis/ovary-sparing, n (%)	
Yes	24 (58.54%)
No	14 (34.15%)
Unknown	3 (7.32%)

[a] One patient had both primary infertility and left sided cryptorchidism

[b] One patient had bilateral cryptorchidism, non-obstructive azoospermia and male infertility

[c] One patient had cryptorchidism, facial and limb deformities—short right femur, hip dysplasia and a syndromic face (Splenogonadal fusion-limb deformity syndrome)

[d] Both patients had cryptorchidism and hypospadias

other reported SGF cases [12, 13, 20, 38]. What made our case unusual was that due to high positions of both testes (in the abdominal cavity), fusion of the left testis to the spleen and the poorly developed and short right spermatic vessel, it would be very difficult and risky to perform routine single stage orchiopexy on either side. Separate two-stage laparoscopic staged Fowler-Stephen orchiopexies for both sides were implemented. First, Stage 1 of the staged Fowler-Stephen orchiopexy for the right side was performed without treating the left side, and post-operative ultrasound visualized the right testis with a normal shape and good blood supply. Stage 2 for the right side (descent of right testis into the scrotum), separation of the left testis from the spleen as well as

Stage 1 for the left side were performed months later, and post-operative ultrasound confirmed that both testes had normal shape and healthy blood supply. Finally, Stage 2 for the left side (descent of the left testis into the scrotum) was performed months after that. This approach reduced the risk of bilateral testicular atrophy associated with orchiopexy, allowed for a potentially more favorable testicular position in the scrotum [48], and spared the patient unnecessary orchiectomy.

Unlike previously reported SGF cases, we performed screening for genetic variant(s) related to disorder of sex development with panel based NGS test using MLPA. The NGS test revealed that the patient carried a missense mutation in SETBP1 (c.2608G>A [p.Gly870Ser]), a causative variation for Schinzel-Giedion syndrome (OMIM #269150). Schinzel-Giedion syndrome is a rare congenital disease characterized by serious intellectual disability, hypertrichosis, characteristic facial gestalt and various congenital malformations [44]. Patients with Schinzel-Giedion syndrome often die within several years after their birth [44]. The patient also carries a frameshift or nonsense mutation in SETBP1 known to cause autosomal dominant mental retardation-29 (OMIM #616078), a disease characterized by severe intellectual disability [45]. Finally, the patient has a mutation in OPHN1 known to cause X-linked mental retardation with cerebellar hypoplasia (OMIM #300486), a rare congenital anomaly characterized by "neonatal hypotonia with motor delay but no obvious ataxia, marked strabismus, early-onset complex partial seizures, and moderate to severe mental retardation" [46]. At the time of writing this article, the patient was a 3-year old who had had normal and healthy physical, cognitive, language and social-emotional development except for having weak eyesight in both eyes. Although visual impairment is one symptom of Schinzel-Giedion syndrome, the patient had not displayed any other symptoms of Schinzel-Giedion syndrome, and as such whether the weak vision displayed by the patient was due to Schinzel-Giedion syndrome is uncertain. Therefore the clinical significance of these mutations remains to be determined. We will follow-up with this patient regularly. Although it has been proposed that SGF is a genetic disorder [33], none of the previous reports on SGF performed panel-based NGS to identify genetic variations potentially related to various congenital disorders. Such testing could potentially allow for early detection and treatment of rare congenital anomalies.

SGF is often an incidental finding during exploration/surgery for scrotal swelling/mass, cryptorchidism or inguinal hernia [1, 5, 12]. In our study, the most common clinical presentations were painful or painless inguinal / scrotal /testicular swelling or mass (68.92%) and cryptorchidism (26.83%) (Table 1). SGF itself does not have characteristic features, its pre-operation diagnosis therefore could be difficult. In addition, lack of awareness of this rare condition could lead to its misdiagnosis [5, 12]. As a result, some patients with SGF underwent unnecessary orchiectomy [12]. In reality, there have been only 4 reported cases of SGF associated with testicular cancer, although cryptorchidism is associated with increased risk of testicular malignancy [6]. Up to 37% of SGF patients underwent unnecessary orchiectomy according to Carragher published in 1990 [3]. In our study, 14 of the 41 cases (34.15%) underwent orchiectomy [6, 8, 9, 12, 14–18, 22, 23, 35, 39], among them, 9 were potentially unnecessary [9, 12, 14–18, 39], reflecting a better awareness and more accurate diagnosis of SGF during the recent years. On the other hand, 21.95% of SGF patients still underwent unnecessary orchiectomy, indicating a continuing need for increasing awareness of this condition and better diagnostic protocols. Li et al. suggested a 3-step diagnostic protocol to rule out malignance and to diagnose and treat SGF when encountering an abnormal gonad [12]. First, SGF should be considered with a testicular mass existing from birth that has being growly slowly for years in a benign fashion [12]. Secondly, imaging techniques such as B-mode ultrasound, computed tomography (CT), MRI and Technicium-99m sulfur colloid liver-spleen scan could be employed to examine the mass for differential diagnosis. Among them, Technicium-99m sulfur colloid liver-spleen scan could detect accessory splenic tissue and thus could help to diagnose SGF when a surgeon has a high pre-operation suspicion of SGF [12]. Meanwhile, MRI is often first choice in detecting the position and shape of the testes and ruling out other congenital anomalies. It is reliable and accurate in detecting/ruling out a testicular or scrotal lesion, localizing the lesion, and differentiating intratesticular and extratesticular lesions [49]. In addition, by using different sequences and administering gadolimium, the pattern of scrotal disorder can be characterized and testicular lesions could be classified [49]. At the same time, it could also detect or rule out anomalies in a patient's other key organs such as liver, spleen, kidneys and brain. However, MRI is expensive and could be hard to perform on infants who need to be sedated. In our case, MRI failed to detect our patient's testes, possibly because too much coats on the infant while being imaged, poor skills of the technician or insufficient bowel preparation. Meanwhile, ultrasound is inexpensive and high-resolution ultrasound employing gray-scale and color-encoded techniques is considered by some to be an accepted standard for scrotal imaging [49]. In our practice, ultrasound is used for the purpose of preliminary screening for congenital anomalies.

It could help to diagnose continuous SGF when a cord connecting the spleen to the testicle is visualized. On the ultrasound, the splenic tissue is usually visualized as a well-encapsulated, extra-testicular homogenous hypoechoic or isoechoic mass [5, 12]. In addition, Doppler ultrasound could monitor blood flow to the testes [50]. In our case, ultrasound visualized both testes in the lower abdominal cavity as well as the upper margin of the left testicle as a hypoechoic mass extending to the spleen indicating an undescended right testis and a possible SGF on the left side. However, it has been suggested that in cases where ultrasound produced inconclusive findings, MRI could be valuable [49]. Li et al. further suggested that the third step was, when unsure, an intra-operation biopsy should be performed to determine the nature of the mass [12]. In any case, diagnostic laparoscopy is recommended as it is safe, reliable and very accurate in diagnosing and treating an impalpable testis [5]. When a definite diagnosis of SGF is made, it is sufficient to completely excise the splenic tissue and preserve the testes especially in young patients [5]. For some, surgery may not even be necessary [12]. In some instances as demonstrated by our case, when routine single stage orchiopexy was not feasible or risky on either the left or the right side, separate two-stage laparoscopic staged Fowler-Stephen orchiopexies on the left and right sides could be performed to prevent unnecessary orchiectomy. Our case report in this sense provides a scenario in which unnecessary orchiectomy could be avoided although whether such treatment strategy could be widely applied could only be determined by future cases.

In conclusion, SGF is a rare congenital anomaly often diagnosed incidentally during exploration/surgery for scrotal swelling/mass, cryptorchidism or inguinal hernia in young patients. Surgeons, especially pediatric surgeons should be aware of this condition to avoid unnecessary, life-altering radical orchiectomy. In some cases, when routine single stage orchiopexy is not feasible or risky for either side, separate two-stage laparoscopic staged Fowler-Stephen orchiopexies could be performed on both the left and right sides to avoid unnecessary orchiectomy.

Abbreviations

SGF: splenogonadal fusion; MRI: magnetic resonance imaging; EMS: External Masculinization Score; NGS: next generation sequencing; MLPA: multiple ligation-dependent probe amplification; SETBP1: SET binding protein 1; OPHN1: oligophrenin-1; IMS: Internal Masculinization Score; CT: computed tomography.

Authors' contributions

GC and DT conceived and designed the study, GC, XW, YZ and LZ collected and assembled the data, GC and XW analyzed and interpreted the data. All authors were involved in drafting the manuscript or revising it critically for important intellectual content and all authors have read and given final approval of the version to be published. Each author has participated sufficiently in the work to take public responsibility for appropriate portions of the content; and each author agreed to be accountable for all aspects of the work in ensuring that questions related to the accuracy or integrity of any part of the work are appropriately investigated and resolved.

Competing interests

The authors declare that they have no competing interests.

References

1. Lin CS, Lazarowicz JL, Allan RW, Maclennan GT. Splenogonadal fusion. J Urol. 2010;184:332–3.
2. Abokrecha A, Almatrfi A. Discontinued splenogonadal fusion and bilateral empty scrotum in an 18-month-old boy. Eur J Pediatr Surg Rep. 2017;5:e1-3.
3. Carragher AM. One hundred years of splenogonadal fusion. Urology. 1990;35:471–5.
4. Putschar WG, Manion WC. Splenicgonadal fusion. Am J Pathol. 1956;32:15–33.
5. Malik RD, Liu DB. Splenogonadal fusion: an unusual case of an acute scrotum. Rev Urol. 2013;15:197–201.
6. Lopes RI, de Medeiros MT, Arap MA, Cocuzza M, Srougi M, Hallak J. Splenogonadal fusion and testicular cancer: case report and review of the literature. Einstein (Sao Paulo). 2012;10:92–5.
7. Xiang X, Jiang Y, Liu JX, Qiu L. A rare content of congenital inguinal hernia: a case report of splenogonadal fusion. BMC Pediatr. 2019;19:422.
8. Speare R, Roberts J, Cohen M, Wales J. Splenogonadal fusion and sex reversal. J Pediatr Endocrinol Metab. 2012;25:541–2.
9. Duhli N, Venkatramani V, Panda A, Manojkumar R. Splenogonadal fusion: pathological features of a rare scrotal mass. Indian J Pathol Microbiol. 2013;56:474–6.
10. Ferrón SA, Arce JD. Discontinuous splenogonadal fusion: new sonographic findings. Pediatr Radiol. 2013;43:1652–5.
11. Celik A, Tiryaki S, Darcan S, Ergun O. Splenogonadal fusion-limb deformity syndrome: a rare but important cause of undescended testis. World J Pediatr. 2016;12:246–8.
12. Li WF, Luan MX, Ma Z, Chen YJ. Splenogonadal fusion: report of four cases and review of the literature. Exp Ther Med. 2013;6:816–8.
13. Liu W, Wu R, Guo Z. The diagnosis and management of continuous splenogonadal fusion in a 6-year-old boy. Int Urol Nephrol. 2013;45:21–4.
14. Croxford WC, Pfistermuller KL, Scott F, Pope AJ. Splenogonadal fusion presenting clinically and radiologically as a seminoma. Urol Case Rep. 2015;3:204–5.
15. Bal K, Ermete M, Balcı U, Dinçel Ç. Splenogonadal fusion: a very rare congenital anomaly in the differential diagnosis of a testicular mass. Turk J Urol. 2014;40:62–4.
16. Harris AM. Splenogonadal fusion: a rare benign testicular mass in a 55-Year-old male. Urol Case Rep. 2016;9:41–2.
17. Karray O, Oueslati A, Chakroun M, Ayed H, Bouzouita A, Cherif M, Ben Slama MR, Derouiche A, Chebil M. Splenogonadal fusion - a rare cause of scrotal swelling: a case report. J Med Case Rep. 2018;12:172.
18. Kocher NJ, Tomaszewski JJ, Parsons RB, Cronson BR, Altman H, Kutikov A, Smith RE. Splenogonadal fusion: a rare etiology of solid testicular mass. Urology. 2014;83:e1-2.
19. Kumar S, Jayant K, Agrawal S, Parmar KM, Singh SK. A rare case of continuous type splenogonadal fusion in a young male with primary infertility. Case Rep Urol. 2014;2014:796761.
20. Lakshmanan PM, Reddy AK, Nutakki A. A surprising content of congenital hernia: complete splenogonadal fusion band. BMJ Case Rep. 2014;2014. pii: bcr2014203640.
21. Sountoulides P, Neri F, Bellocci R, Schips L, Cindolo L. Splenogonadal fusion mimicking a testis tumor. J Postgrad Med. 2014;60:202–4.
22. Zhang Y, Tong Z, Zhang Y. X-ray computed tomography and sonography features of continuous splenogonadal fusion. J Xray Sci Technol. 2013;21:303–8.
23. Shadpour P, Rezaimehr B. "Rosary of testes": splenogonadal fusion in association with bilateral abdominal testes presenting as polyorchidism. Case Rep Urol. 2015;2015:317189.

24. Trottmann M, Marcon J, Mai V, D'Anastasi M, Becker A, Stief C, Reiser M, Clevert DA. Characterization of splenogonadal fusion by contrast-enhanced ultrasound (CEUS) and elastography. Ultraschall Med. 2015;36:97–100.
25. Jayasundara JA, Vithana VH, Lamahewage AK. A case of continuous-type splenogonadal fusion. Singapore Med J. 2013;54:e123–4.
26. Bosnalı O, Cici İ, Moralıoğlu S, Cerrah-Celayir A. Continuous-type splenogonadal fusion: report of a rare case. Turk J Pediatr. 2014;56:680–3.
27. Jakkani R, Alhajri FA, Alteriki A, Almuteri MF, Athyal RP, Hashem KZ. Discontinuous splenogonadal fusion diagnosed on computed tomography. Indian J Radiol Imaging. 2016;26:506–9.
28. Uglialoro AD, Goltzman ME, Niazi M, Lehman D, Silletti J, Bjurlin MA. Splenogonadal fusion presenting as an asymptomatic testicular mass. Urology. 2016;97:1–4.
29. Akama Y, Shimanuki K, Asahi S, Watanabe Y, Ko K, Takano R, Amano H, Kawaguchi T, Uchida E. Incidentally detected splenogonadal fusion in a laparoscopic transabdominal preperitoneal hernia repair operation: A case report. Int J Surg Case Rep. 2017;35:29–32.
30. Huang G, Huang Y, Zeng L, Yuan M, Wu Y, Huang L. Continuous-type splenogonadal fusion: a case report. Exp Ther Med. 2017;13:2019–21.
31. Li X, Ye J, Jiang G. Sonographic diagnosis of splenogonadal fusion in a 2-year-old boy. J Clin Ultrasound. 2017;45:179–82.
32. Preece J, Phillips S, Sorokin V, Herz D. Splenogonadal fusion in an 18-month-old. J Pediatr Urol. 2017;13:214–5.
33. Chiaramonte C, Siracusa F, Li VG. Splenogonadal fusion: a genetic disorder? Report of a case and review of the literature. Urol Case Rep. 2014;2:67–9.
34. Srinivasa Rao RC, Radhakrishna V, Rao N, Rakshit S. Torsion of a Splenule in a case of Splenogonadal fusion mimicking a strangulated inguinal hernia. J Indian Assoc Pediatr Surg. 2018;23:100–2.
35. Shakeri A, Shakeri A, Rasolmali R, Shakeri S. A case of splenogonadal fusion accompanied by accessory spleen in a 4-year-old boy. Urol Ann. 2018;10:406–8.
36. Zhou L, Muthucumaru M, Stunden R, Lenghaus D. Splenogonadal fusion: a rare scrotal mass in a 9-year-old boy. ANZ J Surg. 2018;88:E81–2.
37. Chen CJ, Kavoussi N, Jacobs MA. Splenogonadal fusion: A rare finding during routine orchiopexy. Urol Case Rep. 2019;27:100904.
38. Grosu S, Rübenthaler J, Knösel T, Trottmann M, Marcon J, Clevert DA. Splenogonadal fusion evaluation using contrast enhanced ultrasound and elastography. A case report Med Ultraso. 2019;21:356–8.
39. Mann JA, Ritchie E. Splenogonadal fusion: a case of two lesions. Urol Case Rep. 2019;24:100878.
40. Patre V, Netam S, Luka P, Mandle H. Discontinuous type of splenogonadal fusion syndrome with limb defects. Indian J Urol. 2012;28:94–5.
41. Seager MJ, Alexander S, Muneer A, Walkden M. Splenogonadal fusion: a rare paratesticular lesion and how to recognise it on ultrasound. Ultrasound. 2020;28:54–7.
42. Riley DS, Barber MS, Kienle GS, Aronson JK, von Schoen-Angerer T, Tugwell P, Kiene H, Helfand M, Altman DG, Sox H, Werthmann PG, Moher D, Rison RA, Shamseer L, Koch CA, Sun GH, Hanaway P, Sudak NL, Kaszkin-Bettag M, Carpenter JE, Gagnier JJ. CARE guidelines for case reports: explanation and elaboration document. J Clin Epidemiol. 2017;89:218–35.
43. Ahmed SF, Khwaja O, Hughes IA. The role of a clinical score in the assessment of ambiguous genitalia. BJU Int. 2000;85:120–4.
44. Herenger Y, Stoetzel C, Schaefer E, Scheidecker S, Manière MC, Pelletier V, Alembik Y, Christmann D, Clavert JM, Terzic J, Fischbach M, De Saint MA, Dollfus H. Long term follow up of two independent patients with Schinzel-Giedion carrying SETBP1 mutations. Eur J Med Genet. 2015;58:479–87.
45. Online Mendelian Inheritance in Man. The McKusick-Nathans Institute of Genetic Medicine, Johns Hopkins University School of Medicine. 2017. https://www.omim.org/entry/616078. Accessed 15 May 2019.
46. Online Mendelian Inheritance in Man. The McKusick-Nathans Institute of Genetic Medicine, Johns Hopkins University School of Medicine. 2019. https://www.omim.org/entry/300486. Accessed 15 May 2019.
47. EAU guidelines on paediatric urology. European Association of Urology. 2017. https://uroweb.org/wp-content/uploads/21-Paediatric-Urology_2017_web.pdf. Accessed 02 January 2018.
48. Alam A, Delto JC, Blachman-Braun R, Wayne G, Mittal AG, Castellan M, Kozakowski K, Labbie A, Gosalbez R. Staged Fowler-Stephens and single-stage laparoscopic orchiopexy for intra-abdominal testes: Is there a difference? A single institution experience. Urology. 2017;101:104–10.
49. Mohrs OK, Thoms H, Egner T, Brunier A, Eiers M, Kauczor HU, Hallscheidt P. MRI of patients with suspected scrotal or testicular lesions: diagnostic value in daily practice. AJR Am J Roentgenol. 2012;199:609–15.
50. Elzeneini WM, Mostafa MS, Dahab MM, Youssef AA, AbouZeid AA. How far can one-stage laparoscopic Fowler-Stephens orchiopexy be implemented in intra-abdominal testes with short spermatic vessels? J Pediatr Urol. 2020;16:197.

17

The perils of penile enhancement: Case report of a fulminant penile infection

Nicole Wen Mun Khor[1,2*], Ankur Dhar[1] and Alistair Cameron-Strange[1,2]

Abstract

Background: Penile enhancement with injectable agents is a rising trend and yet has received little scientific attention despite the potential for serious complications. These include cosmetic, functional and systemic complications that may require complex penile reconstructive surgery. We report a case of delayed severe infection following penile filler insertion leading to multi-organ failure and intensive care support.

Case presentation: A 31-year-old man presented with fevers and progressive pain and swelling of the penile shaft, 3 days after unprotected sexual intercourse. The patient received subcutaneous hyaluronic filler injections at a cosmetic clinic for penile enlargement two months prior to presentation. Relevant social history include polysubstance abuse and multiple sexual partners. Physical examination revealed gross penile oedema and erythema, with a ventral curvature of the penile shaft and a superficial abrasion on the distal ventral penile shaft. Within 24 h the patient developed septic shock with anuria, hypotension and fevers to 40 °C, requiring transfer to the Intensive Care Unit (ICU) for vasopressor and inotropic support. Intraoperative penile exploration revealed multiple pus stained fillers which were drained and grew Streptococcus Pyogenes on cultures. There was no abscess or evidence of necrotising fasciitis intraoperatively. The patient improved with intravenous antibiotics and was stepped down from the ICU after four days and discharged on day eight. One month post admission there was significant superficial skin loss to both ventral and lateral aspect of the penis, with healthy granulation tissue at the base. The patient opted for conservative management with regular dressings. He reported normal sexual and urinary function three months post admission.

Conclusion: This is the first published case of sepsis from a penile infection in the context of hyaluronic acid penile fillers. In an era of escalating demand for penile cosmetic procedures, there is an increasing need for early recognition and appropriate management of penile filler infections. We report an unusual case of a localised penile infection rapidly progressing to sepsis with multi-organ failure requiring intensive care support. The case demonstrates early surgical intervention with targeted antimicrobials can result in successful eradication of infection, with satisfactory cosmetic and functional outcomes for patients.

Keywords: Penile diseases, Urologic diseases, Penis, Infections, Hyaluronic acid, Injections, Case report

Background

Penile enhancement with injectable agents is a growing trend and yet has received limited scientific attention, despite the potential of serious complications. We report a case of severe penile cellulitis in a 31-year-old man who underwent subcutaneous penile hyaluronic-acid filler insertion. The localised infection rapidly progressed to septic shock requiring intensive care support and subsequent operative drainage. This is the first reported case of fulminant septic shock with multi-organ failure contributed by hyaluronic-acid penile fillers. The unusual severity and rapid progression of penile cellulitis in this case was multifactorial, due to penile fillers, abnormal scar

*Correspondence: khornicole@gmail.com
[1] Murnaghan Urology Department, Prince of Wales Hospital, Sydney, Australia
Full list of author information is available at the end of the article

tissue from previous hypospadias repair and behavioural risk-factors. This case demonstrates early surgical intervention in conjunction with appropriate antimicrobials and supportive care can result in satisfactory cosmetic and functional outcomes.

Case presentation

A 31-year-old male presented to the emergency department with a 2-day history of progressive pain and swelling of the penile shaft. This was preceded by unprotected sexual intercourse three days prior. The patient subsequently self-administered a single 50 mg dose of oral prednisone the following morning and subsequently developed subjective chills on the same day.

Relevant past medical history included subcutaneous hyaluronic filler injections at a cosmetic clinic for penile girth enhancement two months prior to presentation, distal tubularised hypospadias repair and genital herpes simplex. The patient had multiple behavioural risk factors, including regular self-administered intra-muscular testosterone injections, self-injection of growth hormone to the base of the penis (performed one month prior to penile filler procedure), multiple heterosexual sexual partners, cocaine use, heavy alcohol consumption (22 standard drinks/day) and a 10 pack-year smoking history.

On arrival, the patient was tachycardic to 127, hypotensive to 90/50 and febrile to 40 °C. Physical examination revealed gross penile oedema and erythema of the penile shaft ceasing at the base of the penis, with an associated curvature of the penile shaft towards the 8 o'clock position. There was also a small tender abrasion on the distal ventral aspect of the penile shaft 1 cm proximal to the glans (Fig. 1A). Blood tests showed a white cell count (WCC) of 6.1×10^9/L, creatinine of 95 μmol/L and lactate of 2.3 mmol/L. Urinalysis was negative. The patient was admitted and commenced on intravenous Flucloxacillin for presumed penile cellulitis.

Overnight the patient became increasingly drowsy with a persistent fever > 40 °C and tachycardia. Repeat examination showed new blistering of the penile skin overlying the penile fillers (Fig. 1B). Repeat blood tests showed marked changes with WCC of 25×10^9/L, creatinine of 225 μmol/L and lactate of 6.4 mmol/L, in less than seven hours from initial presentation. He was subsequently transferred to ICU for vasopressor and inotropic support. Antibiotics were changed to intravenous Meropenem, Clindamycin and Vancomycin as empiric therapy towards possible Fournier's Gangrene, on advice from Infectious Diseases specialists. A subsequent Computerised Tomography (CT) of the abdomen and pelvis showed penile oedema and stranding, however excluded intra-pelvic abscess or gas locules (Fig. 2).

The patient was transferred to the operating theatres and an incision was made over the largest blistered site on the penile shaft, which revealed a pus stained filler above Buck's fascia. This filler was removed, albeit with resistance requiring manual pressure to express the filler. The tissue adjacent to the infected filler was inflamed but no further debridement was required. A 21G needle was used to pierce the blistered skin overlying the penile fillers to facilitate drainage of the remaining penile fillers. The wound was dressed with an alginate dressing surrounded by absorbent gauze.

Penile swabs were positive for Streptococcus Agalactiae, Anginosus and Pyogenes, all of which were penicillin sensitive. Operative sample of the penile filler grew Streptococcus Pyogenes (penicillin sensitive). The patient was switched to intravenous Benzylpenicillin on day three on advice from Infectious Disease specialists, and dressings were changed daily. He was weaned off vasopressors and stepped down from ICU on day four.

The patient was subsequently counselled on safe sexual practices and received appropriate drug and alcohol counselling for his polysubstance abuse. A sexually transmitted infection screen showed active intercurrent Herpes Simplex Virus 2 infection for which he was commenced on oral Valaciclovir whilst in hospital. This was decreased to a prophylactic dose on discharge whilst his wounds healed. He was stepped down to oral Amoxicillin on day eight with a plan for three weeks of total antibiotic treatment. On discharge the blisters has flattened with no remaining fluid present, and the penile oedema and erythema had significantly improved.

At his follow up 2-weeks post-discharge, there was superficial skin loss to both the ventral and lateral aspect of the penis, corresponding to the initial blisters overlying his penile fillers with healthy granulation tissue at the base. A small one centimetre area of fibrinous tissue remained at the distal aspect of the shaft (Fig. 3A). There was also a small area of induration at the peno-scrotal junction (Fig. 3B), which expressed a scant amount of purulent discharge that was culture-negative. There was no palpable abscess and ultrasound excluded further penile or scrotal collection.

At his second follow up at five weeks post-discharge, the patient reported ongoing clinical improvement and normal erectile function. Examination revealed significant reduction in the inflammation at the base of penis with no remaining induration. The base of his wounds continued to appear healthy (Fig. 3C, D). The patient was reviewed by a Plastic Surgeon and was offered a split skin graft but was declined by the patient in preference for regular dressings. At three months post-discharged, the patient reported normal sexual and urinary function, and ongoing wound improvement.

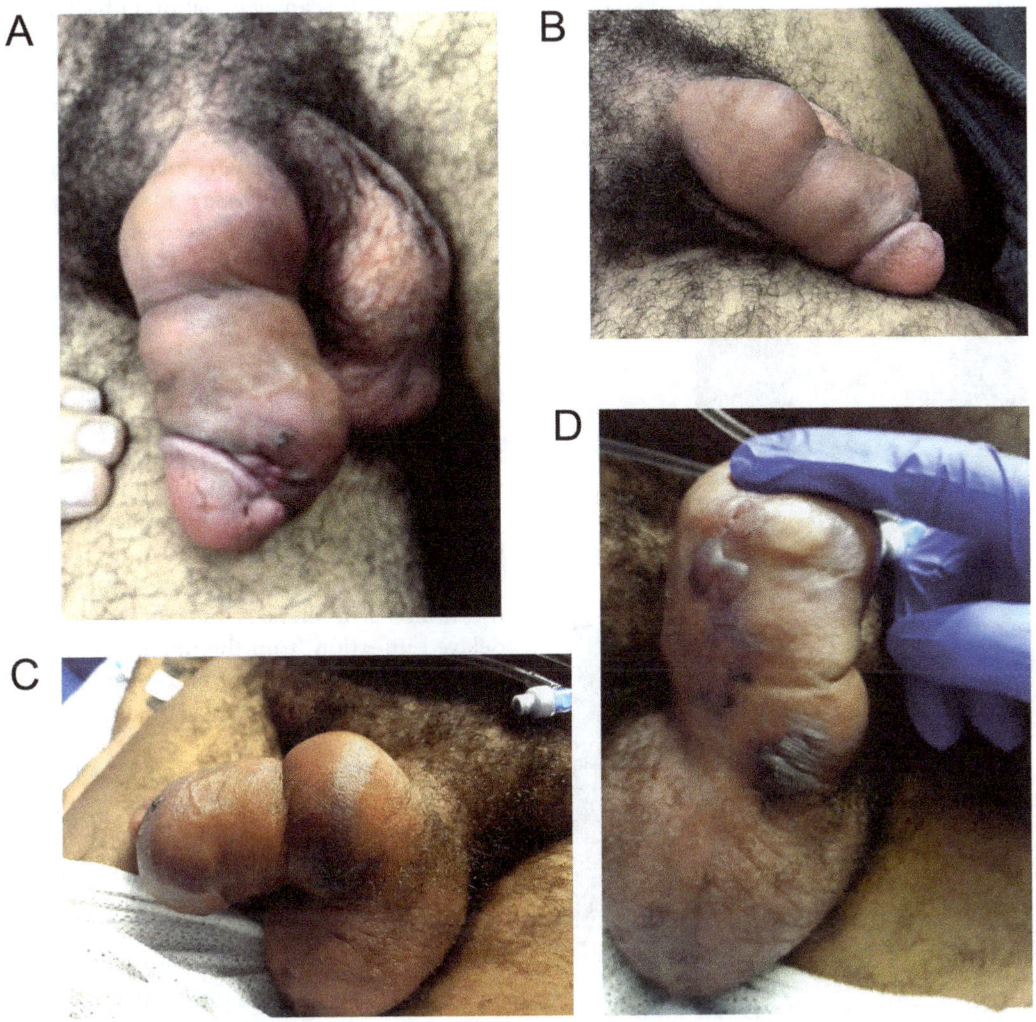

Fig. 1 Penile swelling and erythema on presentation. **A**, **B** Gross penile oedema and erythema with an abrasion on distal ventral penile shaft. Images taken on presentation to Emergency Department. **C**, **D** New blistering overlying cosmetic filler injection sites. Image taken seven hours from initial presentation

Discussion and conclusion

In an era of growing emphasis on physical appearance, there is an increasing demand for penile augmentation procedures [1, 2]. The goal of these procedures is a symmetrical increase in penile girth in both flaccid and erect states [3]. Most men who seek these procedures have physiologically normal penises and undertake these procedures for cosmetic and psychological reasons [1]. Currently there is no recommended indication nor proposed guidelines for penile girth enlargement [2]. The American Urological Association and Sexual Medicine Society of North America have both issued policy statements indicating there is insufficient data to substantiate the safety or efficacy of penile lengthening or girth enhancement surgery [4, 5].

Within the field of penile girth enhancement, there is an increasing utilisation of penile subcutaneous injection therapy as it is seen as simple, safe and minimally invasive [2, 3]. In this case hyaluronic acid, a long-lasting resorbable dermal filler was used. The filler is typically injected in small aliquots above Buck's fascia with a 21G needle after application of topical local anaesthetic cream (lignocaine 25 mg/g and Prilocaine 25 mg/g) and an intra-cavernosal injection to induce a chemical semi-erection [2].

While there is evidence of hyaluronic acid use in cosmetic facial dermatology, evidence of its use in penile girth enhancement is limited. Currently there is no U.S. Food and Drug Administration (FDA) approved injectable filler for the penis, nor is there a review of complications from penile fillers in the literature. However a case

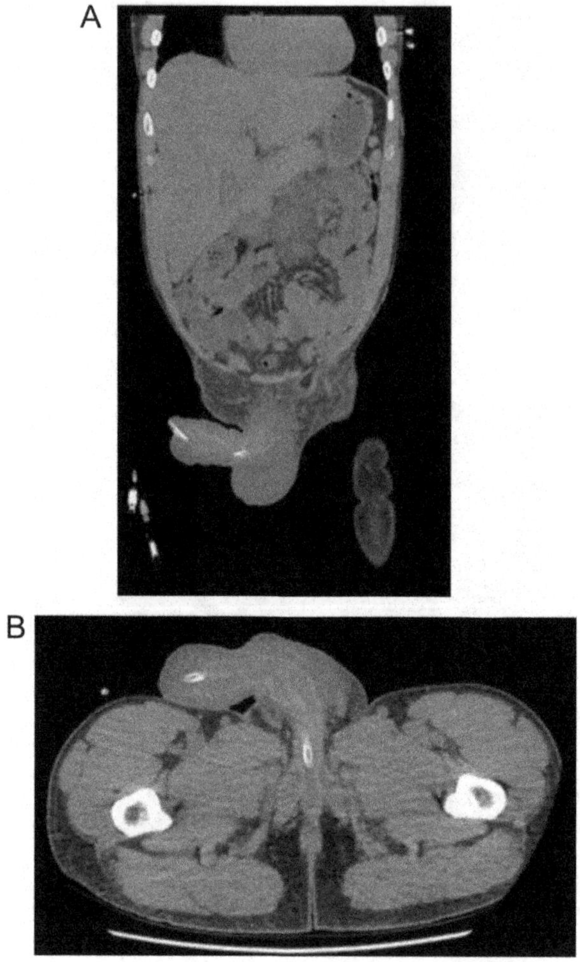

Fig. 2 CT scan of the abdomen and pelvis. **A** Coronal and **B** Axial sections showing indwelling catheter in situ with extensive penile and pre-pubic soft tissue swelling. No identified abscess or gas locules

series of soft-tissue fillers highlight important cosmetic, functional and systemic complications, which can lead to complex penile reconstructive surgery (Table 1) [1, 3, 6]. Fillers used in this study include hyaluronic acid, polymethyl-methacrylate injection, silicone and autologous fat [1, 3, 6].

The role of injectable fillers as a potential immunological barrier and medium for bacterial growth has been established in cosmetic facial hyaluronic acid injections, with a 1% risk of an acute or delayed infection [14]. Dermal facial filler infections can present as acute inflammation or abscess at the site of injection and are typically due to common skin pathogens such as Staphylococcus Aureus or Streptococcus Pyogenes. Delayed or chronic infections tend to affect a more generalised area and may involve atypical organisms such as Escherichia Coli [15]. These infections are related to the formation of bacterial biofilm, which is an aggregation of bacterial cells embedded in a matrix of bacterial macromolecules on the surface of fillers [14].

Eradication of biofilm bacteria is notoriously difficult due to their growth pattern, emergence of resistant phenotypes and resistance to antibiotic penetration. Bacteria within the biofilm exist in a dormant state and can be activated by an immunosuppressed state, trauma, or iatrogenic manipulation [14, 15]. It is reasonable to conclude that penile hyaluronic acid fillers behaves similarly, with a greater likelihood of infection due to extensive bacterial flora and susceptibility to trauma in the urogenital region. This was demonstrated in our case with the appearance of pus-stained fillers intraoperatively and growth of Streptococcus Pyogenes, a common skin coloniser, on operative wound swabs and cultures. In this case, subcutaneous invasion of bacteria likely occurred during sexual intercourse through the abrasion (Fig. 1A) or a herpetic sore, which then invaded the hyaluronic acid fillers. It was considered less likely to be a delayed infection from the initial insertion of penile fillers, due to the onset of symptoms following unprotected intercourse.

Imaging has a limited role in the acutely deteriorating patient. In this case, CT was performed to exclude necrotising fasciitis or a deeper perineal or pelvic collection contributing to the patient's rapid deterioration to guide operative planning and consent. In dermatology, ultrasound is the imaging modality of choice for assessment of cosmetic fillers. High-density hyaluronic acid appears as well delineated, anechoic, pseudocystic structures without internal echoes. CT and MRI may provide limited information to gauge the extent of filler deposits, however do not specifically detect hyaluronic acid deposits [16].

Surgical intervention to remove the potentially infected penile fillers as 'source control' was advocated, given the patient's rapid decline despite aggressive medical management. During pre-operative discussion with the patient's initial cosmetic surgeon it was suggested that routine hyaluronic acid fillers are usually easily expressible after an incision, however, this was not evident due to the inflammatory response of the surrounding tissue. Due to the circumferential location of the penile fillers, there was concern regarding the long term cosmetic and sexual function if multiple incisions were performed. Hence the intra-operative approach was converted to a needle aspiration combined with manual pressure to remove the infected penile fillers.

The diagnostic challenge in these cases lies not in the identification of infection but the assessment of the likely severity and trajectory. Most cases of penile cellulitis rapidly respond to antibiotic therapy [17]. However, there is

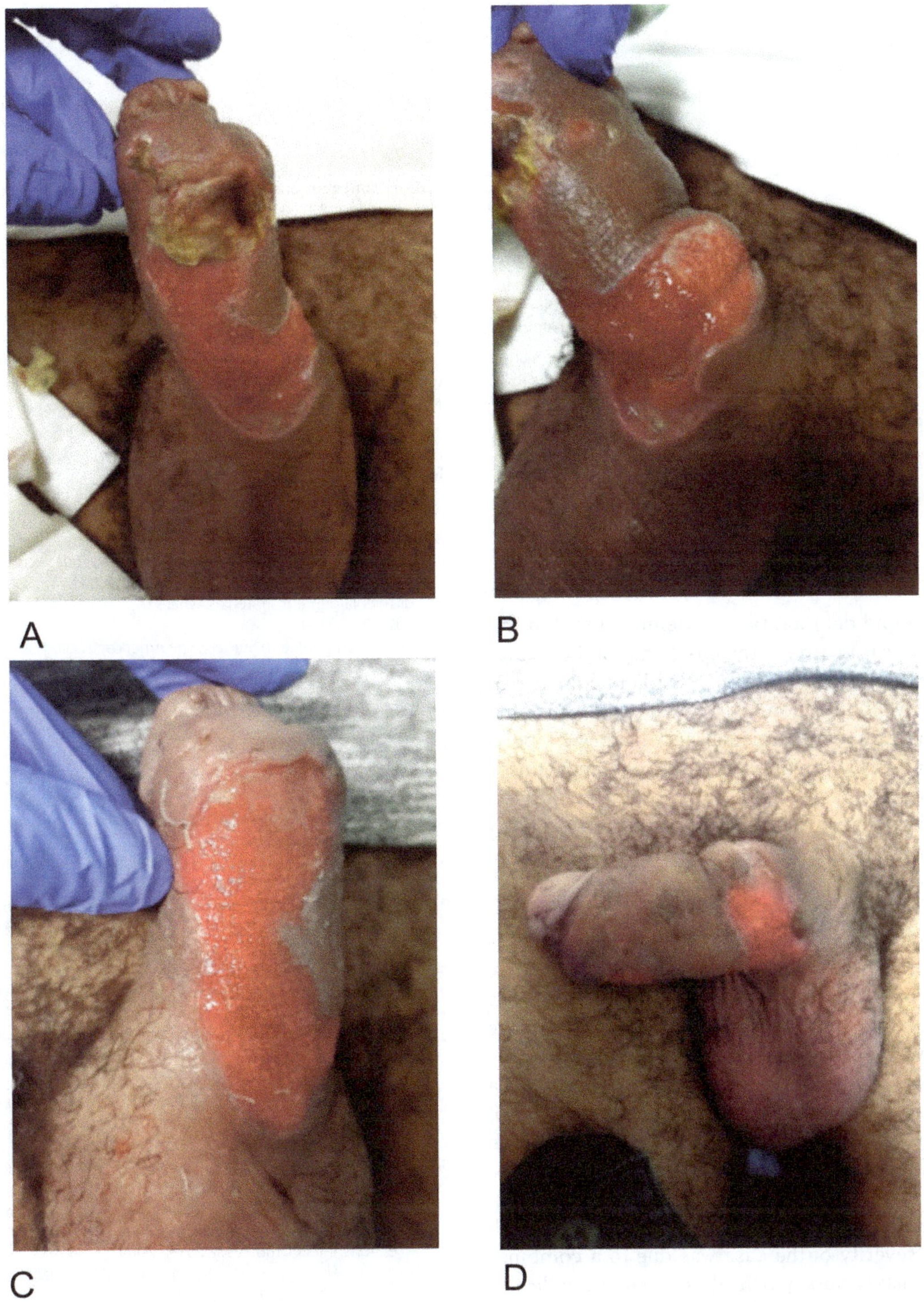

Fig. 3 Follow-up of penile wounds. **A** 2 weeks post discharge, fibrinous tissue at distal edge with otherwise healthy tissue base. **B** 2 weeks post-discharge, induration at base of penis with scant purulent discharge expressed. **C, D** 5 weeks post discharge, significant improvement in inflammation with remaining superficial skin loss

Table 1 Complications of penile filler injections

Cosmetic	Penile distortion, abnormal curvature and asymmetry [3] Nodules—liquified, necrotic, calcified [6] Reabsorption, drifting or distant migration [7] Granulomatous reactions [8]
Functional	Peyronie's disease [3] Erectile dysfunction [6] Male dyspareunia [6] Decreased sensation [9]
Systemic	Venous occlusion and acute hypersensitivity reaction [10] Fat embolism leading to cardiopulmonary collapse and death [11] Silicon embolism, pneumonitis, multi-organ failure and death [12, 13]

potential for rapid deterioration, as demonstrated in this case, where scarring from previous hypospadias repair, combined with hyaluronic acid penile fillers contributed to the severity of infection. Furthermore, the patient's self-administration of prednisone and history of polysubstance abuse likely contributed to a compromised immune state. Indeed active polysubstance abuse in patients undergoing inflatable penile prosthesis surgery has been shown to significantly increase risk of postoperative infection [18]. Clinicians need to assess patient's social history beyond medical comorbidities to adequately assess and predict infection severity.

In an era of growing emphasis on physical appearance and demand of injectable fillers, cosmetic filler infections is more than ever, important to recognise and manage appropriately. There is likely an underestimation of the complications from penile girth enlargement due to a lack of available data. This is the first published case of sepsis from a penile infection contributed by hyaluronic acid penile fillers. In this case, the localised infection rapidly progressed to sepsis with multi-organ failure requiring intensive care support and operative source control. The unusual severity of the case was due to a combination of host risk-factors and hyaluronic-acid penile fillers acting as a foundation for bacterial biofilm formation. This case demonstrates early surgical intervention with targeted antimicrobials can result in successful eradication of infection and satisfactory cosmetic and functional outcomes for patients.

Abbreviations

WCC: White cell count; CT: Computerised tomography; FDA: Food and Drug Administration.

Acknowledgements

Contents of the manuscript was published as part of Volume 125, Issue S1 Special Issue: Abstracts of the Urological Society of Australia and New Zealand 73rd Annual Scientific Meeting, 7–10th March 2020, Sydney, Australia [19].

Authors' contributions

All authors contributed significantly to the manuscript and are in agreement with the content. NK wrote the manuscript in consultation with AD and ACS providing critical feedback including revisions. All authors read and approved the final manuscript.

Competing interests

The authors declare that they have no competing interests.

Author details

[1]Murnaghan Urology Department, Prince of Wales Hospital, Sydney, Australia. [2]Prince of Wales Clinical School, UNSW Medicine, Sydney, NSW, Australia.

References

1. Vardi Y. Is penile enlargement an ethical procedure for patients with a normal-sized penis? Eur Urol. 2006;49(4):609–11.
2. Oates J, Sharp G. Nonsurgical medical penile girth augmentation: experience-based recommendations. Aesthet Surg J. 2017;37(9):1032–8.
3. Hehemann MC, Towe M, Huynh LM, El-Khatib FM, Yafi FA. Penile girth enlargement strategies: what's the evidence? Sex Med Rev. 2019;7(3):535–47.
4. Penile Augmentation Surgery. The American Urological Association. 2018. https://www.auanet.org/guidelines/penile-augmentation-surgery.
5. Penile Lengthening and Girth Enhancement Surgery. Sexual Medicine Society of North America, Inc. 2019 [cited 19 April 2020]. https://www.smsna.org/V1/resources/position-statements.
6. Torricelli FCM, Andrade EM, Marchini GS, Lopes RI, Claro JF, Cury J, et al. Penile enlargement with methacrylate injection: is it safe? Sao Paulo Med J. 2013;131(1):54–8.
7. Shaeer O, Shaeer K. Delayed complications of gel injection for penile girth augmentation. J Sex Med. 2009;6(7):2072–8.
8. Wassermann RJ, Greenwald DP. Debilitating silicone granuloma of the penis and scrotum. Ann Plast Surg. 1995;35(5):505–9.
9. Kwak TI, Oh M, Kim JJ, Moon DG. The effects of penile girth enhancement using injectable hyaluronic acid gel, a filler. J Sex Med. 2011;8(12):3407–13.
10. Coskuner ER, Canter HI. Desire for penile girth enhancement and the effects of the self-injection of hyaluronic acid gel. J Cutan Aesthet Surg. 2012;5(3):198.
11. Zilg B, Råsten-Almqvist P. Fatal fat embolism after penis enlargement by autologous fat transfer: a case report and review of the literature. J Forensic Sci. 2017;62(5):1383–5.
12. Schmid A, Tzur A, Leshko L, Krieger BP. Silicone embolism syndrome: a case report, review of the literature, and comparison with fat embolism syndrome. Chest. 2005;127(6):2276–81.
13. Gurvits GE. Silicone pneumonitis after a cosmetic augmentation procedure. N Engl J Med. 2006;354(2):211–2.
14. Marusza W, Olszanski R, Sierdzinski J, Ostrowski T, Szyller K, Mlynarczyk G, et al. Treatment of late bacterial infections resulting from soft-tissue filler injections. Infect Drug Resist. 2019;12:469.
15. Urdiales-Gálvez F, Delgado NE, Figueiredo V, Lajo-Plaza JV, Mira M, Moreno A, et al. Treatment of soft tissue filler complications: expert consensus recommendations. Aesthetic Plast Surg. 2018;42(2):498–510.
16. Wortsman X. Identification and complications of cosmetic fillers: sonography first. J Ultrasound Med. 2015;34(7):1163–72.
17. Bardapure M, Vaswani NJB. Cellulitis of the penis: a case report. Case Rep. 2009;2009:bcr0120091457.

18. Balen A, Gross MS, Phillips EA, Henry GD, Munarriz RJT. Active polysubstance abuse concurrent with surgery as a possible newly identified infection risk factor in inflatable penile prosthesis placement based on a retrospective analysis of health and socioeconomic factors. J Sex Med. 2016;13(4):697–701.
19. Concurrent Session Presentations. Abstracts of the Urological Society of Australia and New Zealand 73rd annual scientific meeting; March 7–10; Sydney, Australia, vol. 125(S1). . 2020. p. 4–24.

18

Comparison of ureteroscopy (URS) complementary treatment after extracorporeal shock wave lithotripsy failure with primary URS lithotripsy with holmium laser treatment for proximal ureteral stones larger than 10mm

Feng Yao, XiaoLiang Jiang, Bin Xie and Ning Liu*

Abstract

Background: To compare ureteroscopy (URS) complementary treatment following extracorporeal shock wave lithotripsy (SWL) failure with primary URS lithotripsy for proximal ureteral stones > 10 mm, and try to find out acceptable number of SWL sessions followed by safe URS.

Methods: This was a retrospective study following approval from Medical Ethics Committee of People's Hospital of Chongqing Banan District. Patients ($n=340$) who received URS in our hospital for stones > 10 mm from Jan 2015 to June 2020 were divided into two groups according to their previous SWL history. Group 1 consisted of 160 patients that underwent unsuccessful SWL before URS. Group 2 encompassed 180 patients without SWL before URS. Patient's operative outcomes were compared. A logistic regression and receiver operator characteristics (ROC) were used to identify the acceptable number of SWL sessions prior to URS, regarding the intra-operative complications of URS.

Results: The group 1 required more surgery time (41.38 ± 11.39 min vs. 36.43 ± 13.36 min, $p=0.01$). At the same time, more intra-operative (68.1% VS 22.8%, $p<0.05$) and post-operative (35% VS 18.0%, $p=0.001$) complications occurred in group 1. Need more hospital stay in group 1 (2.7 ± 1.2 days vs 1.6 ± 1.1 days, $p<0.05$). More patients in group 1 need further URS (16.3% VS 8.9%, $p=0.029$). After second URS, the SFR of URS in two groups was insignificant differences (82.5% VS 88.9%, $p>0.05$). The median (25–75%) of SWL sessions before URS was 2 (1–3) in group 1. According to the results of logistic regression analysis, patients suffered more SWL failure have an increased risk of complications during URS (OR = 1.995, 95% CI: 1.636–2.434). ROC showed that the optimal number of SWL session followed by URS were 0.5, with a sensitivity of 67.7% and specificity of 71.5%. Intra-operative complication rates of URS treatment were higher in patients who suffered > 1 SWL failure (72.6% vs 57.4%, $p=0.047$).

Conclusion: There was no acceptable number of SWL sessions that could be followed by URS with fewer intra-operative complications. Patients who underwent previous SWL were likely to suffer more intra-operative complications, the average operating time, hospitalization time, and needing further treatment, during URS treatment for proximal ureteral stones larger than 10 mm.

*Correspondence: yaaaa771130@outlook.com
Department of Urology, People's Hospital of Chongqing Banan District, Chongqing 401320, China

Keywords: Ureteral calculus, Ureteroscopy, Lithotripsy, Lasers, Solid-State, Therapeutics

Background

Ureteral calculus is a highly prevalent disease worldwide with a high recurrence rate [1, 2]. Urolithiasis shows variability according to geography, ethnicity, climate, diet and genetics [3]. The occurrence of ureteral stones typically requires ureteroscopy (URS) or extracorporeal shock wave lithotripsy (SWL). SWL has represented the major therapy for ureteral calculi since the 1980s [4]. In comparison to URS, SWL is minimally invasive, has shorter treatment times, fewer complication rates and is cheaper. However, high rates of retreatment are often required, representing a significant weakness in SWL. With advancement in endourology and minimally invasive surgeries with high success rates, the applicability of SWL has decreased. Since 2015, treatment recommendations of the European Association of Urology (EAU) regarding proximal ureteral stones larger than 10 mm have shifted to rigid URS endourologic procedures. SWL has therefore lost its position as a first-line modality, despite its effectiveness [5]. The availability of the equipment dictates the treatment choice, which is often selected based on individually and patient preference. So, in many developing countries, SWL still remains the first-line choice due to its low costs. In our research center, each SWL session costs about 800 RMB, and URS need about 7500 RMB.

It was reported that the stone-free rate (SFR) of retreating ureteral calculi with SWL decreases significantly after the initial treatment [6]. When SWL fails, URS becomes the most commonly used treatments. But some studies mentioned that more complications during URS procedures were seen in patients having already undergone SWL [7, 8]. All these reports reminded us whether there had a number of SWL sessions followed by safe URS especially for large calculus. We performed the study aiming to compare the URS outcomes between complementary URS treatment following SWL failure with primary URS lithotripsy for proximal ureteral stones > 10 mm, and try to find out the acceptable number of SWL sessions followed by safe URS.

Methods

Study population

This was a retrospective study performed from January 2015 to June 2020 following approval from Medical Ethics Committee of People's Hospital of Chongqing Banan District. A total of 340 patients with a single side proximal ureteral stones > 10 mm received URS treatment in our hospital. Group 1 (n = 160) consisted of patients with previous SWL for stones. Group 2 (n = 180) consisted of patients without SWL prior to URS. In our institute, the diameter of proximal ureteral stones less than 15 mm, SWL will be an optional treatment. The treatment procedure was chosen on the basis of the patients' preference.

Kidney function was assessed prior to all surgeries. Patients also received urinalysis kidney-ureter-bladder (KUB) radiography, computerized tomography (CT) and ultrasonography assessments. The proximal ureter was defined as the area of the ureter between the ureteropelvic junction and the upper border of the sacroiliac joint. Exclusion criteria included patients with renal dysfunction, those with an abnormal anatomy, kidney stones, kidney infection, previous URS, Percutaneous nephrostomy, laparoscopy, or open surgical ureterolithotomy. Blood cell counts, biochemical analysis, urinalysis, and aerobic urine cultures were performed post-operation. When present, urinary infections were treated and tested to confirm sterility. All patients were administered antibiotics at induction during operation. Patients with surgical contraindications were not observed. Auxiliary equipment, such as stone baskets and ureteral balloon dilator, were used in the study.

Complications that occurred intraoperatively were graded according to the modified Satava classification system [9]. Those that occurred after operation were classed according to the modified Clavien classification system [10].

SWL procedures

We performed SWL as an outpatient procedure using the Dornier Compact Sigma (EMSE 140f, Dornier MedTech, Germany). Shock waves were delivered at a rate of 60 impulses per minute. The maximum number of shock waves per session was 2000–2500. Pulse levels were set to 4–6. KUB radiography and ultrasound were performed to evaluate stone-free status and hydronephrosis after each session at 1–2 week. SWL failure was considered when the stones persisted or when an increasing degree of hydronephrosis was detected. Prior to the SWL procedure, Ureteral J stent insertion was not performed in any case.

Ureteroscopy technique

URS procedures were performed under general anesthesia using a 8/9.8F and/or 6/7.5F rigid URS (Richard Wolf, Knittlingen, Germany) with a holmium laser

(Generally, 0.5 to 1 J of energy per pulse with a pulse frequency of 10 to 15 Hz). Usually, 10 W [1 J × 10 Hz] and 7.5 W [0.5 J × 15 Hz] settings of holmium laser were performed to break stone dusting and getting popcorn effects. Guidewires (0.035 inch) were placed into the ureteral orifice through the ureteroscope which was delivered directly to the stone following guidewires guidance. The ureteral orifice and ureteral strictures were balloon dilated and stone baskets were employed to subvert stone migration into the renal pelvis. Larger fragments were removed through stone retrieval. If a false intramural route formation, bleeding making the surgical field invisible, inability to reach stone or residual fragments larger than 6 mm, double J stents were implanted, and secondary URS was performed after 2–4 weeks. Percutaneous nephrostomy was performed upon urinary tract perforation occurred, and secondary URS was needed to remove ureteral stones.

Considering a large volume of stones located in the proximal ureter, ureteral injury and edema after operation, double J stents were implanted into all patients in our study. Stents were removed 2 to 4 weeks after surgery. Prior to J stent removal, residual stones were examined by KUB. When the residual stones in the ureteral were larger than 6 mm, second URS sessions were performed. Flexible ureteroscopy procedures were performed when larger than 6 mm residual stones migrated to the renal pelvis. All surgeries were performed by urology surgeons with more than 5 years of ureteroscopy experience. The patient could only be discharged without renal colic, fever and gross hematuria. All 340 patients received oral α-receptor blockers to assist the excretion of stones, and the absence of stones was followed up for 3 months. The SFR (3 months after the last treatment) was determined on the basis of KUB, and any calculi residual fragments were considered as a failure for stone free.

Statistical analysis

Data were analyzed using SPSS25.0 software. Kolmogorov–Smirnov and Probability plots were constructed to verify the normality of the continuous variables. Data are shown as the mean ± SD. The number of cases and percentages were recorded for normally distributed and categorical variables. Intergroup analysis of the continuous variables was performed using a Student-t test. Categorical variables were analyzed with a Chi square test. A logistic regression and receiver operator characteristics (ROC) were performed to identify the acceptable number of SWL sessions followed by safe URS, regarding the intraoperative complications of URS. p values < 0.05 were considered significant.

Results

We included 340 patients in the study. Patients were sub-divided according to SWL history (group 1: 160 patients and group 2: 180 patients). Group 1 encompassed patients with previously unsuccessful SWL prior to URS. Group 2 consisted of patients without SWL prior to URS for the stone. There were insignificant differences between groups in terms of clinical and stone characteristics ($p > 0.05$) (Table 1).

During URS procedure, endoscopic observation revealed edematous inflammation around ureteral calculus, which was defined as impacted ureteral stones. Compared with group 2, group 1 had more impacted ureteral stones ($p < 0.05$). Most of the impacted ureteral stones were at the original site, only 2 was ureteral steinstrasse. Most of findings in the two groups were significant differences (Table 2).

The SFR in group 1 (66.9%) were significantly lower than in group 2 (82.2%) after the first URS session. Deal with some Satava II complications, more patients in group 1 need second URS (26 VS 16; 16.3% VS 8.9%, $p = 0.029$). And15.6% patients in group 1 VS 6.7% patients in group 2 ($p = 0.007$) successfully carried out further URS treatment after placed a double J stent for 2 to 4 weeks. Following the second URS session, the SFR of two groups showed insignificant differences (82.5% VS 88.9%, $p > 0.05$).

Significant differences in intraoperative and postoperative complications were observed between groups ($p < 0.05$). In Satava I, bleeding and proximal stone migration occurred ($p < 0.05$). In Satava II, bleeding making the surgical field invisible and large levels of stone migration to the renal pelvis were observed

Table 1 Comparison in terms of clinical and stone characteristics

	Group 1	Group 2	p value
No. patients, n	160	180	
Age, years, mean (SD)	45.2 (8.8)	46.8 (7.6)	0.083
Gender, n (%)			
Male	76 (47.5)	88 (48.9)	0.442
Female	84 (52.5)	92 (51.1)	
BMI, mean (SD)	24.39 (3.02)	24.68 (2.68)	0.39
Side, n (%)			
Right	68 (42.5)	88 (48.9)	0.142
Left	92 (57.5)	92 (51.1)	
Stone size, mm, mean (SD)	12.6 (1.42)	12.4 (1.39)	0.898
Calcium oxalate stones, n (%)	136 (85)	157 (87.2)	0.331
CT value, Hu, mean (SD)	718.65 (148.30)	739.11 (109.78)	0.159

URS ureteroscopy, *BMI* body mass index, *CT* computed tomography, *SFR* stone-free rate

Table 2 Comparison in terms of URS treatment

	Group 1	Group 2	p value
Impacted ureteral stones fund during URS, n (%)	79 (49.4)	30 (16.7)	<0.05
Energy used for gravel, KJ, mean (SD)	1.459 (0.546)	1.545 (0.606)	0.203
Operation time, minutes, mean (SD)	41.38 (11.39)	36.43 (13.36)	0.01
Using stone baskets, n (%)	113 (70.6)	97 (53.9)	0.001
SFR of URS, n (%)			
After first URS session	107 (66.9)	148 (82.2)	0.001
After second URS session	132 (82.5)	160 (88.9)	0.084
Hospitalization times, days, mean (SD)	2.7 (1.2)	1.69 (1.1)	0.02

URS ureteroscopy, *SFR* stone-free rate

Table 3 Intra-operative complications of URS

Complications	Group 1 (n=160), n (%)	Group 2 (n=180), n (%)	p value
Intra-operative complications	109 (68.1)	52 (28.9)	<0.05
Satava I (Observation)	56 (35.0)	20 (11.1)	<0.05
Bleeding nearly no effect to URS operation	29 (18.1)	10 (5.6)	<0.05
Mucosal tears	6 (3.8)	2 (1.1)	0.107
Stones less than 6 mm migration Renal pelvis	21 (13.1)	8 (4.4)	0.004
Satava II (requiring endoscopic retreatment)	52 (32.5)	32 (17.8)	0.001
Mucosal injury (A false intramural route formation)	3 (1.9)	1 (0.6)	0.269
Bleeding making the surgical field invisible	12 (7.5)	4 (2.2)	0.020
Inability to reach stone requiring secondary URS	1 (0.6)	2 (1.1)	0.544
Residual fragments larger than 6 mm	10 (6.3)	9 (5.0)	0.395
Stones larger than 6 mm migration renal pelvis requiring flexible URS	24 (15.0)	15 (8.3)	0.040
Ureteral perforation requiring percutaneous nephrostomy	2 (1.3)	1 (0.6)	0.456
Satava III (requiring open surgery)	1(0.6)	0	0.471
Urethral stricture	0 (0)	0	
Ureteral avulsion	0 (0)	0	

URS ureteroscopy, *UTI* urinary tract infection

(p < 0.05). There were no significant differences in Satava III (Table 3).

Post-operative complications in group 1 was significantly higher than group 2 (35.0% VS 18.0%, p=0.001). Fever and hematuria in Clavien I were the most frequent postoperative complication in group 1 (9.2% and 20.0%) and group 2 (3.5% and 15.5%) (p < 0.05). There were no significant differences in Clavien II to V.

All 340 participants, which underwent 0, 1, 2, 3, and 4 SWL sessions were 180, 47, 51, 44, and 18, respectively. And, the number of URS intraoperative complications in patients who suffered 0,1, 2, 3, and 4 SWL sessions were 41, 27, 33, 35, and 14, respectively (Fig. 1).

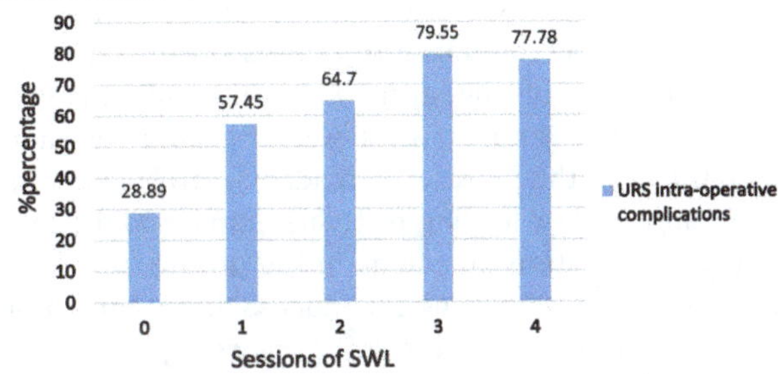

Fig. 1 The percentage of URS intra-operative complications in patients with previous different SWL sessions

According to the results of logistic regression analysis, patients suffered more SWL failure have an increased risk of complications during URS (OR=1.995, 95% CI: 1.636–2.434) (Fig. 2).

The median (25–75%) of SWL sessions was 2 (1–3). ROC showed that the optimal number of SWL sessions followed by safe URS were 0.5, with a sensitivity of 67.7% and specificity of 71.5%. Intraoperative complication rates of URS treatment were higher in patients who suffered > 1 SWL failure (72.6% vs 57.4%, p=0.047).

Variables in the Equation

		B	S.E.	Wald	df	Sig.	Exp(B)	95% C.I. for EXP(B)	
								Lower	Upper
Step 1[a]	sessions	.691	.101	46.433	1	.000	1.995	1.636	2.434
	Constant	-.799	.150	28.165	1	.000	.450		

a. Variable(s) entered on step 1: sessions.

Fig. 2 Logistic regression analysis of the number of SWL sessions to URS intra-operative complications

Discussion

SWL is both non-invasive and more practical than URS, and is widely used in clinical treatment of urinary calculi. In studies by Ziaee et al., patients with proximal ureteral stones that were 10 to 15 mm in size underwent three SWL sessions and achieved 78.6% SFR, which were higher than the 72.5% SFR of URS ($p > 0.05$) [11]. Many shortcomings do however remain for SWL, including the requirement for multiple treatment protocols. The success of SWL has been linked to a number of factors including stone size, location and Hounsfield units, as well as technique and distance of skin to stone [6]. Kenneth et al. showed that the SFR of initial SWL treatment was 68%, which decreased to 46% after re-treatment 1, and they observed a further decrease in the stone-free rate after re-treatment 2 to 31% ($p = 0.001$) [6]. SWL and URS are the most commonly used treatment modalities for proximal ureteral stones [12]. And in cases of SWL failure for proximal ureteral stones, complementary URS treatment is a common procedure.

SWL treatment when compared to URS is considered a less invasive treatment option for ureteral stones. However, SWL can cause tissue damage in the kidney, proximal ureter and adjacent organs [13–15]. The mucosal layer of the ureter was damaged by SWL through the increased number of transitional cells during cytological examination of the urine [13]. The inflammatory response of the target tissues was triggered by shock waves through the release of oxidants, prostaglandins, COX-2 and TNF-α leading to tissue damage and edema [14, 15]. Information on edema in the urothelial mucosa can lead to the small vessels mucosa becoming more fragile, leading to lower levels of hemorrhage. Edema in the urothelial mucosa also complicates subsequent ureteral URS surgery. Holland et al. and Grasso et al. also reported that stone fragments can become embedded in the ureteral mucosa after SWL, occasionally becoming completely submucosal and eventually leading to ureteral stricture [16–18]. All these changes may cause more impacted stones. Severs studies have shown the phenomenon that the impacted stone rates are significantly higher after unsuccessful SWL [19–21], which may cause difficulty and even more complications during URS. In our study, we also found that impacted stones and ureteral inflammation edema were seen predominantly in patients having already undergone SWL.

Complications of URS can occur due to many variables. The size of the stones, stone location, and the size of the ureteroscope used are closely related to the occurrence of complications [8, 22]. In studies by Kilinc et al. [20] and Tugcu et al. [23], insignificant differences were observed between the complication rates of the two groups. However, only proximal and distal-ureteral small stones were investigated in their studies. In Bora et al. study [24], the mean proximal ureteral stone burden was 83.7 ± 57.2 mm^2 and complication rates were significantly higher in patients with previous SWL. The results of this study similarly showed that the complication rates of URS treatment were significantly higher in patients who suffered SWL treatment failure for proximal stones > 10 mm.

In this study, it been found that impacted stone fragments and friable ureter mucosa lead to bleeding easily during URS treatment for patients suffering SWL failure. For improved visibility of the stones, we applied high-pressure saline injections which led to stone/fragment migration to the renal pelvis. To reduce migration, stone baskets were used in both groups. Although a higher number of stone baskets were used in group 1, patient numbers were significantly higher (15.0%) and required flexible ureteroscopes for further treatment to achieve a stone-free status after 2 weeks. Perforation of the ureter is a serious complication during URS procedures [8, 25]. Alapont et al. showed that 68% of their ureteral perforations occurred with stones > 10 mm [25]. Recent research found that the proximal ureter had lower levels of tensile strength which caused ureteral perforation more likely to occur [26]. When stones baskets or balloon dilatation were performed, avulsion and ureteral perforation can occur, particularly in the upper third of the ureter possessing the impacted stones [27, 28]. In this study, perforation was more common in those undergoing SWL failure, despite the differences lacking significance. According to our experience, maintaining good visibility represented an effective method to reduce perforation.

Kilinc et al. [20] and Tugcu et al. [23] respectively reported that URS procedures after SWL failure require longer operation times than direct URS for both distal and proximal ureteral stones. Our results were in accordance with these data. Due to more impacted stones and significant ureteral inflammatory edema, when fragmenting stones occurred, the time taken for laser assessments was extended and the need for extra manipulations and the use of auxiliary equipment prolonged the URS procedure.

Fever and hematuria were the most frequent postoperative complications, which were significantly higher in the previously unsuccessful SWL group. We consider that these complications may be caused by severe ureteral inflammation and injuries. We did observe only cases of sepsis in group 1. The occurrence of fevers and sepsis resolved with antibiotic and antipyretic drugs. Further complications in the unsuccessful SWL group may lead to longer hospitalization times.

In previous studies, the success rates of URS with or without unsuccessful SWL were not statistically significant. The success rates of URS sessions after SWL failure ranged from 73.6%-78.9% [19–21]. In their researches, the stones were less than 10 mm in diameter. It was also reported that the success rates (72.5%) of URS were lower for stones rang from 10 to 15 mm [11]. In our studies, after one URS session, the SFR in group 2 was 82.2% which was in accordance with the 82% SFR of primary URS in the proximal ureteral for stones larger than 10 mm [29]. However, group 1 (66.9%) was significantly lower than group 2. To deal with Satava II intra-operative complications, a double J stent was placed and part of these patients required secondary URS treatment. Following the further URS procedure, the SFR of the two groups showed no significant differences (82.5% VS 88.9%). Although there was insignificant difference in SFR, patients who suffered SWL failure were more likely to need multiple URS treatment.

In developing countries such as China, a large number of treatment centers lack available equipment, and many patients prefer SWL due to its low cost. In our center, even if three SWL sessions cost about 2400 RMB, it is still significantly cheaper than URS, which need about 7500 RMB. The SFR of re-treating ureteral calculi with SWL significantly decreases after the initial treatment and increases the complication rates of URS after unsuccessful SWL. This remind us the question whether acceptable number of SWL sessions can be followed by safe URS, regarding the intra-operative complications of URS. Studies in this area are lacking. We analyzed the influence of SWL on ureteral complications through logistic regression analysis, and showed that the more SWL sessions before URS followed by the higher risk of intra-operative complications. We calculated the optimal number of SWL sessions followed by safe URS as 0.5 with a sensitivity of 67.7% and specificity of 71.5%. We further showed that the complication rates of URS were higher in patients who suffered more than a single SWL (72.6% vs 57.4%, $p=0.047$). These results suggest that no acceptable number of SWL sessions for safe URS to treat large stones in the proximal ureter currently exist. And patients who underwent more previous SWL were more likely to suffer intra-operative complications during URS complementary treatment. To get lower complications, it was suggested that URS procedures should be delayed 2–3 weeks after unsuccessful SWL [24].

This study had some limitations, including its retrospective nature that led to selection shifts. Moreover, different surgeons, the small number of patients, unpublished and missing data may have resulted in bias. However, this study was the first to identify whether acceptable number of SWL sessions exist that can be followed by safe URS for proximal ureter stones > 10 mm.

Conclusions

The average operating time, hospitalization time, and needing further URS in complementary treatment for patients suffering SWL failure were significantly higher than primary URS lithotripsy treatment in proximal ureteral stones larger than 10 mm. There was no acceptable number of SWL sessions that could be followed by URS with fewer intra-operative complications.

Abbreviations

URS: Ureteroscopy; SWL: Extracorporeal shock wave lithotripsy; EAU: European Association of Urology; KUB: Kidney-ureter-bladder; CT: Computerized tomography; IVU: Intravenous urography; SFR: Stone-frees rate.

Acknowledgements

The authors thank the Department of Urology, WEST CHINA SCHOOL OF MEDICINE SICHUAN UNIVERSITY for their support.

Authors' contributions

FY: Study design, Manuscript writing. NL: Data collection, Data management, Manuscript editing. BX: Project development, Manuscript writing. XL J: Data collection. All authors read and approved the final manuscript.

Competing interests

The authors declare that they have no competing interests.

References

1. Sorokin I, Mamoulakis C, Miyazawa K, et al. Epidemiology of stone disease across the world. World J Urol. 2017;35(9):1301–20.
2. Liang L, Li L, Tian J, et al. Androgen receptor enhances kidney stone-CaOx crystal formation via modulation of oxalate biosynthesis & oxidative stress. Mol Endocrinol. 2014;28(8):1291–303.
3. Hesse A, Brandle E, Wilbert D, Kohrmann KU, Alken P. Study on the prevalence and incidence of urolithiasis in Germany comparing the years 1979 vs 2000. Eur Urol. 2003;44:709.
4. Torricelli FCM, Danilovic A, Vicentini FC, et al. Extracorporeal shock wave lithotripsy in the treatment of renal and ureteral stones. Rev Assoc Med Bras (1992). 2015;61(1):65–71.
5. Türk C, Petřík A, Sarica K, et al. EAU guidelines on interventional treatment for urolithiasis. Eur Urol. 2016;69(3):475–82.

6. Pace KT, Weir MJ, Tariq N, et al. Low success rate of repeat shock wave lithotripsy for ureteral stones after failed initial treatment. J Urol. 2000;164(6):1905–7.
7. Strohmaier WL, Schubert G, Rosenkranz T, et al. Comparison of extracorporeal shock wave lithotripsy and ureteroscopy in the treatment of ureteral calculi: a prospective study. Eur Urol. 1999;36(5):376–9.
8. Fuganti PE, Pires S, Branco R, et al. Predictive factors for intraoperative complications in semirigid ureteroscopy: analysis of 1235 ballistic ureterolithotripsies. Urology. 2008;72(4):770–4.
9. Tepeler A, Resorlu B, Sahin T, et al. Categorization of intraoperative ureteroscopy complications using modified Satava classification system. World J Urol. 2014;32:131–6.
10. Mandal S, Goel A, Singh MK, et al. Clavien classification of semirigid ureteroscopy complications: a prospective study. Urology. 2012;80:995–1001.
11. Ziaee SA, Halimiasl P, Aminsharifi A, et al. Management of 10–15-mm proximal ureteral stones: ureteroscopy or extracorporeal shockwave lithotripsy? Urology. 2008;71(1):28–31.
12. Ceylan Y, Ucer O, Bozkurt O, et al. The effect of SWL and URS on health-related quality of life in proximal ureteral stones. Minim Invasive Ther Allied Technol. 2018;27(3):148–52.
13. Mustafa M, Pancaroglu K. Urine cytology to evaluate urinary urothelial damage of shock-wave lithotripsy. Urol Res. 2011;39:223–7.
14. Lildal SK, Norregaard R, Andreassen KH, et al. Ureteral access sheath influence on the ureteral wall evaluated by cyclooxygenase-2 and tumor necrosis factor-α in a porcine model. J Endourol. 2017;31:307–13.
15. Clark DL, Connors BA, Evan AP, et al. Effect of shock wave number on renal oxidative stress and inflammation. BJU Int. 2014;107:318–22.
16. Holland R, Margel D, Livne PM, et al. Retrograde intrarenal surgery as second-line therapy yields a lower success rate. J Endourol. 2006;20:556–9.
17. Grasso M, Liu JB, Goldberg B, et al. Submucosal calculi: endoscopic and intraluminal sonographic diagnosis and treatment options. J Urol. 1995;153(5):1384–9.
18. Dretler SP, Young RH. Stone granuloma: a cause of ureteral stricture. J Urol. 1993;150(6):1800–2.
19. Osti AH, Hofmockel G, Frohmüller H. Ureteroscopic treatment of ureteral stones: only an auxiliary measure of extracorporeal shockwave lithotripsy or a primary therapeutic option? Urol Int. 1997;59(3):177–81.
20. Kilinc MF, Doluoglu OG, Karakan T. Ureteroscopy in proximal ureteral stones after shock wave lithotripsy failure: is it safe and efficient or dangerous? Can Urol Assoc J. 2015;9(9–10):E718–22.
21. Philippou P, Payne D, Davenport K, et al. Does previous failed ESWL have a negative impact of on the outcome of ureterorenoscopy? A matched pair analysis. Urolithiasis. 2013;41(6):531–8.
22. Fernandez DMS, Noldus J, Huland H. Ureterorenoscopy (URS) in treatment of ureteral calculi. I. Safety and effectiveness of URS as auxiliary treatment after ESWL. Urologe A. 1999;38(2):128–32.
23. Tugcu V, Gürbüz G, Aras B, et al. Primary ureteroscopy for distal-ureteral stones compared with ureteroscopy after failed extracorporeal lithotrips. J Endourol. 2006;20(12):1025–9.
24. Irer B, Sahin MO, Erbatu O, et al. Impact of previous SWL on ureterorenoscopy outcomes and optimal timing for ureterorenoscopy after SWL failure in proximal ureteral stones. World J Urol. 2020;38(3):769–74.
25. Alapont AJM, Broseta RE, Pontones MJL, et al. Complications of ureterorenoscopy. Actas Urol Esp. 2003;29:692–9.
26. Shilo Y, Pichamuthu JE, Averch TD, et al. First prize: evaluation of the tensile strength of the human ureter-preliminary results. J Endourol. 2014;28(12):1470–3.
27. Chotikawanich E, Korman E, Monga M. Complications of stone baskets: 14-year review of the manufacturer and user facility device experience database. J Urol. 2011;185(1):179–83.
28. Kuntz NJ, Neisius A, Tsivian M, et al. Balloon dilation of the ureter: a contemporary review of outcomes and complications. J Urol. 2015;194(2):413–7.
29. Turk C, Knoll T, Petrik A, et al. European Association of Urology Guidelines on Urolithiasis, 2012. www.uroweb.org/gls/pdf/20_Urolithiasis_LR%20March%2013%202012.pdf. Accessed 19 April 2013.

19

Appropriate timing of performing abdominal ultrasonography and termination of follow-up observation for antenatal grade 1 or 2 hydronephrosis

Akihiro Nakane[1,2,3], Kentaro Mizuno[4*], Taiki Kato[3], Hidenori Nishio[4], Hideyuki Kamisawa[3], Satoshi Kurokawa[3], Tetsuji Maruyama[3], Takahiro Yasui[3] and Yutaro Hayashi[4]

Abstract

Background: Most cases of antenatal the Society of Fetal Urology (SFU) grade 1or 2 hydronephrosis (HN) improve or resolve spontaneously with conservative treatment. However, there is no consensus on the duration of follow-up for cases of grade 1or 2 HN. The aim of this study was to determine the need for continuous follow-up period and new management of children with antenatal grade 1or 2 HN.

Methods: Subjects underwent ultrasonographic assessment for HN according to the SFU classification. We retrospectively evaluated 112 patients with postnatal grade 1 HN and 69 with grade 2 HN using abdominal ultrasonography between January 2010 and December 2017. We examined the change in HN grade on repeat ultrasonography. Kaplan–Meier method was used to show the effect of HN grade on the rate of HN changes.

Results: The mean follow-up duration was 44.9 ± 36.4 months (range 12–274). Initial SFU grade 1 HN disappeared in 47.0% of cases at 12 months, 66.4% at 24 months and 73.2% at 48 months. Initial SFU grade 2 HN showed improvement in grade in 74.7% of cases at 12 months, 88.3% at 24 months and 89.5% at 48 months. However, 14.6% of SFU grade 1 and 2.8% of SFU grade 2 cases increased in grade and of the 17 cases, 16 cases worsened within the first 6 months. No cases with increased grade required pyeloplasty. Initial disappearance and later reappearance of HN occurred in 40.5% of SFU grade 1 and 2 cases. The mean duration of later reappearance of HN was 39.1 ± 36.2 months (range 12–137). No cases showed reappearance of HN after more than 1 year.

Conclusions: Ultrasonography within the first 6 months was necessary for management of children with antenatal grade 1or 2 HN, because some patients showed worsening. After that, it is considered safe to spread the follow-up interval for stable cases. Most cases of grade 1or 2 HN resolved spontaneously, however a few cases reappeared within 1 year. Therefore, ultrasonography after 1 year was necessary in children with HN that spontaneously disappeared. The appropriate time to end the follow-up was considered to have been after 1 year or more has passed since the disappearance was confirmed.

Keywords: Antenatal hydronephrosis, Ultrasonography, Continuous follow-up period

*Correspondence: kmizuno@med.nagoya-cu.ac.jp
[4] Department of Pediatric Urology, Nagoya City University Graduate School of Medical Sciences, 1 Kawasumi, Mizuho-cho, Mizuho-ku, Nagoya 467-8601, Japan
Full list of author information is available at the end of the article

Background

Fetal hydronephrosis (HN) is the most common anomaly detected on antenatal ultrasonography, with an estimated prevalence of approximately 2–5.5% [1–3]. In most cases, HN is diagnosed in the absence of urinary tract obstruction, when the anteroposterior diameter of the renal pelvis is just above the normal range for gestational age [4]. Studies have shown that most cases of antenatal HN improve or resolve spontaneously with conservative treatment [2, 3]. The cases of 98% in the Society of Fetal Urology (SFU) grade 1or 2 HN improve or resolve in a systematic review of seven articles meta-analysis [5]. The resolution rate of SFU grade 1 and 2 are reported to be 98–99% and 60–98% in two prospective studies [6, 7]. However, some patients do not show improvement or increase grade of HN, and a few cases need operation [8, 9]. The detection and postnatal follow-up of persistent antenatal HN is believed to help in the early recognition and prevention of progressive renal damage [3, 10–12]. There is no consensus on the duration of follow-up for cases of grade 1or 2 HN [13]. In patients with SFU grades 1 and 2 HN, a more abbreviated follow-up may be warranted and could save costs [14]. However, It has been pointed out that SFU grade 1 and grade 2 show different natural course [7], and there is concern whether similar follow-up may be acceptable for SFU grade 1 and grade 2. The aim of this study is to examine the hypothesis that there are different continuous follow-up period and new management for children with antenatal SFU grade 1or 2 HN.

Methods

Patient characteristics

Ultrasonographic assessments of HN grade were performed according to the SFU classification [15]. We let patients hydrate and test the patient's bladder when it was not full. All patients visited our institutions from 48 h after birth within 1 month of age and assessed to divide their HN groups as a baseline. We retrospectively evaluated 112 antenatally-detected HN patients with grade 1 unilateral HN and 69 with grade 2 unilateral HN using abdominal ultrasonography at our institutions between January 2010 and December 2017. There were 11 excluded patients who had repeated febrile urinary tract infections or hydroureter and those who were diagnosed with symptomatic vesicoureteral reflux on voiding cystourethrography or diagnosed with ureterovesical junction obstraction on magnetic resonance imaging. Seven cases (2 in grade 1 and 5 in grade 2) had hydroureter and were excluded prior to the initial follow-up of this study. Four cases in grade 2 were excluded during this follow-up due to repeated febrile urinary tract infections. These cases are not added to the total number of each grade. Patient characteristics at baseline were shown in Table 1.

Table 1 Patient characteristics at baseline (between 48 h after birth and 1 month of age)

Parameter	Number	Percentage (%)
Total	181	100
Gender		
Male	148	81.8
Female	33	18.1
Laterality		
Right	70	38.7
Left	111	61.3
SFU grade		
Grade 1	112	61.9
Grade 2	69	38.1
Excluded patients		
Total	11	100
Urinary tract infection	5	45.5
Hydroureter	6	54.5

Follow-up surveillance

The patients were followed up according to the grade of HN, and ultrasonography was performed once every 1–3 months and diagnosed HN of SFU grade by several pediatric urologists. Single pediatric urologists (AN) reviewed all Ultrasonography as a second blinded reviewer and if the first several urologist and the second single reviewer disagreed, the diagnosis of the second reviewer was adopted to minimize inter and intra-rater reliability [16]. In the process of adopting the opinion of the second reviewer, 3 cases in grade 2 were upgraded from grade 2 to 3. The term "resolved" indicated a change in the SFU grade to grade 0, and includes all the final resolutions; "improved" indicated a decrease in the SFU grade at the final evaluation by one or more levels, and this included resolved cases; "no change" indicated no change in the initial SFU grade; and "worsened" indicated an increase in the SFU grade, includes temporary upgrade. In the further follow-ups, repeat ultrasonography was performed for low (1–2) SFU grade HN, while renal nuclear medicine studies using dynamic scanning modes were performed for HN that progressed to a high (3–4) SFU grade [17]. Of the resolved cases, 42 cases were followed up every 1–6 months to examine whether the condition of resolution was stable.

All these procedures were performed after obtaining informed consent for clinical care of follow-ups form the parents. These clinical data were obtained as a retrospective study. Additionally, the procedures were performed as a clinical trial at our institution after obtaining institutional review board approval (approved by Ethical Committee of the Gamagori City Hospital, approval no. Gamabyo 500-4). All statistical analyses were performed using SPSS Statistics Ver. 22 (IBM, Armonk, NY, USA). Values are shown as mean ± SD (range minimum–maximum). Kaplan–Meier method was used to show the effect of HN grade on the rate of HN changes and compared with the use of the log-rank test. All tests were 2-sided. A p value of less than 0.05 was considered statistically significant.

Results

The mean follow-up duration was 44.9±36.4 months (range 12–274). Patients' characteristics at baseline was shown in the Table 1. The rate of time to resolution or improvement in SFU grade 1 or 2 were determined using Kaplan–Meier method (Fig. 1). Initial SFU grade 1 HN resolved in 47.0% of cases at 12 months, 66.4% at 24 months and 73.2% at 48 months. The median of time to resolution was 14 months (95% confidence interval (CI) 9.49–18.51). Initial SFU grade 2 HN showed improvement in grade in 74.7% of cases at 12 months, 88.3% at 24 months and 89.5% at 48 months. The median of time to resolution was 7 months (95% CI 6.15–7.85). Initial SFU grade 2 HN resolved in 20.9% of cases at 12 months, 45.9% at 24 months and 72.9% at 48 months. The median of time to resolution was 25 months (95% CI 14.71–35.29). The rate of resolution in grade 1 HN or improvement of grade 2 HN was significantly higher in SFU grade 2 than grade 1 (log-rank test, $\chi^2=14.679$, $P=0.00013$). However, the rate of resolution of HN was significantly higher in SFU grade 1 than grade 2 (log-rank test, $\chi^2=3.839$, $P=0.05$). On the other hand, 14.6% of SFU grade 1 (15 cases) and 2.8% of SFU grade 2 (2 cases) increased in grade, including cases of temporary upgrade. Of the 17 cases, 16 cases worsened within the first 6 months and only one case of SFU grade 1 showed beyond 6 months (at the 13 months). The rate of time to worsening in SFU grade 1 or 2 were determined using Kaplan–Meier method (Fig. 2). The rate of worsening of HN was significantly higher in SFU grade 1 than grade 2 (log-rank test, $\chi^2=6.227$, $P=0.013$). None of the patients underwent pyeloplasty due to deterioration of renal function. We followed up on 42 cases that HN resolved. The mean additional follow-up duration was 39.1±36.2 months (range 12–137). Initial disappearance

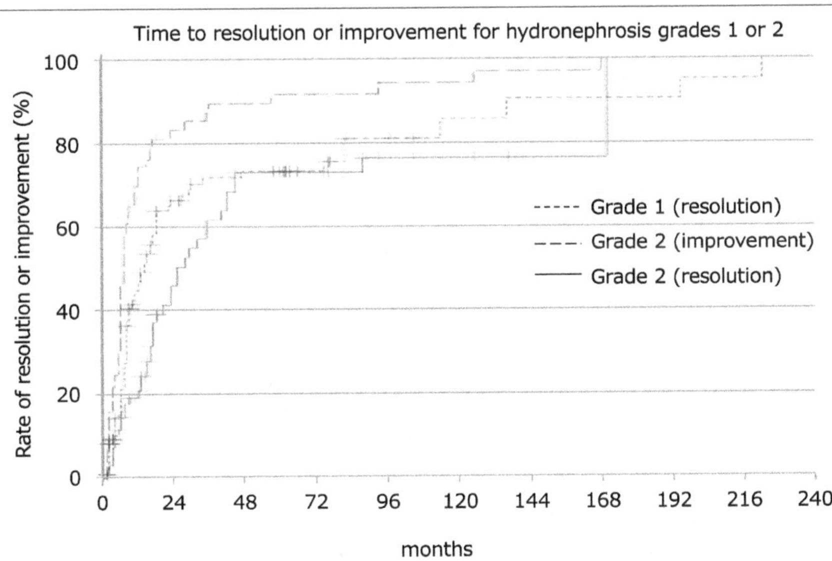

Number of patients at risk

Month	baseline	2	4	6	12	24	36	48	72	96	144	168	170	233
Grade 1 (resolution)	112	95	85	78	49	27	20	19	12	6	2	2	2	0
Grade 2 (improvement)	69	61	55	39	17	8	5	5	4	2	1	0	-	-
Grade 2 (resolution)	69	67	62	55	47	24	17	11	11	4	1	1	0	-

Rate of resolution or inmprovement of hydronephrosis

Month	2	4	6	12	24	36	48	72	96	144	168	170	233
Grade 1 (resolution)	8.2	14.2	21.3	47.0	66.4	71.8	73.2	75.5	80.9	90.5	90.5	90.5	100
Grade 2 (improvement)	16.6	25.2	46.8	74.7	83.3	89.5	89.5	91.6	94.4	97.2	100	-	-
Grade 2 (resolution)	2.9	10.1	14.5	20.9	45.9	61.7	72.9	72.9	76.3	76.3	76.3	100	-

Fig. 1 Rate of time to resolution or improvement of hydronephrosis in grade 1 or 2. Kaplan–Meier method. Points displayed as crosses shows censored cases. The upper table in this figure shows the number of affected patients at risk at each observational point. The lower table in this figure shows the rate (%) of resolution or improvement of hydronephrosis at each observational point. The rate of resolution or improvement of hydronephrosis was significantly higher in grade 2 than grade 1 (log-rank test, $\chi^2=14.679$, $P=0.00013$). However, the rate of resolution of HN was significantly higher in SFU grade 1 than grade 2 (log-rank test, $\chi^2=3.839$, $P=0.05$)

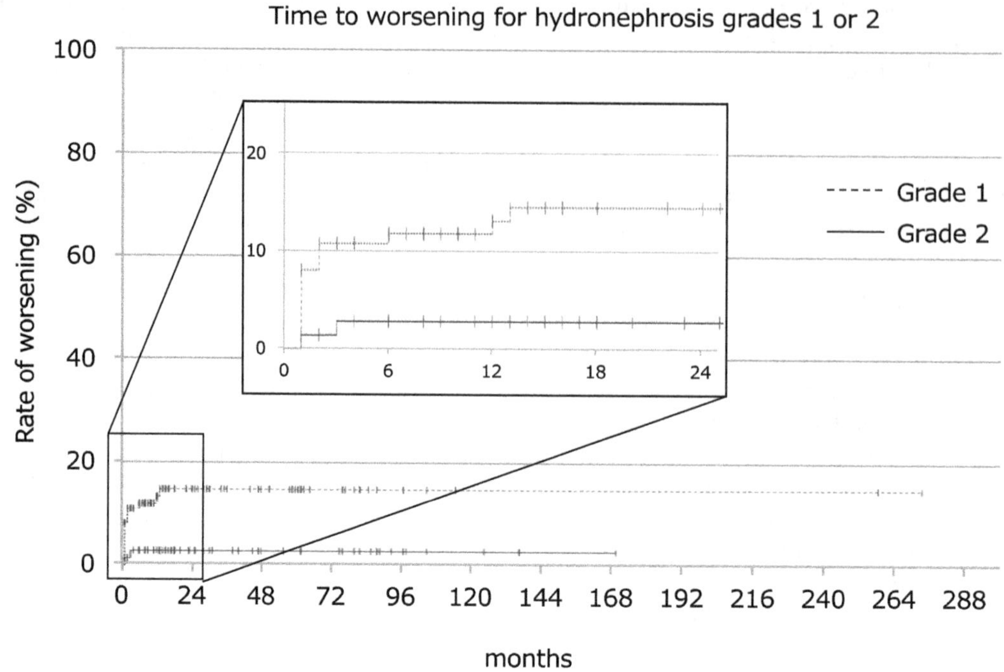

Number of patients at risk

Month	baseline	2	4	6	8	10	12	13	24	48	96	170	274
Grade 1	112	95	89	85	77	70	60	58	40	25	5	2	0
Grade 2	69	64	62	59	57	55	53	47	31	18	7	0	-

Rate of worsening for hydronephrosis (%)

Month	2	4	6	8	10	12	13	24	48	96	170	274
Grade 1	10.8	10.8	11.8	11.8	11.8	13.1	14.6	14.6	14.6	14.6	14.6	14.6
Grade 2	1.4	2.8	2.8	2.8	2.8	2.8	2.8	2.8	2.8	2.8	2.8	-

Fig. 2 Rate of time to worsening of hydronephrosis in grade 1 or 2. Kaplan–Meier method. Points displayed as crosses shows censored cases. The upper table in this figure shows the number of affected patients at risk at each observational point. The lower table in this figure shows the rate (%) of worsening of hydronephrosis at each observational point. The rate of worsening of hydronephrosis was significantly higher in grade 1 than grade 2 (log-rank test, $\chi^2=6.227$, $P=0.013$). There were 14.6% of grade 1 and 2.8% of grade 2 cases increased in grade. Then, 99.3% of these cases worsened within the first 6 months, only one case of grade 1 worsened at the 13 months over the study period

and later reappearance of HN occurred in 40.5% (17 cases). The mean duration of later reappearance of HN was 6.4±3.5 months (range 1–11). The rate of time to reappearance of HN was determined using Kaplan–Meier method (Fig. 3). No cases showed reappearance of HN after more than 1 year. Reappeared HN resoluved again in 10 cases. Reappeared HN of SFU grade 1 or 2 remained in 7 cases. However, none of the patients underwent pyeloplasty during the observation period.

Discussion

Most cases of antenatal HN improve or resolve spontaneously with conservative treatment [2, 3]. However, some patients do not show improvement without treatment. No consensus currently exists regarding the optimal schedule and duration of follow-up with SFU grade 1 or 2 HN. It is unclear which neonates require postnatal evaluation, when postnatal evaluation for HN should be performed, how long follow-up should be continued, how long an examination should be performed [13].

The timing of postnatal resolution of HN is quite variable, occurring over the first few years of life. Despite variabilities in the underlying diagnoses, mild grades of HN generally show early resolution, with most cases of SFU grade 1–2 HN resolving within 12–18 months of age [8, 18, 19]. In our study, most cases of SFU grade 1–2 HN showed natural improvement or resolution within 4 years of age. In particular, since SFU grade 2 HN resolve more slowly than grade 1 on the early follow-up, the follow-up period is likely to be longer for many cases. However,

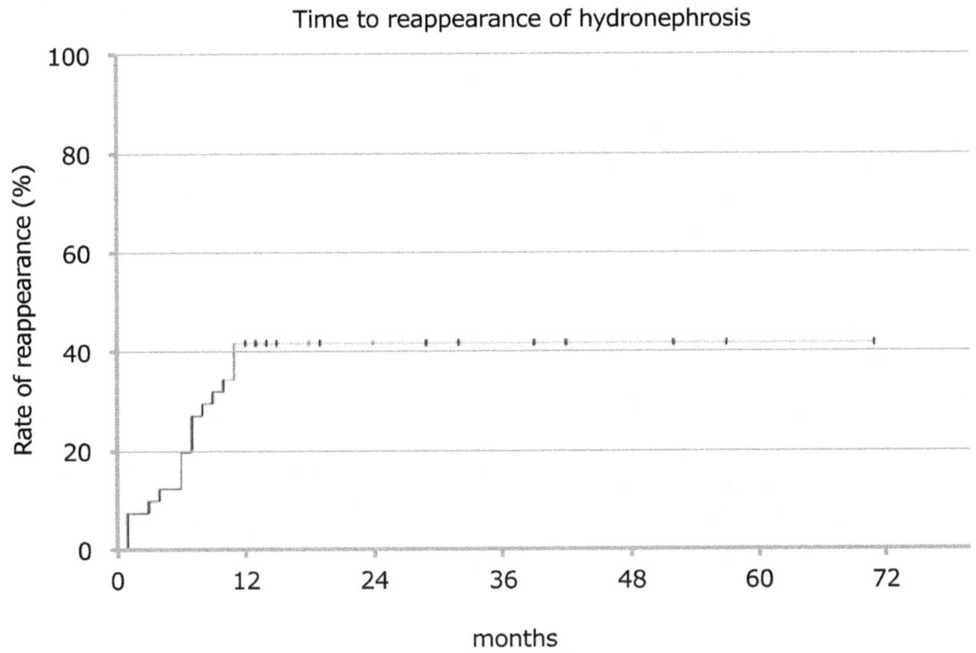

Number of patients at risk

Month from resolution baseline		1	3	4	6	10	11	12	24	48	71
Grade 1 or 2	42	41	39	38	34	28	25	20	10	5	0

Rate of reapearance of hydronephrosis (%)

Month from resolution	1	3	4	6	10	11	12	24	48	71
Grade 1 or 2	7.1	9.5	11.9	19.0	33.3	40.5	40.5	40.5	40.5	40.5

Fig. 3 Rate of time to reappearance of hydronephrosis. Kaplan–Meier method. Points displayed as crosses shows censored cases. The upper table in this figure shows the number of affected patients at risk at each observational point. The lower table in this figure shows the rate (%) of reapearance of hydronephrosis at each observational point. No cases showed reappearance of hydronephrosis after more than 1 year

A small number of cases showed worsening from SFU grade 1 to 2 or SFU grade 2 to 3, and this worsening was mainly noted within 6 months of age in our study. In SFU grade 2, the HN grade that increased within 6 months was a change to the higher risk SFU grade 3, so careful observation may be required for SFU grade 2 during this period. A previous study reported the need for surgical intervention in a small percentage of cases of mild-grade HN [20]. In another previous report, of 225 kidneys with SFU grade 2 HN, 3 showed worsening of HN to a severe grade [8]. Furthermore, following SFU grade 3 cases, there are cases that finally required surgery [21], so it is concluded that more closely monitoring is required than SFU grade 2 [17]. Previous study has been suggested that SFU grade 1 may be more physiologic in nature [22]. If SFU grade 1 persists in perpetuity without need for intervention, perhaps it does not need to be followed as aggressively. We think that 6 months and 1 years SFU grade 1 patients should undergo ultrasonography at the time when the grade of HN may worse. After that, it is considered safe to stop close follow-up and spread the follow-up interval to about 1 year for stable cases. On the other hand, in SFU grade 2 patients, there is a possibility of worsening high grade of HN at 6 months or less, so it is considered necessary to perform serial ultrasonography. However, after that period, it will be possible to spread the follow-up interval as with SFU grade 1.

Operative repair was not required in all cases in our study. Since there were no patients who finally had surgery, it was thought that the follow-up interval could be spreaded. However, our study showed that there is a high probability that HN will reappeare immediately after it disappears. It is considered that reappearance of HN needs to be noted as a new finding against the question of whether it is sufficient to confirm the disappearance of HN once at the end of follow-up. In our study, once HN disappeared for more than 1 year, no case had reappearance of HN. It was suggested that follow-up could be completed if there was no reappearance for more than 1 year. In our study, there were 7 cases that remained recurrent. Although no cases have been operated on, it is not possible at this time to describe what kind of natural history these cases have and new prospective studies are needed to determine its natural history.

Chertin et al. reported that 50% of cases requiring surgical intervention undergo surgery within the first 2 years and almost all cases undergo surgery within the first 4 years [23]. These authors recommended evaluation every 3–6 months during the abovementioned period [23]. Some authors have proposed that further evaluation is unnecessary for SFU grade 1 or 2 [14, 24]. Others have advised serial US until decrease or resolution of HN, or until patients are old enough to communicate symptoms of renal colic [25, 26]. Taken together the above results, we propose the end of follow-up when it can be confirmed that HN disappearance continues after 1 year, or when low grade of HN remains stable for more than 4 years (enough to communicate symptoms) while the follow-up interval is spreaded.

Our study had some limitations. This was a retrospective study. Additionally, follow-up indications were not standardized across the participating physicians. The evaluation grade of HN was SFU classification only, anterior–posterior diameter measurement [27] and UTD classification [28] are not performed. Furthermore, this cohort may have not only ureteropelvic junction obstructon but also other complicating malformations, including asymptimatic vesicoureteral reflux, because we do not routeinly do voiding cystourethrography or magnetic resonance imaging on asymptomatic HN patients. SFU grading system has problems with inter and intra-rater reliability [16, 29]. We tried to minimize the problems by adopting a second single blinded reviewer to minimize bias from the treating physician, however the other problem remains that reliability for grade 2 and 3 is rather low [16, 30]. In this study, the cases requiring arbitration when the first reviewer and the second blinded reviewer disagreed were not evaluated by a third blinded arbitrator. Further studies are needed to overcome these limitations and confirm the findings of the present study.

Conclusions

Ultrasonography within the first 6 months was necessary for management of children with SFU grade 1or 2 HN, because some patients showed worsening. After that, it is considered safe to stop close follow-up and spread the follow-up interval for stable cases. Most cases of perinatal SFU grade 1or 2 HN resolved spontaneously with conservative treatment. However, a few cases reappeared within 1 year. Therefore, ultrasonography after 1 year was necessary in children with HN that spontaneously disappeared. The appropriate time to end the follow-up was considered to have been after 1 year or more has passed since the disappearance was confirmed.

Abbreviations

CI: Confidence interval; HN: Hydronephrosis; SFU: The Society of Fetal Urology.

Authors' contributions

Conception and design: AN and YH; enrollment of patients and acquisition of data: AN, KM, and HN; drafting of the manuscript: AN, KM, and YH; statistical analysis: AN and HK; analysis and interpretation of data: TK, SK, and TM; manuscript editing: AN, KM, HN and TY; supervision: TY. We confirm that all authors read and approved the final manuscript.

Competing interests

The authors declare that they have no competing interests.

Author details

[1] Education and Research Center for Community Medicine, Nagoya City University Graduate School of Medical Sciences, Nagoya, Japan. [2] Department of Urology, Gamagori City Hospital, Gamagori, Japan. [3] Department of Nephro-urology, Nagoya City University Graduate School of Medical Sciences, Nagoya, Japan. [4] Department of Pediatric Urology, Nagoya City University Graduate School of Medical Sciences, 1 Kawasumi, Mizuho-cho, Mizuho-ku, Nagoya 467-8601, Japan.

References

1. Livera LN, Brookfield DS, Egginton JA, Hawnaur JM. Antenatal ultrasonography to detect fetal renal abnormalities: a prospective screening programme. BMJ. 1989;298:1421–3.
2. Blyth B, Snyder HM, Duckett JW. Antenatal diagnosis and subsequent management of hydronephrosis. J Urol. 1993;149:693–8.
3. Gunn TR, Mora JD, Pease P. Antenatal diagnosis of urinary tract abnormalities by ultrasonography after 28 weeks' gestation: incidence and outcome. Am J Obstet Gynecol. 1995;172:479–86.
4. Scott JE, Wright B, Wilson G, Pearson IA, Matthews JN, Rose PG. Measuring the fetal kidney with ultrasonography. Br J Urol. 1995;76:769–74.
5. Sidhu G, Beyene J, Rosenblum ND. Outcome of isolated antenatal hydronephrosis: a systematic review and meta-analysis. Pediatr Nephrol. 2006;21:218–24.
6. Braga LH, McGrath M, Farrokhyar F, Jegatheeswaran K, Lorenzo AJ. Society for Fetal Urology classification vs Urinary Tract Dilation grading system for prognostication in prenatal hydronephrosis: a time to resolution analysis. J Urol. 2018;199:1615–21.
7. Kohata E, Kimata T, Onuma C, et al. Natural course of isolated mild congenital hydronephrosis: a 2-year prospective study at a single center in Japan. Int J Urol. 2019;26:643–7.
8. Madden-Fuentes RJ, McNamara ER, Nseyo U, Wiener JS, Routh JC, Ross SS. Resolution rate of isolated low-grade hydronephrosis diagnosed within the first year of life. J Pediatr Urol. 2014;10:639–44.
9. Rigas A, Karamanolakis D, Bogdanos I, Stefanidis A, Androulakakis PA. Pelvi-ureteric junction obstruction by crossing renal vessels: clinical and imaging features. BJU Int. 2003;92:101–3.
10. Dhillon HK. Prenatally diagnosed hydronephrosis: the Great Ormond Street experience. Br J Urol. 1998;81:39–44.
11. Stocks A, Douglas R, Frentzen B, Richard G. Correlation of prenatal renal pelvic anteroposterior diameter with outcome in infancy. J Urol. 1996;155:1050–2.
12. Podevin G, Mandelbrot L, Vuillard E, Oury JF, Aigrain Y. Outcome of urological abnormalities prenatally diagnosed by ultrasound. Fetal Diagn Ther. 1996;11:181–90.
13. Nguyen HT, Herndon CD, Cooper C, et al. The Society for Fetal Urology consensus statement on the evaluation and management of antenatal hydronephrosis. J Pediatr Urol. 2010;6:212–31.
14. Akhavan A, Schnorhavorian M, Garrison LP, et al. Resource utilization and costs associated with the diagnostic evaluation of nonrefluxing primary hydronephrosis in infants. J Urol. 2014;92:919–24.
15. Fernbach SK, Maizels M, Conway JJ. Ultrasound grading of hydronephrosis: introduction to the system used by the Society for Fetal Urology. Pediatr Radiol. 1993;23:478–80.
16. Keays MA, Guerra LA, Mihill J, et al. Reliability assessment of Society for

Fetal Urology ultrasound grading system for hydronephrosis. J Urol. 2008;180:1680–3.
17. Kohno M, Ogawa T, Kojima Y, et al. Pediatric congenital hydronephrosis (ureteropelvic junction obstruction): medical management guide. Int J Urol. 2020;27:369–76.
18. Mallik M, Watson AR. Antenatally detected urinary tract abnormalities: more detection but less action. Pediatr Nephrol. 2008;23:897–904.
19. Koff SA. Postnatal management of antenatal hydronephrosis using an observational approach. Urology. 2000;55:609–11.
20. Noe HN, Magill HL. Progression of mild ureteropelvic junction obstruction in infancy. Urology. 1987;30:348–51.
21. Ericson BA, Maizels M, Shore RM, et al. Newborn society of fetal urology grade 3 hydronephrosis is equivalent to preserved percentage differential function. J Pediatr Urol. 2007;3:382–6.
22. Zee RS, Herndon CDA, Cooper CS, et al. Time to resolution: a prospective evaluation from the Society for Fetal Urology hudronephrosis registry. J Pediatr Urol. 2017;13(316):e1-5.
23. Chertin B, Pollack A, Koulikov D, Rabinowittz R, Hain D, Hadas-Halpren I. Conservative treatment of ureteropelvic junction obstruction in children with antenatal diagnosis of hydronephrosis: lessons learned after 16 years of follow-up. Eur Urol. 2006;49:734–8.
24. Riccabona M, Avni FE, Blickman JG, et al. Imaging recommendations in paediatric uroradiology: minutes of the ESPR workgroup session on urinary tract infection, fetal hydronephrosis, urinary tract ultrasonography and voiding cystourethrography, Barcelona, Spain, June 2007. Pediatr Radiol. 2008;38:138–45.
25. Gantti JM, Broecker BH, Scherz HC, et al. Antenatal hydronephrosis with postnatal resolution: how long are postnatal studies warranted? Urology. 2005;57:1178i-iii.
26. Matui F, Shimada K, Matsumoto F, et al. Late recurrence of symptomatic hydronephrosis in patients with prenatally detected hydronephrosis and spontaneous improvement. J Urol. 2008;180:322–5.
27. Alconcher LF, Tombesi MM. Natural history of bilateral mild isolated antenatal hydronephrosis conservatively managed. Pediatr Nephrol. 2012;27:1119–23.
28. Nguyen HT, Benson CB, Bromley B, et al. Multidisciplinary consensus on the classification of prenatal and postnatal urinary tractdilation (UTD classification system). J Pediatr Urol. 2014;10:982–98.
29. Chalmers DJ, Meyers ML, Brodie KE, Palmer C, Campbell JB. Inter-rater reliability of APD, SFU and UTD grading systems in fetal sonography and MRI. J Pediatr Urol. 2016;12(305):e1-5.
30. Rickard M, Easterbrook B, Kim S, et al. Six of one, half a dozen of the other: Ameasure of multidisciplinary inter/intra-rater reliability of the society for fetal urology and urinary tract dilation grading systems for hydronephrosis. J Pediatr Urol. 2017;13(80):e1-5.

20

Anti-reflux endoscopic injection therapy in post-pubertal patients via techniques adopted for the dilated ureteral orifice

Tetsuji Maruyama[1], Kentaro Mizuno[2], Hidenori Nishio[2], Taiki Kato[1], Takashi Hamakawa[1], Yosuke Ikegami[1], Takahiro Yasui[3] and Yutaro Hayashi[2*]

Abstract

Background: To investigate the efficacy and safety of endoscopic injection therapy for vesicoureteral reflux in post-pubertal patients with dilated ureteral orifice via modified hydrodistension implantation techniques.

Methods: We retrospectively reviewed medical records including operational procedure and clinical course of all consecutive patients over 12 years old with a history of injection therapy. Endoscopic injection of dextranomer/hyaluronic acid copolymer was performed under hydrodistension implantation technique with some modifications in order to inject through dilated ureteral orifice align with the intramural ureter. Technical selections were done according to hydrodistension grade of the ureteral orifice. Voiding cystourethrography was evaluated at 3 months postoperatively. Hydronephrosis was evaluated using ultrasonography preoperatively until 6 months postoperatively.

Results: From 2016 to 2019, 12 patients (all female, 16 ureteral units; median age 32 [range 15–61] years) underwent endoscopic injection therapy at one of our institutions. We have identified grade II vesicoureteral reflux in 5 ureters, grade III in 8, and grade IV in 3 ureters. Grade 3 ureteral-orifice dilation were presented in 12 ureters (75%), grade 2 in 3 and grade 1 in 1 ureter in the present cases. Postoperatively, vesicoureteral reflux was diminished to grade 0 in 12 ureteral units (75%), decreased to grade I in 3 (9%), and remained grade III in 1 (6%). Three patients reported dull flank pain for several days postoperatively and there was 1 case of acute pyelonephritis. Temporary hydronephrosis was confirmed in 3 ureteral units (19%) at 1 month postoperatively. Median follow-up duration was 23 (range 13–63) months long. Although, 3 patients were experienced f-UTI 1–2 times, repeated VCUG showed no VUR recurrence.

Conclusions: According to hydrodistension grade of the ureteral orifice, endoscopic injection therapy via modified hydrodistension implantation technique is an effective and safe treatment for vesicoureteral reflux in post-pubertal female patients with dilated ureteral orifice. While ureteral deformities or a history of anti-reflux surgery may increase the risks, these can be managed with appropriate methods that ensure sufficient mound appearance and height.

Keywords: Dextranomer/hyaluronic acid copolymer, HIT, STING, Urinary tract infection, Vesicoureteral reflux

*Correspondence: yutaro@med.nagoya-cu.ac.jp
[2] Department of Pediatric Urology, Nagoya City University Graduate School of Medical Sciences, 1 Kawasumi, Mizuho-cho, Mizuho-ku, Nagoya 467-8601, Japan
Full list of author information is available at the end of the article

Background

Vesicoureteral reflux (VUR) is major cause of febrile urinary tract infection (f-UTI) in children and sometimes adolescent and young adult females [1, 2]. For ureteral reimplantation, open surgery is the gold standard procedure owing to its reliably high success rate (more than 95%) [3, 4]. However, the development of a less invasive approach such as laparoscopic or robot-assisted surgery would be highly arising in the field [5]. In addition, the use of endoscopic injection therapy has increased since the injectable agents and techniques have been refined, resulting in subureteral transurethral injection (STING), hydrodistension implantation technique (HIT), and double-HIT procedure [6–8]. Currently, this minimally invasive therapy is a new option for the treatment of VUR in children [9].

In adult patients, less invasiveness is also eligible so that impact of the surgery to their active social life are sever. However, there is little information regarding the clinical utility of the therapy partially due to the limited number of patients or such technical difficulties associated with large-caliber ureter or might be pathological stiffness originated from chronic inflammation in the adult ureter.

The present study investigated the efficacy and safety of endoscopic injection therapy for VUR in adults via modified HIT techniques adopted for large-caliber ureters. The primary objective was the successful treatment of VUR defined as the absence of VUR at 3-month follow-up by voiding cystourethrography (VCUG). The secondary objectives were complications including ureteral obstruction or occurrence of comorbidity such as flank pain or renal failure caused by hydronephrosis or f-UTI. And also estimated were factors that might contribute to the successful treatment so that grade and timing of VUR and hydrodistention (HD) grade [7].

Methods

Preoperative evaluation

After institutional review board approval (20-04-330), we retrospectively reviewed medical records of all consecutive patients over 12 years old who were referred to one of our facilities (Nagoya City East Medical Center) between 2016 and 2019 underwent endoscopic injection therapy for VUR. All patients were referred from our tertiary center (Nagoya City University) and were willing to undergo injection therapy after discussion of all surgical options (open, laparoscopic, and robot-assisted-surgery) along with their advantages and disadvantages [10, 11]. After explaining the possible outcomes, complications, and comorbidities associated with each procedure, written informed consent was obtained from all patients before the surgery. In case of subjects are under 18, the written informed consent was also obtained from a parent and/or legal guardian.

All patients presented with several episodes of f-UTI were include in the study. Patients with a history of any anti-reflux surgery were not excluded. Exclusion criteria were grade V VUR, grade I VUR without contralateral VUR, ureterocele, posterior urethral valves, obstructed megaureter and ectopic ureters, and presence of voiding dysfunction. The reflux grade was based on the results of preoperative VCUG, according to the International Classification System (International Reflux Study Committee), which was also evaluated postoperatively. We re-evaluated VCUG before surgery to confirm grade and timing (i.e., filling or voiding). Hydronephrosis was evaluated using ultrasonography preoperatively and until 6 months postoperatively. The hydronephrosis was graded according to the Society for Fetal Urology. None of the patients in this series exhibited voiding dysfunction at the time of injection, as confirmed by uroflowmetry just before and after surgery.

Surgical procedure

All procedures were performed at one facility by a single surgeon (TM) using one material; dextranomer/hyaluronic acid copolymer (Dx/HA). The surgeon had previously conducted endoscopic injection surgery using another material (Teflon) with two of the other authors (TY, YH) [12].

Cystography was conducted first under general or lumbar anesthesia. If reflux was observed, cystography was repeated intraoperatively. A pediatric urethral cystoscope with an offset lens (8-12Fr, 13 cm long; KARL STORZ K27030KA) was placed in position and the configuration of the ureteral orifice recorded. Subsequently, HD was performed to grade the dilation of the ureteral orifice under irrigation 40 cm above the patient's position but not exceeded 50% of the expected bladder capacity [7]. HD technique was originally introduced by Kirsh et al. [7], which direct a pressure stream of irrigation fluid into the ureter (hydrodistension) to define the site of injection within ureteral submucosa. HD grade was recorded according to the definition [13]. Briefly, H3 is defined as 'orifice opens and extramural ureter evident', H2; orifice opens and intramural tunnel evident, H1; orifice opens and intramural tunnel not evident, H0; no orifice distention evident. Although we recorded the contralateral HD grade, we did not perform prophylactic injection for single-sided VUR as is not approved by the Japanese healthcare insurance. Endoscopic injection was performed via STING [6], HIT [7], or double-HIT [8] methods, with some modifications adopted for large -caliber adult ureter (described below).

Injection method was selected according to HD grade. Briefly, in cases determined to be grade H3 when the cystoscope could be inserted through the intramural ureter, injection was performed confirming direction of injection needle align with the ureter and punctured at the proximal and distal portion without withdrawing the scope (referred to as inserting HIT/I-HIT) (Fig. 1) until a

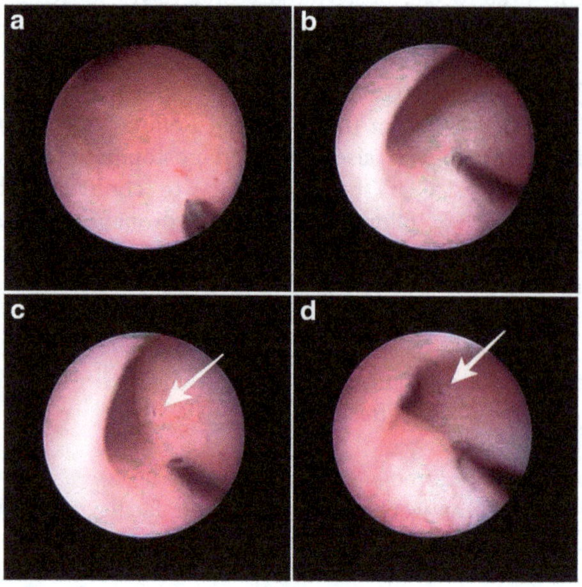

Fig. 1 Intraoperative photographs of inserting hydrodistension implantation technique (I-HIT). (**a**) First injection inside intramural ureter, (**b**) after small amount injected, (**c**) second injection near the first (arrow), (**d**) after second injection

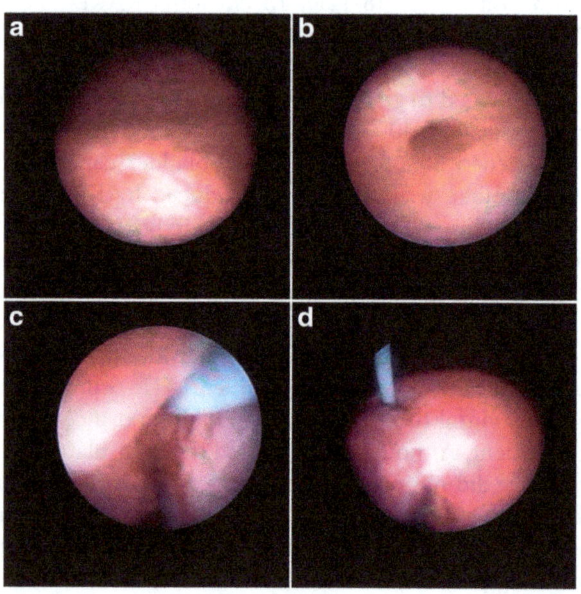

Fig. 2 Intraoperative photograph of guide-wired hydrodistension implantation technique (G-HIT). (**a**) The ureteral orifice looked like horseshoe and (**b**) Hydrodistension grade 2 appearance under hydrodistension, (**c**) injection using guidewire, (**d**) combined subureteral injection technique after the injection

high mound formed. In cases graded as H2, a guide wire was used to inject align to ureteral direction at the distal portion (referred to as guide-wired HIT/G-HIT) (Fig. 2). To create a volcano-like mound [14], Dx/HA was added in cases where STING was performed. In all procedures, the total injection volume was kept below 3.0 ml per ureter.

Postoperative evaluation

Success was defined as the absence of VUR as on VCUG at the 3-month follow-up. Following successful treatment of VUR by Dx/HA injection, antibiotic prophylaxis was discontinued, and patients were followed-up with regular urinalysis and ultrasound until 1 year postoperatively. A repeat VCUG was performed after successful endoscopic treatment when the patient had previously experienced at least one episode of f-UTI or repeated afebrile UTIs. Other adverse events including flunk pain, low abdominal pain, dysuria, or low- or high-grade fever were evaluated.

Statistical analysis

The Chi-square test or Fisher's exact test were used to compare two groups with respect to a dichotomous endpoint. The Mann–Whitney test was used to compare two groups with respect to a continuous endpoint such as injection time or volume. The Kruskal–Wallis H-test was used for comparisons between three groups. Statistical significance was set as P-value < 0.05. All reported p values are two-sided. All statistical analyses were performed using R statistical software (version 3.2.3, The R Foundation for Statistical Computing, Vienna, Austria).

Results

Preoperative evaluation

Twelve post-pubertal patients (all female, a total of 16 ureteral units) with a median age of 32 (range 15–61) years underwent endoscopic injection therapy at Nagoya East Medical Center (Table 1). Four patients had bilateral VUR, the other 8 exhibited single-sided VUR. The VUR was evaluated to be grade II in 5 ureters, grade III in 8 and grade IV in 3. Two patients had a history of anti-reflux surgery; one had undergone collagen injection remained single-sided grade III VUR, the other had undergone laparoscopic implantations by extravesical approach remained single -sided grade II VUR.

The HD grades of the ureteral orifice in relation to VUR grade and timing are summarized in Table 2. H3-dilation were presented in 12 ureters (75%) in the present cases. The portion of H3 ureters were increased as VUR grade increasing as VUR II: 40%; VUR III: 88%; 100%: VUR IV. Where filling VUR were pointed, H3 ureters were more evident: 78%; H2: 11%; H1; 11%.

Table 1 Patients data

Age (y), median (range)	32 (15–61)
Gender, n (%)	
Female	12 (100)
Male	0 (0)
Affected side, n	
Right	8
Left	8
Laterality, n	
Single side	8
Bilateral	4
VUR grade, n [ureteral units]	
II	5
III	8
IV	3
Indications for operation, n (%)	
Recurrent urinary tract infection	10 (83)
Failed anti-reflux operation	2 (17)
Post-op hospital stays (d), median (range)	3 (2-5)
Follow-up (m), median (range)	22 (13-63)

VUR vesico ureteral reflux

Table 2 Numbers of affected ureters for each grade of hydrodistension and vesicoureteral reflux

HD grade	VUR grade			
	II	III	IV	Total
	(n = 5)	(n = 8)	(n = 3)	(n = 16)
H1	0 [0]	1 [1]	0 [0]	1 [1]
H2	3 [1]	0 [0]	0 [0]	3 [1]
H3	2 [0]	7 [4]	3 [3]	12 [7]
Total	5 [1]	8 [5]	3 [3]	16 [9]

HD hydrodistension grade, *VUR* vesicoureteral reflux

Vesicoureteral reflux timing is presented in brackets as, n [filling vesicoureteral reflux]

Surgical procedure

The injection methods used in relation to HD grade and VUR grade were summarized in Table 3. I-HIT combined with STING method were conducted in 10 ureters (63%), following G-HIT combined with STING in 4 ureters (25%). The median number of injection sites (range) were, 4(3–6) points, 4(3–5) points, 3 points and 2 points, respectively. The median volume (range) were, 2.5 (1.2–3.0) ml, 2.0 (2.0–3.0) ml, 1.5 ml and 0.6 ml. These showed no significant differences between these 2 methods ($P = 0.203$ and $P = 0.102$, respectively). Exceptionally, in 2cases of H3 dilated ureter, G-HIT combined with STING method were used owing to distal ureteral deformities. In 1 case of H2 dilated ureter, was added the Dx/HA by the STING.

Surgical results

The flow chart of patients' progress is presented in Fig. 3. Postoperatively, VUR was diminished to grad 0 in 12 ureters (75%) and decreased to grade I in 3 ureters (19%). In patients-based words, 9 (75%) cases succeeded and 11 (92%) cured after the-first operation. Only one case, who underwent the first operation via I-HIT combined with STING method, remained as VUR grade III perceived successful second injection therapy; no patients required a third injection.

The success rates of each injection methods in terms of HD and VUR grades were summarized in Table 4. I-HIT combined with STING method, only conducted in H3 dilated ureters, succeeded in 7 (70%) ureters. G-HIT combined with STING method was successed in 3 (75%), G-HIT: 1 (100) % and STING: 1 (100%) ureter. There was no statistical difference ($P = 0.588$).

As for H3 dilated ureters, all of grade IV VUR were diminished apart from those in which the 'filling reflux' was present preoperatively, though 1 failed and 2 downgraded ureters with grade III VUR were exist. In 1

Table 3 Numbers of ureters according to selected injection methods for each grade of hydrodistension and vesicoureteral reflux

Injection method	HD grade			VUR grade		
	H1	H2	H3	II	III	IV
	(n = 1)	(n = 3)	(n = 12)	(n = 5)	(n = 8)	(n = 3)
I-HIT + STING			10	2	6	2
G-HIT + STING		2	2	2	1	1
G-HIT		1		1		
STING	1				1	

HD hydrodistension grade, *VUR* vesicoureteral reflux, *I-HIT* inserting hydrodistension implantation technique, *G-HIT* guide-wired hydrodistension implantation technique, *STING* subureteral transurethral injection

Intraoperative cystography showed VUR, in 3 of 4 cases of bilateral VUR confirmed preoperatively and 4 ipsilateral ureters from 8 patients with single-sided VUR. There were no cases of intraoperative VUR that had not been diagnosed preoperatively. There was not apparent correlation between postoperative and intraoperative VUR grade (data not shown)

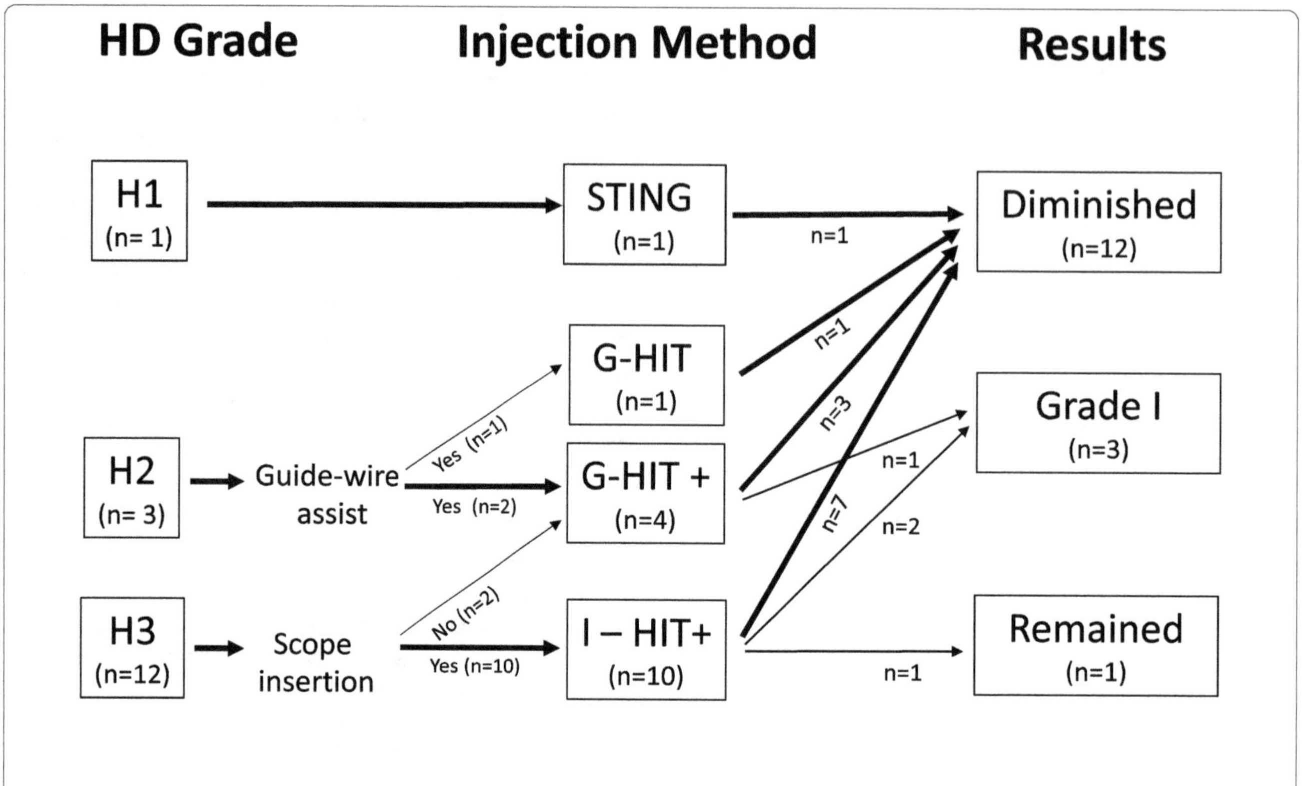

Fig. 3 Flowchart of patient progress during the study. *HD* hydrodistension grade, *VUR* vesicoureteral reflux, *I-HIT* inserting hydrodistension implantation technique, *G-HIT* guide-wired hydrodistension implantation technique, *STING* subureteral transurethral injection

Table 4 Numbers of succeeded ureters, n (%) according to each injection methods for each grade of hydrodistension and vesicoureteral reflux

Injection method	HD grade			VUR grade			*p* value [#]
	H1	H2	H3	II	III	IV	
	(n = 1)	(n = 3)	(n = 12)	(n = 5)	(n = 8)	(n = 3)	
I-HIT + STING			7 (70)*	2 (100)	3 (50)*	2 (100)	0.588
G-HIT + STING		1 (50)**	2 (100)	1 (50)**	1 (100)	1 (100)	
G-HIT		1 (100)		1 (100)			
STING	1 (100)				1 (100)		

HD hydrodistension grade, *VUR* vesicoureteral reflux, *I-HIT* inserting hydrodistension implantation technique, *G-HIT* guide-wired hydrodistension implantation technique, *STING* subureteral transurethral injection

*One failed 'dropped' ureter, 1 downgraded 'dropped' ureter, and 1 downgraded ureter after collagen injection therapy

** One downgraded 'kinked' ureter

Calculated by Fisher's exact test

bilateral case with 1 failed and 1 downgraded ureter, initially diagnosed as grade III VUR with H3 dilation, treatment of both sides was carried out via this method; one side remained grade III and another was downgraded to grade I postoperatively. Intraoperative cystoscopy had showed bilateral deformity of the distal ureter ('dropped ureters') because of large myoma or flaccid bladder. In the second operation, these were treated successfully via the same method, but injecting into more lateral portion of the intramural ureter where a sufficient mound was formed due to the softness of the tissue. The other case remained grade I VUR ureter exhibited insufficient mound height due to tissue stiffness owing to a history of collagen injection therapy. Another 2 cases with H3 dilated 'dropped ureter', one with grade IV and one with grade III VUR, were exceptionally treated via G-HIT combined with STING in order to inject into lateral portion of the distal ureter, where softness of the tissue was suspected, and resulted successful outcomes.

As for H2 cases, 1 patient had a history of laparoscopic implantations by extravesical approach and had remained grade II VUR was treated successfully via G-HIT combined with STING method. Although the other remained grade I VUR case, lateral lifting ('kinking') of the H2 dilated ureter due to deviation of the uterus lead to insufficient mound height.

Complications and comorbidity

Temporary postoperative mild HN (G1 or G2) occurred in three ureteral units (19%) at 1 month postoperatively. These HN disappeared until 3 months without any urinary-tract infection. Dull flank pain was reported by three patients for several days postoperatively, which was safely managed with painkillers like acetaminophen. Only one case experienced acute left-sided pyelonephritis requiring antibiotic infusion for 3 days before discharge. In this case, contralateral right-side ureter was treated first, although intraoperative cystography showed grade I VUR in left side. During follow-up duration; median 23 (range 13–63) months long, 9 patients were suffered no f-UTI. Although, 3 patients were experienced f-UTI 1–2 times, repeated VCUG showed no VUR recurrence.

In one of 12 cases (6%), contralateral VUR (i.e., occult VUR) newly recognized grade IV was detected after 1.5 years of follow-up without any f-UTI, while intraoperative cystoscopy had detected H2 dilation of ureteral orifices and lateral positioning.

Discussion

The present study demonstrates that endoscopic injection therapy is an effective and safe treatment for VUR in post-pubertal female patients. Conducted via modified HIT techniques adopted for dilated ureteral orifice, we achieved successful results in 75% of patients and over 90% of patients were cured after the first operation. In the present study, although post-pubertal female patients had some risks to injection therapy i.e. ureteral deformity or history of anti-reflux surgery that cause tissue stiffness, our meticulous method to select adequate site in the dilated ureter overcame those risks.

A previous meta-analysis has shown that refinement of injection materials and methods has led to the present success rate over 70% in children [15]. Recently, by a single experienced pediatric urologist, HIT has been reported to have a high success rate in adult [16], although this was among patients with mainly low-grade VUR. The present study demonstrates high success rates even in grade IV filling VUR applying modified HIT techniques adopted for adult ureters.

Reported predictors for success include a volcano-like mound appearance [17], mound height (as assessed by ultrasound) [18] and injection volume [19]. Moreover, VUR grade [20] and timing of VUR are suspected predictors [21]. And also, HD grade could be another predictor, seeing the fact HD grade is reported to have high correlation with VUR grade [13], in accordance with our present results. In adult ureter, additional risks are exist seeing the present study, like that the deformity ('dropped' or 'kinked') and the pathological stiffness owing to historical change more evident in adult ureters.

To manage these requirements, the injection must be conducted carefully with the needle align with the ureter puncturing at the adequate location where good tissue-softness guaranteed, so as to ensure enough mound appearance and height. We used two kinds of methods, I-HIT or G-HIT, with technique-selection according to HD grade adopted for large-caliber adult ureter. As a result, we found high success rate even in grade IV VUR. The flow chart that we developed and is presented here may provide a guide for the selection of injection technique.

In the present study, we found ureteral deformities or a history of anti-reflux surgery were associated with reduced success of outcomes. Anatomical anomalies like complete duplicated ureter pose a challenge to injection [22]; therefore, ureterocele and Hutch diverticulum are considered contraindications for endoscopic injection therapy [23]. In these complicated ureters, care must be taken to inject with an adequate volume to create sufficient mound height. These risks may be ameliorated using meticulous methods like I-HIT or G-HIT.

In the present study, we have experienced one case of acute pyelonephritis requiring antibiotic infusion before discharge. In this case, single sided VUR confirmed by intraoperative cystography may lead to subsequent f-UTI. Maintaining bladder volume and considering the intraoperative VUR could result in better outcomes. In this meaning, intraoperative cystography has some benefit.

This study showed the prevalence of occult VUR to be considerable postoperatively (6%). Although intraoperative cystography is not recommended for detection of occult VUR owing to its low sensitivity [24], other methods to predict occult VUR are needed. Alternatively, protective injection according to HD grade could be recommended [25], so that VUR grade is reported to have high correlation with HD grade [21] as mentioned in the former section.

We recommend 6 months of follow-up including ultrasound examination after surgery, based on our finding that temporary postoperative HN until 3 months occurred in nearly 20% of patients. One of the risks of obstruction, the beak sign of ureterovesical junction [16], may have contributed to any case of persistent HN.

The present study had some limitations which should be acknowledged. First, this was a retrospective study with a small sample size. However, we included all consecutive patients, and all operations were performed by a single urologist at a single institution, thereby reducing bias relating to the cohort. Secondly, not all patients underwent repeated VCUG after successful treatment. Although late recurrence was reported in 20% of cases over the 2 years [26–28]. Three-month postoperative VCUG examinations are widely performed while late VCUG is not routinely performed due to the radiation exposure involved [29]. We performed regular urinalysis and ultrasound postoperatively and would recommend that repeated VCUG is performed in cases where at least one episode of f-UTI or repeated afebrile UTI are experienced. Long-term follow-up including ultrasound or dimercaptosuccinic acid examination of growth and blood pressure is important for patients with renal scarring [30]. Further randomized clinical trials with larger cohorts evaluating long-term clinical outcomes, prevention of f-UTI, and renal function are required to fully confirm the efficacy and safety of injection therapy in adult patients.

Conclusions

In this study, we have showed that endoscopic injection therapy can achieve a high success rate with few complications even in post-pubertal female patients. While ureteral deformities or a history of anti-reflux surgery may increase the risks, these can be managed with appropriate methods that ensure sufficient mound appearance and height. Via modified HIT techniques according to HD grade of the ureteral orifice, endoscopic injection therapy is an effective and safe treatment for VUR in post-pubertal female patients.

Abbreviations

Dx/HA: Dextranomer/hyaluronic acid copolymer; f-UTI: Febrile urinary tract infection; HIT: Hydrodistension implantation technique; HD: Hydrodistension; STING: Subureteral transurethral injection; VUR: Vesicoureteral reflux; VCUG: Voiding cystourethrography.

Acknowledgements

We would like to thank Editage for English language editing.

Authors' contributions

Conception and design: TM and YH; enrollment of patients and acquisition of data: TM, TH, and YI; drafting of the manuscript: TM, KM, and YH; statistical analysis: TM, HN, and TK; analysis and interpretation of data: TM, KM, TH, and YI; manuscript editing: TM, KM, HN, TK, and YH; supervision: TY. We confirm that all authors read and approved the final manuscript.

Competing interests

The authors declare that they have no competing interests.

Author details

[1]Department of Urology, Nagoya City East Medical Center, 2 Wakamizu-cho, Chikusa-ku, Nagoya 464-8547, Japan. [2]Department of Pediatric Urology, Nagoya City University Graduate School of Medical Sciences, 1 Kawasumi, Mizuho-cho, Mizuho-ku, Nagoya 467-8601, Japan. [3]Department of Nephro-Urology, Nagoya City University Graduate School of Medical Sciences, 1 Kawasumi, Mizuho-cho, Mizuho-ku, Nagoya 467-8601, Japan.

References

1. Antoine EK, Darius JB. Management strategies for vesicoureteral reflux. In: Partin AW, editor. Campbell-Walsh-Wein Urology. 12th ed. Philadelphia: Elsevier; 2020. p. 490.
2. Chand DH, Rhoades T, Poe SA, et al. Incidence and severity of vesicoureteral reflux in children related to age, gender, race and diagnosis. J Urol. 2003;170:1548–50.
3. Hubert KC, Kokorowski PJ, Huang L, et al. Durability of antireflux effect of ureteral reimplantation for primary vesicoureteral reflux: findings on long-term cystography. Urology. 2012;79:675–9.
4. Routh JC, Bogaert GA, Kaefer M, Manzoni G, et al. Vesicoureteral reflux: current trends in diagnosis, screening, and treatment. Eur Urol. 2012;61:773–82.
5. Kurtz MP, Leow JJ, Varda BK, et al. The decline of the open ureteral reimplant in the United States: national data from 2003 to 2013. Urology. 2017;100:193–7.
6. O'Donnell B, Puri P. Treatment of vesicoureteral reflux by endoscopic injection of Teflon. Br Med J (Clin Res Ed). 1984;289:7–9.
7. Kirsch AJ, Perez-Brayfield M, Smith EA, et al. The modified sting procedure to correct vesicoureteral reflux: improved results with submucosal implantation within the intramural ureter. J Urol. 2004;171:2413–6.
8. Kirsch AJ, Arlen AM, Lackgren G. Current trends in dextranomer hyaluronic acid copolymer (Deflux) injection technique for endoscopic treatment of vesicoureteral reflux. Urology. 2014;84:462–8.
9. Miyakita H, Hayashi Y, Mitsui T, et al. Guidelines for medical management of pediatric vesicoureteral reflux. Int J Urol. 2020;27:480–90.
10. Kojima Y, Mizuno K, Umemoto Y, et al. Ureteral advancement in patients undergoing laparoscopic extravesical ureteral reimplantation for treatment of vesicoureteral reflux. J Urol. 2012;188:582–7.
11. Hayashi Y, Mizuno K, Kurokawa S, et al. Extravesical robot-assisted laparoscopic ureteral reimplantation for vesicoureteral reflux: initial experience in Japan with the ureteral advancement technique. Int J Urol. 2014;21:1016–21.
12. Yasui T, Akita H, Sasaki S, et al. Endoscopic injection of Teflon for correction of primary vesicoureteral reflux in children. Int J Urol. 1997;4:349–51.
13. Kirsch AJ, Kaye JD, Cerwinka WH, et al. Dynamic hydrodistension of the ureteral orifice: a novel grading system with high reproducibility and clinical correlation in children with vesicoureteral reflux and urinary tract infection. J Urol. 2009;82:688–92.
14. Lavelle MT, Conlin MJ, Skoog SJ, et al. Subureteral injection of Deflux for correction of reflux: analysis of factors predicting success. Urology. 2005;65:564–7.
15. Elder JS, Diaz M, Caldamone AA, et al. Endoscopic therapy for vesicoureteral reflux: a meta-analysis. I. Reflux resolution and urinary tract infection. J Urol. 2006;175:716–22.
16. Moore K, Bolduc S. Treatment of vesicoureteral reflux in adults by endoscopic injection. Urology. 2011;77:1284–7.
17. Chertin B, Mele E, Kocherov S, et al. What are the predictive factors leading to ureteral obstruction following endoscopic correction of VUR in the pediatric population? J Pediatr Urol. 2018;14(538):1–7.
18. Zambaiti E, Pensabene M, Montano V, et al. Ultrasonographic mound height as predictor of vesicoureteral reflux resolution after endoscopic treatment in children. J Pediatr Surg. 2016;51:366–9.
19. Yucel S, Gupta A, Snodgrass W. Multivariate analysis of factors predicting success with dextranomer/hyaluronic acid injection for vesicoureteral reflux. J Urol. 2007;177:1505–9.

20. Routh JC, Reinberg Y. Predicting success in the endoscopic management of pediatric vesicoureteral reflux. Urology. 2010;76:195–8.
21. Han DS, Cambareri G, Alagiri M, et al. Reflux timing is a predictor of successful endoscopic treatment of vesicoureteral reflux. Urology. 2019;124:237–40.
22. Miyakita H, Ninan GK, Puri P. Endoscopic correction of Vesico-ureteric reflux in duplex systems. Eur Urol. 1993;24:111–5.
23. Routh JC, Kramer SA, Inman BA, et al. Utility of dextranomer hyaluronic acid injection in setting of bladder and ureteral anomalies. Urology. 2008;71:03–11.
24. López PJ, Reed F, Ovalle A, et al. Intraoperative cystography pre- and post-endoscopic treatment for vesicoureteral reflux: guaranteed success? J Pediatr Urol. 2014;10:831–4.
25. Cerwinka WH, Kaye JD, Traci L, et al. Selective endoscopic treatment of the non-refluxing contralateral ureter prevents new contralateral vesicoureteral reflux. J Pediatr Urol. 2013;9:51–6.
26. Holmdahl G, Brandstrom P, Lackgren G, et al. The Swedish reflux trial in children II: vesicoureteral reflux outcome. J Urol. 2010;184:280.
27. Sedberry-Ross S, Rice DC, Hans G, et al. Febrile urinary tract infections in children with an early negative voiding cystourethrogram after treatment of vesicoureteral reflux with dextranomer/hyaluronic acid. J Urol. 2008;180:1605.
28. Hunziker M, Mohanan N, D'Asta F, et al. Incidence of febrile urinary tract infections in children after successful endoscopic treatment of vesicoureteral reflux: a long-term follow-up. J Pediatr. 2012;160:1015–20.
29. Palmer L. The role of intraoperative cystography following the injection of dextranomer/hyaluronic acid copolymer. J Urol. 2008;179:1118–21.
30. Peters CA, Skoog SJ, Arant BS Jr, et al. Summary of the AUA guideline on management of primary vesicoureteral reflux in children. J Urol. 2010;184:1134.

21

Ureteral polyps protruding from the urethra

Zhi-Wei Sun, Jian-Kang Ge, You Wu and Ye-Qing Huang*

Abstract

Background: Ureteral fibro-epithelial polyp (UFP) is a rare benign ureteral tumor, and surgical removal of the polyps is still the preferred solution. Although many cases have reported polyps extending to the bladder, our case was the first to report a huge UFP that underwent endoscopic laser resection to highlight the urethra and cause severe end hematuria permanently.

Case presentation: In 2019, a 37-year-old woman came to the hospital because of hematuria and a dark red extraurethral mass. CTU inspection showed: filling defect between the right ureter and the bladder at the entrance of the bladder. After ureteroscopy, it was found that the ureteral mass came out of the urethral orifice. Then, under the direct view of the ureteroscope, a Ho:YAG laser was used to remove the tumor by cutting off along the its base, and the patient was discharged 3 days after the operation.

Conclusion: Urethral polyps from the ureter should be considered in the differential diagnosis of urethral neoplasms. Ho:YAG laser resection under ureteroscopy is an effective option for treating UFP, but be careful of ureteral stricture after surgery.

Keywords: Ureteral fibro-epithelial polyp, Protrusion through urethra, Ureteroscopy, Case report

Background

Ureteral fibro-epithelial polyp (UFP) is a rare benign ureteral tumor that causes symptoms, such as hematuria, low back pain, frequent urination, and difficulty in urinating. Various factors, including congenital malformation, obstruction, trauma, irritation, infection, and specific-derived hormone imbalance, contribute to this disease [1]. Its specific etiological mechanism is still unknown. Ludwig reported that the median size of UFP was 4 cm, and no statistical difference was observed for the occurrence on both sides [2]. Moreover, the upper part of the ureter was the most common origin of these polyps. In this case, we report a severe lower end ureteral polyp in middle-aged women with severe terminal hematuria and permanent protrusion of the urethra from the polyp. Reports of such a large UFP outside the urethra are rare.

*Correspondence: qingye3@126.com
Department of Urology, Affiliated Hospital of Nantong University, No. 20 Xisi Road, Nantong, China

Case presentation

A 37-year-old female patient experienced intermittent hematuria with dysuria for 10 days, with dark red vegetation prolapsed from the urethra during urination. The patient had no evident urinary urgency, pyuria, waist discomfort, or fever. During the physical examination, a dark red strip-shaped mass protruded from the urethral orifice. This mass was soft, and its root could not be explored (Fig. 1). Ultrasound showed a 36 mm × 17 mm mild hydronephrosis in the right kidney, and other echoes were observed at the opening of the bladder in the lower part of the right ureter (Fig. 2a). The inner diameter of the lower end of the right ureter was 8 mm, and the inner diameter of the upper segment was 6 mm. Computed tomography urography (CTU) examination showed a strip filling defect at the entrance of the bladder on the right ureter (Fig. 2b). The filling of the bladder was satisfactory, and a nodular filling defect was observed on the posterior wall (Fig. 2c). Afterwards, the patient received ureteroscopy diagnosis under general anesthesia. During operation, the exposed

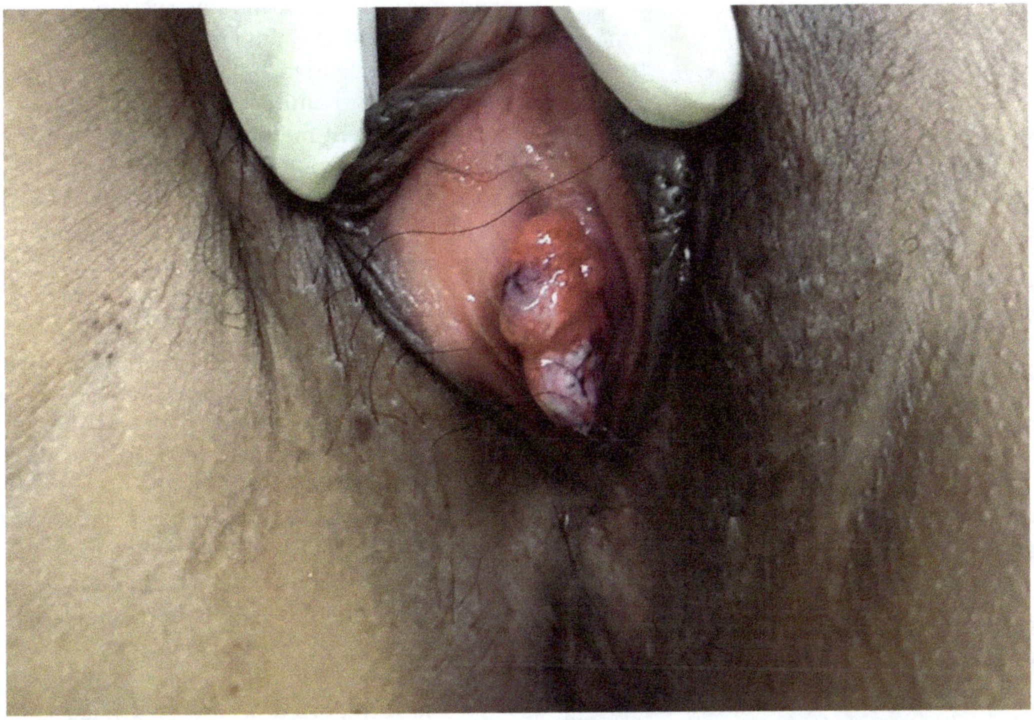

Fig. 1 Long mass protruding from the urethral opening

mass was held with tissue forceps, and the tension was slightly maintained. A ureteroscope was used to examine the bladder through the urethra (Fig. 3a), and the mass was seen protruding from the right ureteral opening (Fig. 3b). The silk and ureteroscope were utilized to assess the right ureter, and the base of the mass was found in the middle and lower section of the right ureter (Fig. 3d). The mass was strip-shaped, the surface was smooth, and no obvious hemorrhage and necrosis were observed. The basal mucosa of the mass showed edema, and the tumor tissue did not completely block the ureteral cavity (Fig. 3c). Then, under the direct view of the ureteroscope, a 200 mm Ho:YAG laser fiber with an energy setting of 1 J and a frequency of 15 Hz was used to remove the tumor by cutting off along the its base. The tissue was clamped out of the tumor, and the right ureter was placed with an F5 double J tube. The long grape-shaped mass was 12 cm in length with a smooth surface. The diameter of the tube was approximately 0.8–1.8 cm, and the edema was translucent (Fig. 4a). Combined with hematoxylin and eosin staining (Fig. 4b) and immunohistochemical nucleus Gata3 (+) (Fig. 4c), CK20 (−) in the cytoplasm (Fig. 4d) was diagnosed as a polyp formed by ureteric epithelial proliferation. The double J tube was removed 3 months after the operation by ureteroscopy which was performed to review the wound. The patient received the urinary system B-ultrasound 6 months after the operation, indicating no ureteral stenosis or hydronephrosis.

Discussion and conclusion

UFPs are rare benign ureteral tumors, accounting for 1% of all urogenital tumors. The proximal ureter is the most common origin of these polyps [3], and polyps from the lower urinary tract are uncommon. The symptoms of UFP depend on the size and condition of the polyp. The typical symptoms include hematuria, low back pain, frequent urination, and dysuria [2]. Although this patient has hematuria and mild hydronephrosis, but she came

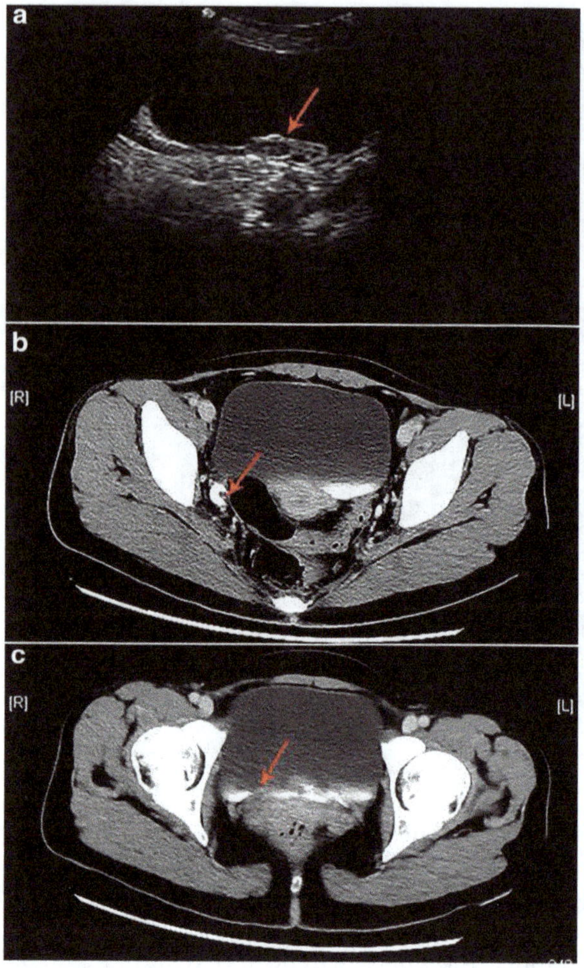

Fig. 2 **a** First-class echo at the bladder opening in the lower ureter. **b** Filling defect between the right ureter and the bladder at the entrance of the bladder. **c** Filling of the bladder is acceptable, and no nodular filling defect is observed in the posterior wall. (shown by the red arrow)

to the hospital due to an unknown mass protruding from the urethra.

Imaging studies can help diagnose UFP. Intravenous pyelography or CTU can show filling defects and can also reveal the possibility of hydronephrosis, which suggests the patient's renal function status. Most importantly, distinguishing UFP from transitional cell carcinoma based on imaging findings alone may be difficult [4]. Thus, ureteroscopy is also needed for patients suspected of UFP assessed by intravenous pyelography, computed tomography or retrograde urography for diagnosis and treatment. The shape, number of tumors, the base diameter, and the location of the obstruction can be determined simultaneously by ureteroscopy. Preliminary judgments about benign and malignant tumors will be noted.

To date, no uniform standard is available for the main treatment methods for ureteral polyps, and surgical removal of polyps is still the preferred solution. In this case, ureteroscopy reveals that the single polyp is extremely long and originated from the lower part of the ureter. The strip-shaped mass has a smooth surface with no obvious hemorrhage and necrosis. The mucosa at the base of the mass is edema. For ureteral polyps, the surgical field of the basal floor is clear, and then intraluminal resection is selected. At the same time, a Double-J stent is placed to prevent ureteral stricture after surgery. Endoscopic resection has minimal trauma to the patient but with rapid post-operative recovery and minimizes the risk of ureteral stenosis and renal impairment [5]. For patients with malignant and multiple tumors, poor ureteroscopy is unable to expose the base of the polyp, which is not suitable for endoscopic resection. In this case, laparoscopic or open surgery can be opted.

We have reported a case of a huge UFP originating from a 12 cm UFP distal to the right ureter, which completely protrudes from the urethral opening, and the polyps were removed by laser under ureteroscopy. In 2013, Ali Momenzadeh et al. reported a case of large UFP presenting a vegetative bladder mass excised ureteroscopically and recommended further assessment for any mass juxtaposed vesicoureteral junction and also suggest ureteroscopically approach to distal UFPs, it was the first report from IRAN [6]. At present, the literature has reported many similar cases of ureteral polyps extending into the bladder cavity, only one case report a UFPs with permanent extension beyond the bladder cavity through the urethra, this 19-year-old patient had two UFPs from the distal left ureter, they used cautery to remove the entire polyp under the endoscope [7]. According to the Ludwig D.J, due to advances in technology, more UFP cases had been treated by electrocautery or YAG laser through ureteroscopy since 1980s, with no reported recurrence. Abdominal CTU after 3 months and urinary system ultrasound after 1 year to detect possible recurrence (ureteral stenosis and hydronephrosis) were recommended during the surveillance of this pathology [2]. Our case reports a huge UFP with permanent extension beyond the bladder cavity through the urethra, which is the first case in China. Simultaneously, immunohistochemistry assay was performed to strong evidence for our diagnosis.

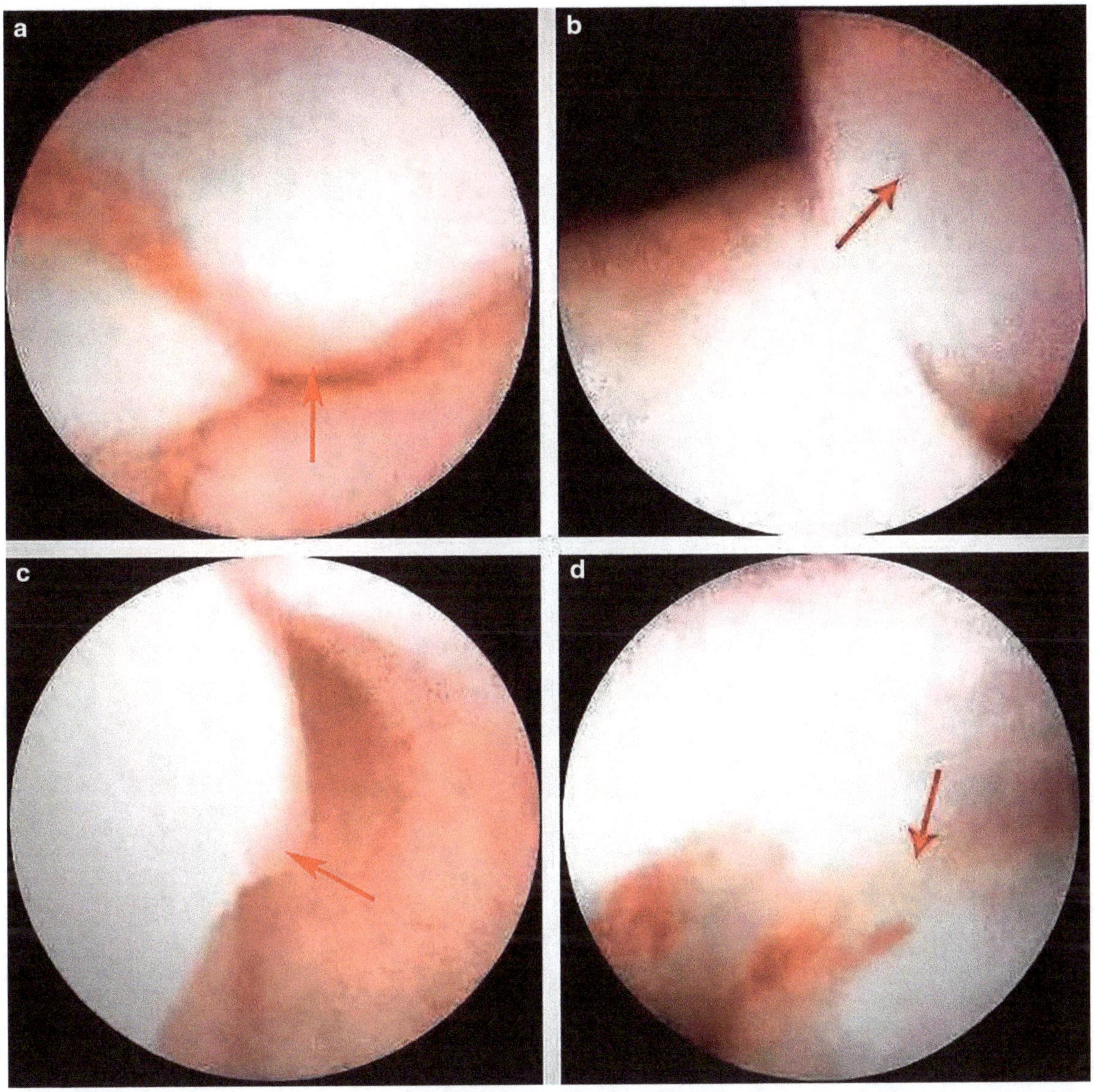

Fig. 3 Ureteroscopy during surgery. **a** Sees the tumor protruding through the urethra; **b** sees the tumor protruding from the opening of the right ureter; **c** does not completely block the ureteral cavity; **d** sees the base of the tumor (shown by the red arrow)

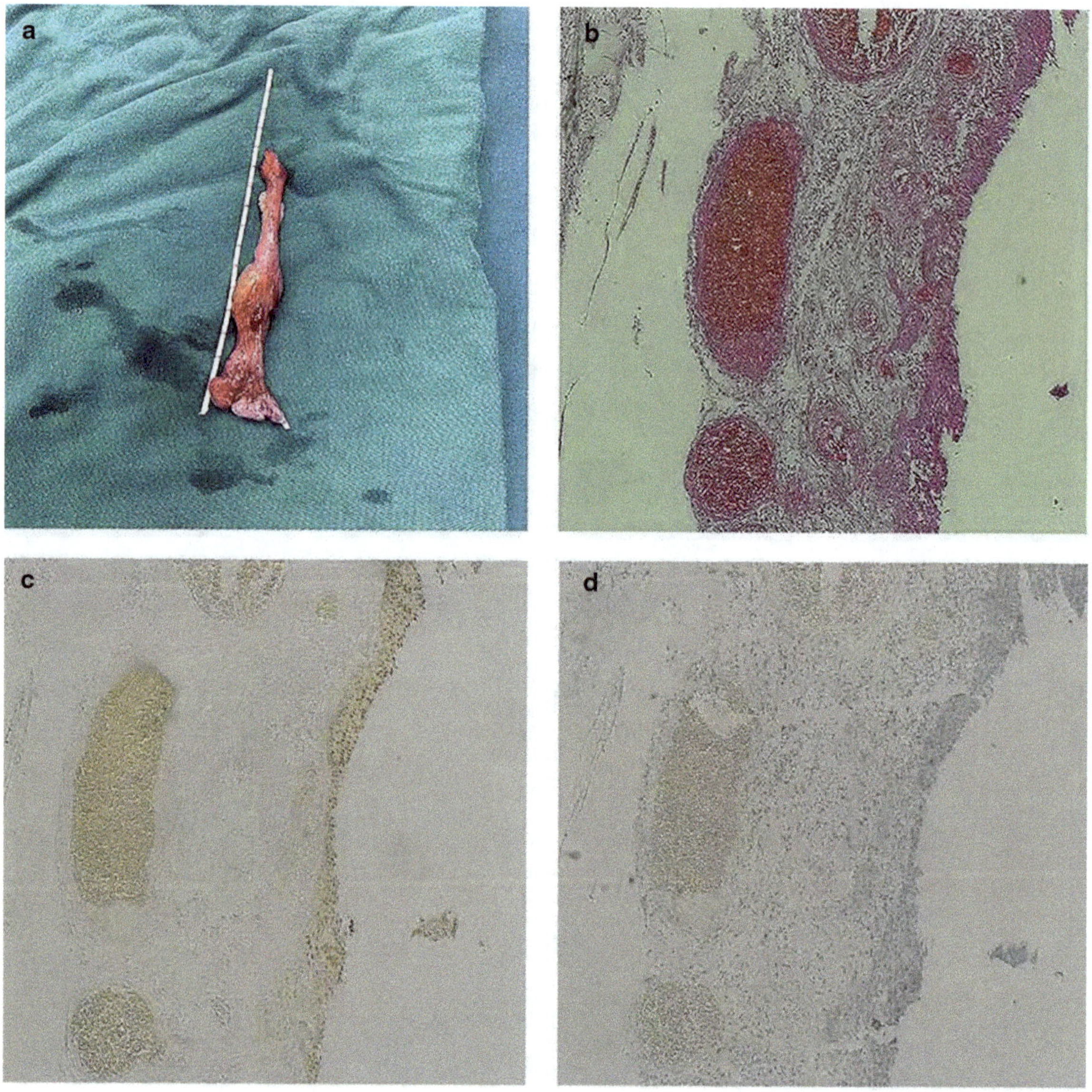

Fig. 4 **a** Gross specimens and pathology after surgery. The total length of the tumor is approximately 12 cm, the surface is smooth, the diameter of the tube is approximately 0.8–1.8 cm, the cut surface is grayish red, and the edema is translucent. **b** H & E staining (× 100) showed that urothelial hyperplasia conformed to polypoid changes, but no dysplasia or malignancy. **c** Immunohistochemistry indicates positive Gata3 nucleus. **d** Immunohistochemistry indicates negative CK20 cytoplasm

Abbreviations

UFP: Ureteral fibro-epithelial polyp; CTU: Computed tomography urography.

Authors' contributions

ZWS: Design and drafting of the article, and final approval of the version to be submitted. JKG: Data acquisition, drafting of the article, and final approval of the version to be submitted. WY: Data acquisition, critical revision of the article, and final approval of the version to be submitted. YQH: Critical revision of the article, and final approval of the version to be submitted. All authors read and approved the final manuscript.

Competing interests

The authors declare that they have no competing interests.

References

1. Ye L, Zhao LJ, Yue F, Song XS, Wei W, Jiang XJ, et al. Large ureteral fibroepithelial polyp lacking epithelium due to ischemic infarction. Kaohsiung J Med Sci. 2012;28:457–61.
2. Ludwig DJ, Buddingh KT, Kums JJ, Kropman RF, Roshani H, Hirdes WH. Treatment and outcome of fibroepithelial ureteral polyps: A systematic literature review. Can Urol Assoc J. 2015;9:E631–7.
3. Piovesan AC, Torricelli FC, Borges LL, Chambo JL, Mesquita JL, Srougi M. Ureteral fibroepithelial polyps in a pregnant woman: case report. Sao Paulo Med J. 2009;127:238–40.
4. Patheyar V, Venkatesh SK, Siew EP, Consiglieri DT, Putti T. MR imaging features of fibroepithelial ureteral polyp in a patient with duplicated upper urinary tract. Singapore Med J. 2011;52:e45–7.

5. Hubosky SG, Bagley DH. Laser Resection of Fibroepithelial Polyps with Digital Ureteroscopy. J Endourol Case Rep. 2015;1:36–8.
6. Momenzadeh A, Sarrafzadeh F, Nourbala MH, Saburi A, Telkabadi Z. Giant ureteral fibroepithelial polyp presenting as a bladder mass resected ureteroscopically: a case report. Nephrourol Mon. 2013;5:706–8.
7. Abdessater M, Kanbar A, Khoury JE, Hachem CE, Halabi R, Boustany J, et al. Endourologic treatment for a fibroepithelial ureteral polyp protruding from the urethra. J Surg Case Rep. 2019;2019:rjz320.

22

Lateral herniation during treatment with collagenase Clostridium histolyticum (Xiaflex) for Peyronie's disease

Margaret K. Gannon* and Amy M. Pearlman

Abstract

Background: Collagenase Clostridium histolyticum (CCH), also know as Xiaflex, with penile modeling is considered to be the gold standard non-surgical option for management of Peyronie's disease and is known to be safe and efficacious. Corporal rupture is a rare but known adverse event of CCH treatment, however there are limited studies describing corporal herniation without rupture. Here we present a patient who experienced a rare complication following CCH injections for Peyronie's disease: lateral herniation of the tunica albuginea in the setting of a dorsal penile plaque.

Case presentation: A 58-year-old male presented to our clinic seeking treatment for Peyronie's disease. On exam, he was found to have a palpable dorsal plaque and > 30 degrees leftward curvature of the penis. He was deemed an appropriate candidate for and patient decided to proceed with CCH and modeling. He received 2 cycles of CCH injections (4 total CCH injections) with in-office and at-home penile modeling, per manufacturer's protocol. Two weeks following in-office modeling during his second CCH cycle, the patient reported a painless, soft swelling involving the left side of his penile shaft only occurring with erection. Exam and history were suggestive of lateral herniation rather than corporal rupture. CCH was discontinued. Patient declined further evaluation with penile ultrasound.

Conclusions: This is the first case report detailing lateral herniation with CCH injections. Symptoms and exam that should raise suspicion of corporal herniation are a soft, painless mass with erection.

Keywords: Xiaflex, Herniation, Peyronie's disease, Collagenase, Collagenase Clostridium histolyticum

Background

Peyronie's disease is a penile condition characterized by pain, curvature, and/or shortening of the penis and is often associated with erectile dysfunction and difficulty engaging in sexual intercourse [1]. Disorganized and excessive deposition of collagen likely results in the formation of a fibrous penile plaque within the tunica albuginea [2], most commonly observed in the dorsal midline [3].

Collagenase Clostridium histolyticum (CCH), also known as Xiaflex, injections with in-office and at-home penile modeling is an effective treatment option for reducing penile curvature for patients with Peyronie's disease who meet specific inclusion criteria [4]. Common adverse events include penile hematoma formation (50.2%), pain (33.5%), and swelling (28.9%), however, these often resolve without intervention [1]. One of the most serious adverse events is corporal body rupture/penile fracture (0.9%) which may be related to modeling, resumption of sexual intercourse prior to recommended hiatus, or the injection itself [5].

Here, we present a patient who experienced a rarely reported complication following CCH injections for

*Correspondence: margegannonmd@gmail.com
Department of Urology, Carver College of Medicine, University of Iowa, Iowa City, IA, USA

Peyronie's disease: a lateral herniation following injection of a dorsal penile plaque.

Case presentation

A 58-year-old Caucasian male with history of hyperlipidemia and recurrent nephrolithiasis presented to our clinic with treatment naive Peyroni's disease. The patient reported a stable, leftward penile curvature that had been present for 3 years. The patient denied pain with erections or erectile dysfunction, however the curvature was affecting his ability to have intercourse. Using a goniometer to measure his curvature in the erect state, he was noted to have 20 and 32 degrees of leftward curvature at proximal one third and distal one third of penile shaft, respectively. A dorsal penile plaque was palpated approximately 2 cm distal to the penopubic junction. After discussing treatment options, the patient decided to proceed with CCH injections and penile modeling.

The patient received 0.58 mg intralesional CCH injection at the side of maximal curvature (the distal 1/3 of the penile shaft for this patient) on 2 occasions 1 day apart followed by in-office modeling 6 days after the second CCH injection, per protocol. He performed regular at-home penile modeling for 6 weeks. The patient then repeated the above injections, in-office modeling procedure, and daily at-home stretches, per protocol, for 2 total cycles. Other than transient ecchymosis, there were no complications or adverse events following either of the CCH cycles.

The patient returned to clinic 6 weeks after completion of his second round of CCH injections to receive the first injection of his third cycle, however, he reported painless swelling on the left side of his penile shaft that he noticed 2 weeks after the second CCH injection of his second cycle. He denied engaging in intercourse, experiencing penile trauma or hearing any "popping" associated with the onset of the swelling. On exam, the flaccid penis did not have a palpable corporal defect, tunical thickening, or hematoma, and appeared grossly normal. Exam following a 20 mcg alprostadil injection showed a small amount of swelling was noted on the left side of the penile shaft distal to the base of the penile shaft (Figs. 1, 2). The swelling was soft and nontender without any overlying skin changes. The third cycle of CCH was deferred and the patient was instructed to wrap the penis in Coban and return to clinic in 1 week to reassess the swelling. At time of follow up, the patient reported continued outpouching of his left erectile body with erections. A repeat exam following a 20 mcg alprostdil injection was consistent with his previous exam. The patient declined further investigation of the swelling with Doppler ultrasound.

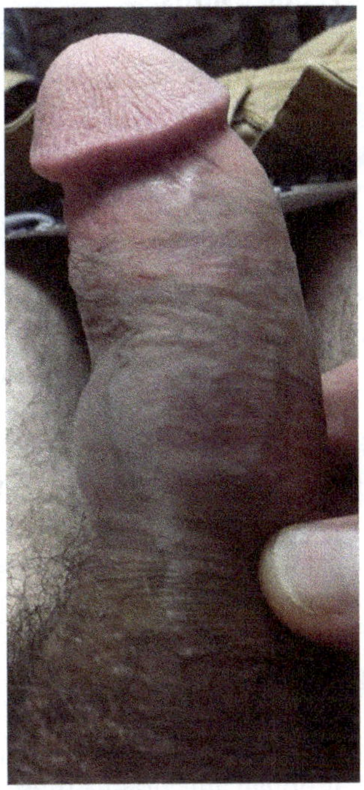

Fig. 1 Lateral penile swelling following second cycle of Xiaflex/penile modeling; superior view

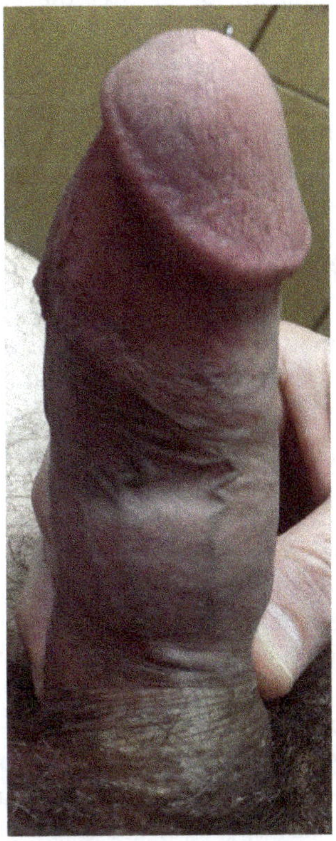

Fig. 2 Lateral penile swelling following second cycle of Xiaflex/penile modeling; lateral view

Discussion and conclusions

This case illustrates a rarely reported complication of lateral herniation following CCH injections and penile modeling.

CCH with penile modeling is considered to be the gold standard non-surgical option for management of Peyronie's disease [6]. The safety and efficacy of CCH has been demonstrated in large scale well-designed clinical trials [4, 5] and the adverse events of the treatment are well-known. Most patients (~93%) treated with CCH and modeling report at least one treatment associated adverse event, most commonly penile hematoma (≥25% of patients) [5]. Although most patients do experience treatment related adverse events, the vast majority are only mild or moderate in severity [5]. The minority of patients (~10%) who experience severe treatment related adverse events most commonly experience a severe penile hematoma (3.7%).

Corporal rupture or penile fracture is also a known treatment related serious adverse event of CCH and modeling. Large scale clinical trials have reported rates of less than 1%, although anecdotally there is controversy among experts about the prevalence of corporal rupture with CCH treatments. One study surveying providers reported a rupture rate of 34%, and found that most occurred after the second CCH cycle (28%) and 16% of those ruptures did not occur over the plaque/injection site [7].

The unique aspect of this case is that our patient's adverse event described above was not consistent with a corporal rupture but rather lateral herniation, not well characterized in the existing literature. In fact, only one published case report has ever described this phenomenon [8]. Similar to our patient, this case report describes a painless, soft penile mass present only during erections. Doppler penile ultrasound confirmed the mass was vascular and upon surgical exploration, the patient was found to have local tunical attenuation and an aneurysmal dilation of the corpora. Tunica herniation was briefly mentioned in Brant et al. as a complication seen when injecting CCH into lateral penile plaques. In fact, the authors recommend avoiding CCH injections for lateral plaques in order to prevent herniation or microrupture of the tunica based on their anecdotal experience [9]. Although studies citing lateral herniation of the tunica following CCH are limited, it may be that this complication happens more than is currently appreciated in the current literature.

This case highlights a tunical herniation that did not occur at the site of the plaque or previous CCH injections. We can only speculate about the etiology of this complication. We do know that the lateral tunica thickness is less than that of the dorsal/ventral tunica (0.8 mm vs 2.2 mm), making it more susceptible to injury [10]. At-home modeling protocol involves stretching of the penis in its flaccid state, as well as straightening of the penis when erect, as per recommended protocol. It is possible that the patient may have caused trauma to the tunica during modeling though the patient denied any known occurrence of trauma. It is possible that the Peyronie's disease complex of disordered collagen deposition and scar tissue formation had weakened the tunica in locations other than where a palpable plaque was formed. Alternatively, a CCH injection into healthy tissue or extravasation of the medication with manipulation of the needle in and out of the plaque could have compromised the surrounding tunica, although injections for our patient were localized to his plaque according to detailed procedure notes.

This is the first case report detailing lateral herniation following CCH injections and penile modeling for a palpable dorsal plaque. Symptoms of corporal herniation are a soft, painless mass with erection, and diagnosis can be confirmed with imaging or surgical exploration. Although this condition is rare, it is important to characterize such injuries so we can better understand how to prevent and manage them.

Abbreviation

CCH: Collagenase Clostridium histolyticum.

Authors' contributions

MG and AP both contributed to the writing and editing of the case report. All authors have read and approved the manuscript for publish.

Competing interests

Amy Pearlman is a consultant for Endo Pharmaceuticals.

References

1. Shin D, Shah T, Sadeghi-Nejad H. Xiaflex for treatment of Peyronie's disease. Eur Urol Focus. 2018;4(3):302–3.
2. Brock G, Hsu GL, Nunes L, et al. The anatomy of the tunica albuginea in the normal penis and Peyronie's disease. J Urol. 1997;157:276–81.
3. Mulhall JP, Schiff J, Guhring P. An analysis of the natural history of Peyronie's disease. J Urol 2006;175:2115–8; discussion 8.
4. Gelbard M, Goldstein I, Hellstrom WJ, et al. Clinical efficacy, safety and tolerability of collagenase Clostridium histolyticum for the treatment of Peyronie disease in 2 large double-blind, randomized, placebo controlled phase 3 studies. J Urol. 2013;190:199–207.
5. Carson CC 3rd, Sadeghi-Nejad H, Tursi JP, Smith TM, Kaufman GJ, Gilbert K, Honig SC. Analysis of the clinical safety of intralesional injection of collagenase Clostridium histolyticum (CCH) for adults with Peyronie's disease (PD). BJU Int. 2015;116(5):815–22.
6. Abdel Raheem A, Johnson M, Ralph D, Garaffa G. Collagenase clostridium histolyticum: a novel medical treatment for Peyronie's disease. Minerva Urol Nefrol. 2018;70(4):380–5.
7. Yafi FA, Anaissie J, Zurawin J, Sikka SC, Hellstrom WJ. Results of SMSNA survey regarding complications following intralesional injection therapy with collagenase Clostridium histolyticum for Peyronie's disease. J Sex Med. 2016;13(4):684–9.
8. Watson DL, Morgentaler A. Spontaneous corporeal herniation of the penis: a new abnormality of the tunica albuginea? J Urol. 1995;153(3 Pt 1):737–40.
9. Brant WO, Reed-Maldonado A, Lue TF. Injection therapy for Peyronie's disease: pearls of wisdom. Transl Androl Urol. 2015;4(4):474–7.
10. Hsu GL, Brock G, Martínez-Piñeiro L, von Heyden B, Lue TF, Tanagho EA. Anatomy and strength of the tunica albuginea: its relevance to penile prosthesis extrusion. J Urol. 1994;151(5):1205–8.

23

Optimal timing of ureteroscopic lithotripsy after the initial drainage treatment and risk factors for postoperative febrile urinary tract infection in patients with obstructive pyelonephritis

Yoshitaka Itami[1,2], Makito Miyake[2*], Takuya Owari[1,2], Takashi Iwamoto[2], Daisuke Gotoh[2], Hitoshi Momose[1], Kiyohide Fujimoto[2] and Shuya Hirao[1]

Abstract

Background: A history of preoperative obstructive pyelonephritis has been reported as a risk factor for febrile urinary tract infection (fUTI) after ureteroscopic lithotripsy (URSL). But there is no clear evidence of risk factors for developing fUTI including the optimal timing of URSL after obstructive pyelonephritis treatment.

Methods: Of the 1361 patients, who underwent URSL at our hospital from January 2011 to December 2017, 239 patients had a history of pre-URSL obstructive pyelonephritis. The risk factors were analyzed by comparing the patients' backgrounds with the presence or absence of fUTI after URSL. The factors examined were age, gender, body mass index, comorbidity, presence or absence of preoperative ureteral stent, stone position, stone laterality, stone size, Hounsfield unit (HU) value on computed tomography scan, history of sepsis during obstructive pyelonephritis, period from antipyresis to URSL, ureteral stenting period, operation time, and presence or absence of access sheath at URSL. In addition, the stone components and renal pelvic urinary culture bacterial species during pre-URSL pyelonephritis were also examined.

Results: Post-URSL fUTI developed in 32 of 239 patients (13.4%), and 11 of these 32 cases led to sepsis (34.4%). Univariate analysis showed that stone position, stone maximum HU value, presence of sepsis during obstructive pyelonephritis, period from antipyresis to URSL, pre-URSL ureteral stent placement, operation time were risk factors of fUTI. Stone components and urinary cultures during pyelonephritis were not associated with risk of fUTI. Multivariate analysis showed that renal stone position, pre-URSL ureteral stent placement > 21 days, and operation time > 75 min were independent risk factors of fUTI following the URSL.

Conclusions: F-UTI following the URSL could be avoided by ureteral stent placement period 21 days or less and operation time 75 min or less in patients with obstructive pyelonephritis.

Keywords: Ureteroscopic lithotripsy, Febrile urinary tract infection, Obstructive pyelonephritis, Preoperative ureteral stent placement period, Operation time

*Correspondence: makitomiyake@yahoo.co.jp
[2] Department of Urology, Nara Medical University, 840 Shijo-cho, Kashihara, Nara 634-8522, Japan
Full list of author information is available at the end of the article

Background

Obstructive pyelonephritis related to ureteral stones can be a fatal urological emergency [1, 2]. Obstructive pyelonephritis is often severe and can lead to severe sepsis and disseminated intravascular coagulation [3]. The mortality rate of patients with sepsis due to acute complicated pyelonephritis has been reported to be about 2% [4]. Emergency urinary drainage using a ureteral stent or nephrostomy and subsequent stone treatment is crucial in treating these patients [1, 2]. However, a history of preoperative obstructive pyelonephritis and ureteral stent placement has been reported as a risk factor for febrile urinary tract infection (fUTI) after ureteroscopic lithotripsy (URSL) [5, 6].

It has not been established whether URSL can be safely performed after renal drainage; there are concerns that URSL may cause post-URSL fever or sepsis due to increased renal pressure. Furthermore, the optimal timing of URSL after drainage and risk factors for post-URSL fUTI has not been established. The elucidation of patient-, stone-, and operative-factors associated with increased risk of post-URSL fUTI is important to be able to identify high-risk patients, advise on individual risks before operation, and reduce the incidence of fUTI. The purpose of this study is to establish the optimal timing of URSL and risk factors for fUTI following URSL in patients with obstructive pyelonephritis.

Methods

Patient data collection

The methods and procedures for this study were approved by the Ethics Committee of Hirao Hospital (project identification code: 2019–4). The retrospective analyses evaluated data from 1361 patients who underwent URSL at Hirao Hospital from January 2011 to December 2017. There was no history of pre-URSL pyelonephritis, ureteral stone of ileal conduit, or transplant renal stone in 1122 of these patients, leaving 239 patients with a history of pre-URSL obstructive pyelonephritis eligible for this study. All patients underwent urinary drainage by insertion of a ureteral stent or nephrostomy.

The diagnosis of obstructive pyelonephritis was based on computed tomography (CT) and laboratory data, such as bacteriuria and leukocyturia. According to criteria established by the American College of Chest Physicians/Society of Critical Care Medicine Consensus Conference Committee [7], systemic inflammatory response syndrome (SIRS) was defined by the presence of ≥ 2 of the following features: (1) body temperature lower than 36 °C or higher than 38 °C (2) heart rate > 90 beats per minute; (3) respiratory rate > 20 breaths per minute or $PaCO_2$ less than 32 mmHg; (4) a white blood cell count higher than 12,000 per mm^3 or lower than 4,000 per mm^3. In this study, fUTI accompanied with SIRS were defined as sepsis based on an international definition [8].

Treatment policy of obstructive pyelonephritis

The first line treatment for obstructive pyelonephritis is urinary drainage, which is mainly performed by ureteral stenting. Retrograde placement of a 6 Fr ureteral stent was performed using a flexible cystoscope under transurethral local anesthesia. In case with highly viscosity of the renal pelvic urine, we used a single J stent that can clean the renal pelvis because of a high risk of ureteral stent occlusion. If retrograde placement was not possible, nephrostomy using an 8.3 Fr pigtail stent (Jinro, Boston Scientific, Tokyo, Japan) was performed under ultrasound and fluoroscopy. In most cases, renal pelvic urine cultures were submitted, and empirical antibiotic treatment was administered for at least 14 days. The period between pyelonephritis treatment and URSL was based on the judgment of each physician. The day of antipyresis was defined as the first day of body temperature less than 37 °C, which continued for two or more days.

URSL procedure

All URSLs were performed under general anesthesia in the lithotomy position. Ureteral stent was removed at the beginning of URSL. A semi-rigid 6.4/7.8 Fr ureteroscope (Olympus, Tokyo, Japan) was inserted into the ureter along with a flexible 0.035 inch guidewire. If there were only distal ureteral stones, they were broken up with a holmium: yttrium–aluminum-garnet laser (VersaPulse; Lumenis, Tel Aviv, Israel) using a semi-rigid ureteroscope and collected with basket forceps. If there were renal stones, a ureteral access sheath (UAS) (Flexor, 12/14 Fr, COOK, Tokyo, Japan; Bi-Flex, 12/14 Fr or 10/12 Fr, ROCAMED, Mclean, VA, USA) was inserted into the proximal ureter along with the guidewire under fluoroscopy. A part of upper ureteral stones were pushed back into the renal pelvis during URSL, and a UAS was inserted to perform intrarenal surgery. The flexible ureteroscope (URF-P5, Olympus) was then inserted through the UAS, and stones were crushed by the same methods of semi-rigid ureteroscopy. Ureteral stents and urethral catheters were placed after all ureteroscopic procedures. If there was no fever after URSL, urethral catheters were removed the day after operation, and ureteral stents were removed 7–14 days after operation outpatiently. Pre-URSL antibiotic prophylaxis was based on the judgment of each physician. Mostly perioperative antibiotics were infused with second or third generation cephems for 3 days from the operation date. Based on the results of preoperative renal pelvic urine culture, the antibiotic was appropriately changed to a sensitive antibiotic. Post-URSL fUTI was defined as a fever of 38 °C or higher accompanied by pyuria or bacteriuria within 7 days of surgery.

Analysis of potential risk factors

The parameters investigated as potential risk factors included age, sex, body mass index (BMI), comorbidity (diabetes, hypertension, hyperlipidemia), presence or absence of pre-URSL ureteral stent, stone position at

Table 1 Patients characteristics of URSL with or without post-URSL fUTI

Variables	fUTI − (N = 207)	fUTI + (N = 32)	p value
Age			
Median (range), years	66 (19–89)	66 (35–90)	0.97
Gender			
Male/female (%)	110/97 (53.1)	13/19 (40.6)	0.19
Body mass index			
Median (range), kg/m^2	23.5 (14.3–41.8)	23.9 (15.9–37.9)	0.74
Comorbidities			
Diabetes yes/no (%)	49/158 (23.7)	5/27 (15.6)	0.31
Hypertension yes/no (%)	88/127 (42.5)	15/17 (46.9)	0.64
Hyperlipidemia yes/no (%)	30/177 (14.5)	6/26 (18.8)	0.53
Pre-URSL sepsis			
Yes/no (%)	69/138 (33.3)	17/15 (53.1)	0.01
Stone position at URSL			
Lower/mid/upper ureter/renal (%)	48/14/89/56 (23.2)/(6.8)/(43.0)/(27.0)	0/3/10/19 (0)/(9.3)/(31.2)/(59.5)	0.002
Stone laterality			
Right/left/bilateral (%)	90/113/4 (43.5)/(54.6)/(1.9)	14/16 /2 (43.7)/(50.0)/(6.3)	0.54
Stone size (maximal diameter)			
Median (range), mm	7.7 (2.5–49.2)	9.5 (5.5–44.6)	0.98
Maximal hounsfield unit value			
Median (range), HU	651 (163–1999)	875 (320–1593)	0.034
Pre-URSL renal pelvic urine culture			
Positive/negative/not evaluated (%)	83/104/20 (40.1)/(50.2)/(9.7)	13/18/1 (40.6)/(56.3)/(3.1)	0.4
Pre-URSL blood culture			
Positive/negative/not evaluated (%)	23/63/121 (11.1)/(30.4)/(58.5)	4/13/15 (12.5)/(40.6)/(46.9)	0.45
Pre-URSL prophylactic antibiotics			
Yes/no (%)	39/168 (18.8)	8/24 (33.3)	0.41
Operation time			
Median (range), min	57.0 (14–220)	81.5 (21–147)	< 0.001
Pre-URSL ureteral stenting			
Yes/no (%)	192/15 (92.8)	30/2 (93.8)	0.41
Pre-URSL nephrostomy			
Yes/no (%)	15/192 (7.2)	2/30 (6.2)	0.66
Period from antipyresis to URSL			
Median (range), days	13.5 (1–83)	21.0 (2–90)	0.043
Pre-URSL ureteral stenting placement period			
Median (range), days	20 (0–124)	28.5 (2–117)	0.003
Using access sheath during URSL			
Yes/no (%)	124/83 (59.9)	25/7 (78.1)	0.047
Initial stone free rate			
Yes/no (%)	188/19 (90.8)	29/3 (90.6)	0.97

fUTI febrile urinary tract infection, *CT* computed tomography, *URSL* ureteroscopic lithotripsy

URSL, stone laterality, stone size, Hounsfield unit (HU) value, history of sepsis during obstructive pyelonephritis, renal pelvic urine culture at urinary drainage, period from antipyresis to URSL, pre-URSL ureteral stent placement period, operation time, and presence or absence of UAS at URSL. In addition, the stone components and renal pelvic urinary culture bacterial species at urinary drainage during pre-URSL pyelonephritis were also examined.

Table 2 Patients characteristics of URSL according to stone position, ureteral or renal stones

Variables	Ureteral stone (N = 164)	Renal stone (N = 75)	p value
Age			
Median (range), years	65 (26–90)	69 (19–89)	0.011
Gender			
Male/female (%)	88/76 (53.7)	35/40 (46.7)	0.32
Body mass index			
Median (range), kg/m^2	23.5 (14.3–37.2)	23.6 (15.9–41.8)	0.4
Comorbidities			
Diabetes yes/no (%)	30/134 (18.3)	24/51 (32.0)	0.019
Hypertension yes/no (%)	61/103 (37.2)	42/33 (56.0)	0.006
Hyperlipidemia yes/no (%)	22/142 (13.4)	14/61 (18.7)	0.29
Pre-URSL sepsis			
Yes/no (%)	51/113 (31.1)	33/42 (44.0)	0.05
Stone laterality			
Right/left/bilateral (%)	64/94/6 (39.0)/(57.3)/(3.7)	40/35 /0 (53.3)/(46.6)/(0)	0.044
Stone size (maximal diameter)			
Median (range), mm	7.2 (2.5–36.3)	11.2 (3.1–49.2)	< 0.0001
Maximal hounsfield unit value			
Median (range), HU	618 (163–1593)	843 (293–1999)	< 0.0001
Pre-URSL renal pelvic urine culture			
Positive/negative/not evaluated (%)	64/87/13 (39.0)/(53.0)/(8.0)	32/35/8 (42.7)/(46.7)/(10.7)	0.6
Pre-URSL blood culture			
Positive/negative/not evaluated (%)	14/56/94 (8.5)/(34.1)/(57.3)	13/20/42 (17.3)/(27.1)/(56.0)	0.11
Pre-URSL prophylactic antibiotics			
Yes/no (%)	30/134 (18.3)	17/58 (22.7)	0.43
Operation time			
Median (range), min	50.0 (14–220)	72.0 (25–147)	< 0.0001
Pre-URSL ureteral stenting			
Yes/No (%)	149/15 (91.5)	73/2 (97.3)	0.07
Pre-URSL nephrostomy			
Yes/no (%)	15/149 (8.5)	2/73 (2.7)	0.07
Period from antipyresis to URSL			
Median (range), days	13.0 (1–79)	17.0 (3–90)	0.018
Pre-URSL ureteral stenting placement period			
Median (range), days	20 (0–124)	24 (2–117)	0.11
Using access sheath during URSL			
Yes/no (%)	74/90 (45.1)	75/0 (100)	< 0.0001
Post-URSL futi			
Yes/no (%)	13/151 (7.9)	19/56 (25.3)	< 0.0001
Initial stone free rate			
Yes/no (%)	158/6 (96.3)	59/16 (78.7)	< 0.0001

fUTI febrile urinary tract infection, *CT* computed tomography, *URSL* ureteroscopic lithotripsy

Table 3 Risk factors for fUTI following URSL performed after obstructive pyelonephritis treatment

Variables	Univariable analysis[a]			Multivariable analysis[a]		
	Odds ratio	95% CI	p value	Odds ratio	95% CI	p value
Gender						
Male	1					
Female	1.66	0.78–3.53	0.19			
Pre-URSL sepsis						
No	1			1		
Yes	2.75	1.29–5.86	0.009	2.08	0.89–4.83	0.089
Stone position						
Ureter	1					
Renal	3.94	1.83–8.51	< 0.001	2.91	1.29–6.58	0.01
Maximal Hounsfield unit value (HU)[b]						
< 750	1			1		
≥ 750	2.79	1.13–6.87	0.026	1.15	0.49–2.68	0.74
Period from antipyresis to URSL (days)[b]						
< 20	1					
≥ 20	2.23	1.02–4.86	0.043			
Pre-URSL ureteral stent placement period (days)[b]						
< 21	1			1		
≥ 21	4.22	1.65–10.8	0.003	2.77	1.12–6.8	0.028
Operation time (min)[b]						
< 75	1			1		
≥ 75	6.75	3.05–14.9	< 0.001	3.37	1.45–7.84	0.005
Using access sheath during URSL						
No	1					
Yes	2.39	0.99–5.78	0.053			

fUTI febrile urinary tract infection, *CT* computed tomography, *HU* hounsfield unit, *URSL* ureteroscopic lithotripsy

[a] Logistic analysis

[b] Cutt off value of continuous variable is calculated from ROC curve

Statistical analysis

Data are shown as bar charts or dot plots and were evaluated using the Student t-test, the Mann–Whitney U test, or the χ^2 test, as appropriate. Multivariate analyses were used to identify independent prognostic variables based on logistic analysis ($p < 0.05$ in the univariate analyses). Multivariate analyses were performed using StatMate (version 5.0; Tokyo, Japan) and other data were analyzed using PRISM software (version 7.00; San Diego, CA, USA). A p value < 0.05 was considered statistically significant.

Results

Of the 239 patients with pre-URSL obstructive pyelonephritis, 222 (92.9%) had a ureteral stent, of which 205 were double J stents and 17 were single J stents, and 17 (7.1%) had a nephrostomy during urinary drainage. Pre-URSL pyelonephritis with concurrent sepsis was detected in 86 of 239 patients (36.0%). Post-URSL fUTI developed in 32 of 239 patients (13.4%). Post-URSL fUTI led to sepsis in 11 of these 32 patients (34.4%). Table 1 shows the perioperative characteristics of the 239 patients and a comparison between those with post-URSL fUTI and those without. 8 patients had stones with a diameter of 2 cm or more and recommended PNL, but URSL was performed due to patient preferences such as limited hospital stay for work. There were no significant differences in age, sex, BMI, comorbidities, or stone size between the two groups. 149 patients used UAS during URSL, 140 patients (94.0%) were 12/14 Fr, 9 patients (6.0%) were 10/12 Fr, and there was no significant difference in post-URSL

Table 4 Risk factors for fUTI in renal stones following URSL performed after obstructive pyelonephritis treatment

Variables	Univariable analysis[a]			Multivariable analysis[a]		
	Odds ratio	95% CI	p value	Odds ratio	95% CI	p value
Gender						
Male	1					
Female	1.99	0.69–5.75	0.20			
Pre-URSL sepsis						
No	1					
Yes	2.13	0.74–6.11	0.24			
Maximal Hounsfield unit value (HU)[b]						
<750	1					
≥750	1.12	0.39–3.17	0.84			
Period from antipyresis to URSL (days)[b]						
<20	1					
≥20	0.9	0.31–2.64	0.85			
Pre-URSL ureteral stent placement period (days)[b]						
<21	1			1		
≥21	4.3	1.13–16.4	0.033	5.16	1.28–20.8	0.021
Operation time (min)[b]						
<75	1			1		
≥75	3.35	1.11–10.1	0.032	4.00	1.25–12.8	0.020

curvefUTI febrile urinary tract infection, *CT* computed tomography, *HU* hounsfield unit, *URSL* ureteroscopic lithotripsy

[a] Logistic analysis

bCutt off value of continuous variable is calculated from ROC

fUTI incidence with UAS size. The fUTI group presented with renal stones at URSL, had a higher maximal HU value, higher incidence of concurrent sepsis during obstructive pyelonephritis, longer period from antipyresis to URSL, longer period of pre-URSL ureteral stent placement, and longer operation time than the non-fUTI group. However, the initial stone-free rate was similar between the two groups (90.8% versus 90.6%). There was no significant difference in the number of patients administered pre-URSL prophylactic antibiotics between the two groups. Furthermore, there was no

Table 5 Renal pelvic urinary culture bacterial species at drainage during pre-URSL pyelonephritis with or without post-URSL fUTI

	fUTI −		fUTI +	
	n	%	n	%
Negative	104	50.2	18	56.3
Escherichia coli	35	17.2	4	12.5
Enterococcus faecalis	18	8.7	1	3.1
Pseudomonas aeruginosa	9	4.3	2	6.3
Staphylococcus aureus	7	3.4	0	0
Klebsiella pneumoniae	6	2.9	1	3.1
Proteus mirabilis	5	2.4	2	6.3
Streptococcus agalactiae	4	1.9	0	0
Morganella morganii	1	0.5	0	0
Others	18	8.7	4	12.5
Total	207		32	

URSL ureteroscopic lithotripsy, *fUTI* febrile urinary tract infection

Table 6 Stone component with or without post-URSL fUTI

	fUTI −		fUTI +	
	N	%	n	%
Ca oxalate	136	65.7	22	68.8
Ca phosphate	10	4.8	3	9.4
NH4MgPO4	24	11.6	2	6.3
Carbonate apatite	2	1	2	6.3
Uric acid	7	3.4	0	0
Not evaluated	28	13.5	3	9.4
Total	207		32	

URSL ureteroscopic lithotripsy, *fUTI* febrile urinary tract infection

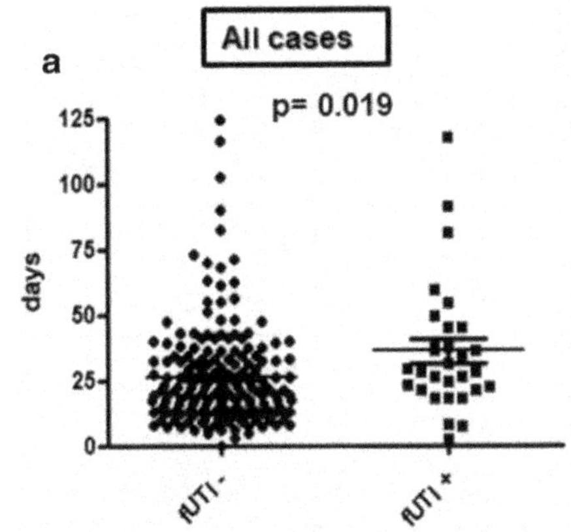

Ureteral stenting period (days)	fUTI-	fUTI+ (sepsis)	%
56-	13	4 (1)	23.5 (5.9)
35-56	28	8 (2)	22.2 (5.6)
28-35	23	5 (2)	17.9 (7.1)
21-28	26	7 (3)	21.2 (9.1)
14-21	46	3 (0)	6.1 (0)
7-14	42	2 (1)	4.5 (2.3)
0-7	7	1 (0)	12.5 (0)

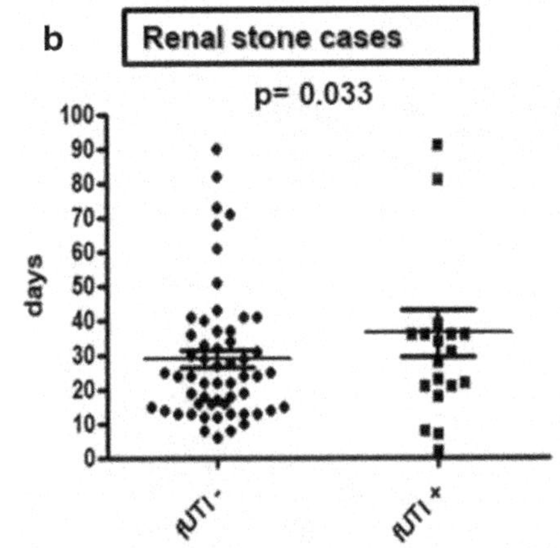

Ureteral stenting period (days)	fUTI-	fUTI+ (sepsis)	%
56-	6	3 (1)	33.3 (11.1)
35-56	9	3 (1)	25.0 (8.3)
28-35	8	3 (2)	27.3(18.2)
21-28	8	4 (3)	33.3 (25)
14-21	12	1 (0)	7.7 (0)
7-14	10	2 (1)	16.7 (8.3)
0-7	1	1 (0)	50 (0)

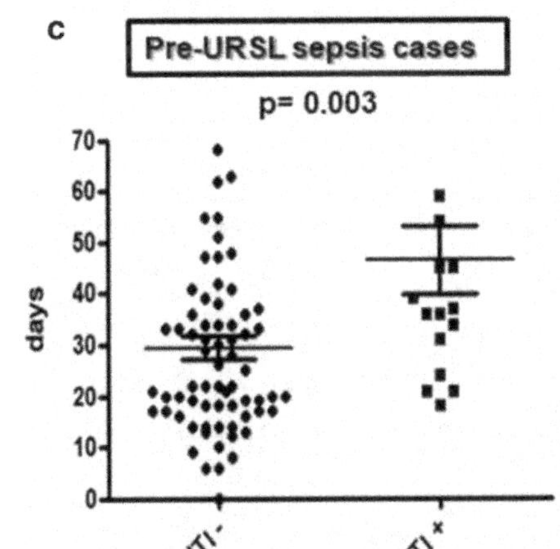

Ureteral stenting period (days)	fUTI-	fUTI+ (sepsis)	%
56-	5	4 (2)	44.4(22.2)
35-56	14	7 (1)	33.3 (4.8)
28-35	13	2 (1)	13.3 (6.7)
21-28	8	3 (0)	27.3 (0)
14-21	21	1 (0)	4.5 (0)
7-14	6	0 (0)	0 (0)
0-7	2	0 (0)	0 (0)

Fig. 1 Post-URSL fUTI incidence depending on pre-URSL ureteral stent placement period. **a** Comparison of pre-URSL ureteral stent placement periods with or without post-URSL fUTI and post-URSL fUTI incidence according to pre-URSL ureteral stent placement in all cases except seven cases when insertion was unknown. **b** Same examination as (**a**) in renal stone cases. **c** Same examination as (**a**) in pre-URSL with sepsis cases. *fUTI* febrile urinary tract infection, *URSL* ureteroscopic lithotripsy

significant difference in fUTI between nephrostomy or ureteral stent, and also between single J stent or double J stent. Table 2 compares the perioperative characteristics of 239 patients, divided into ureteral and renal stones. 164 patients (68.6%) had ureteral stones and 75 patients (31.4%) had renal stones. UAS was used in all 75 cases of renal stones. In 74 of 99 cases of upper ureteral stones, the stones were pushed back into the renal pelvis from the ureter and were performed intrarenal surgery. Patients with renal stones were significantly older, and had more DM and HT comorbidities, higher stone sizes and HU values than those with ureteral

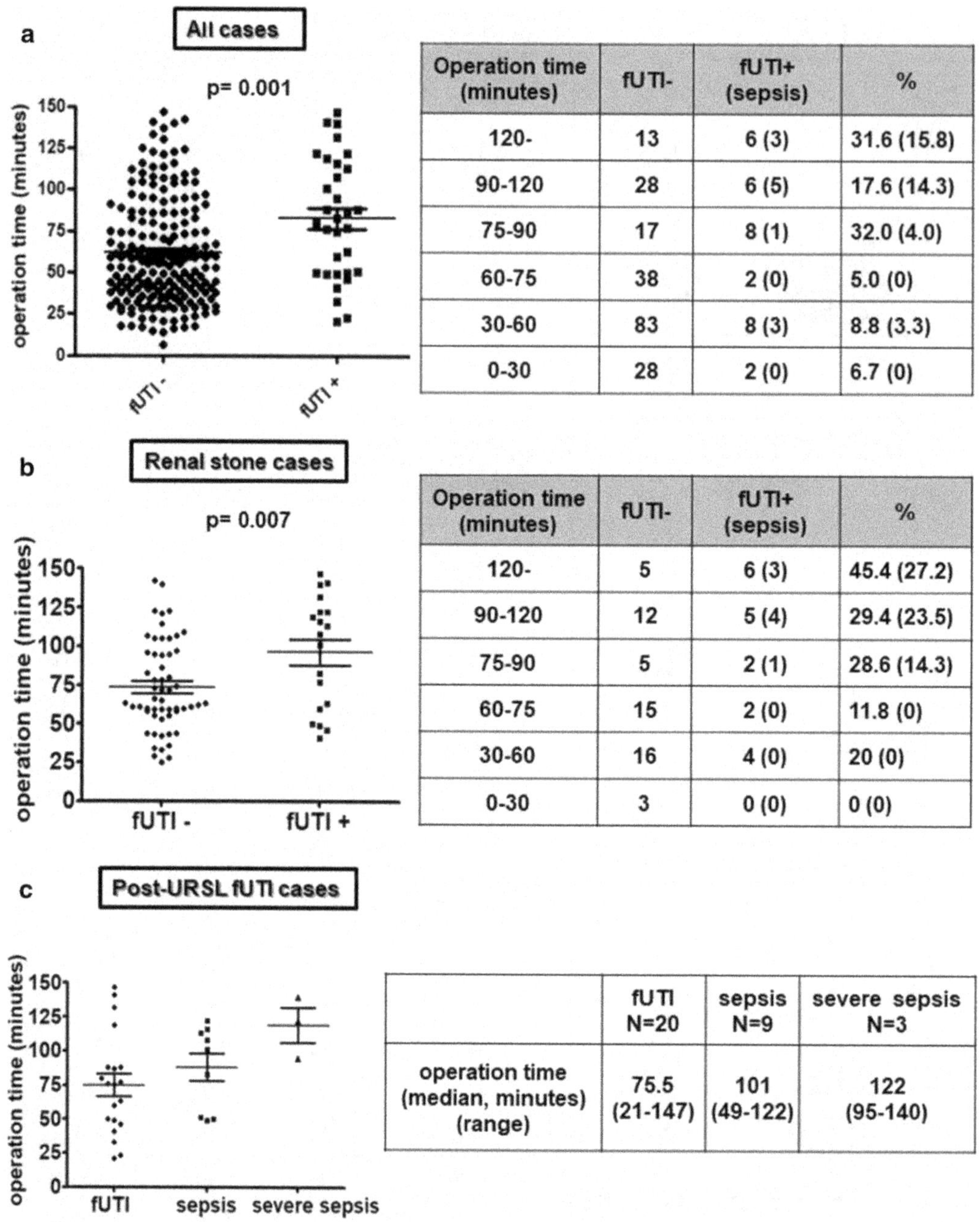

a

Operation time (minutes)	fUTI-	fUTI+ (sepsis)	%
120-	13	6 (3)	31.6 (15.8)
90-120	28	6 (5)	17.6 (14.3)
75-90	17	8 (1)	32.0 (4.0)
60-75	38	2 (0)	5.0 (0)
30-60	83	8 (3)	8.8 (3.3)
0-30	28	2 (0)	6.7 (0)

b

Operation time (minutes)	fUTI-	fUTI+ (sepsis)	%
120-	5	6 (3)	45.4 (27.2)
90-120	12	5 (4)	29.4 (23.5)
75-90	5	2 (1)	28.6 (14.3)
60-75	15	2 (0)	11.8 (0)
30-60	16	4 (0)	20 (0)
0-30	3	0 (0)	0 (0)

c

	fUTI N=20	sepsis N=9	severe sepsis N=3
operation time (median, minutes) (range)	75.5 (21-147)	101 (49-122)	122 (95-140)

Fig. 2 Post-URSL fUTI incidence depending on operation time. **a** Comparison of operation time with or without post-URSL fUTI and post-URSL fUTI incidence according to operative time. **b** Same examination as (**a**) in renal stone cases. **c** Comparison of operation time by severity in post-URSL fUTI cases. Severe sepsis was defined as concurrent disseminated intravascular coagulation (DIC) or as a condition requiring a vasopressor. *fUTI* febrile urinary tract infection, *URSL* ureteroscopic lithotripsy

stones. Moreover, operation time of URSL was significantly longer for renal stones than for ureteral stones. The initial stone-free rate of renal stones was significantly lower than ureteral stones (78.7% versus 96.3%).

Multivariate analysis in all patients showed that renal stone position at URSL, pre-URSL ureteral stent placement period > 21 days, and operation time > 75 min were independent risk factors (Table 3). In Table 2, it was shown that the operation time was significantly longer in renal stone patients than in ureteral stone patients, so the risk factors were examined only in renal stone patients. Similar to Table 3, pre-URSL ureteral stent placement

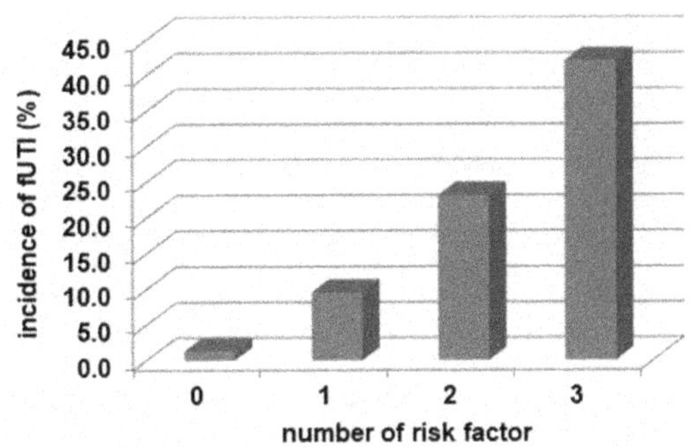

number of risk factor	0	1	2	3
fUTI+/ total	1 / 78	7 / 73	16 / 69	8 /19
incidence of fUTI (%)	1.3	9.6	23.2	42.1

Fig. 3 Post-URSL fUTI incidence stratified by three risk factors, renal stone position at URSL, pre-URSL ureteral stent placement period > 21 days, and operation time > 75 min. The number of risk factors were defined as the point. *URSL* ureteroscopic lithotripsy, *fUTI* febrile urinary tract infection

period > 21 days, and operation time > 75 min were independent risk factors for renal stone patients only (Table 4).

The bacterial species found in renal pelvic urinary cultures at urinary drainage during obstructive pyelonephritis and the stone components were not associated with post-URSL fUTI (Tables 5 and 6).

The pre-URSL ureteral stent placement period both in all cases and renal stone cases was significantly longer in the post-URSL fUTI group (Fig. 1a, b). Furthermore, the incidence of post-URSL fUTI significantly increased when the stent placement period was over 21 days. Similarly, in cases with pre-URSL concurrent with sepsis, the incidence of fUTI increased significantly after 21 days, and increased further after 35 days. No post-URSL fUTI with sepsis was found within 28 days of stent placement (Fig. 1c).

With respect to the duration of the operation both in all cases and renal stone cases, the frequency of post-URSL fUTI increased significantly after an operation > 75 min, and post-URSL fUTI with sepsis increased following an operation > 90 min (Fig. 2a, b). The length of the operation showed a correlation with the severity of post-URSL fUTI (Fig. 2c).

Three risk factors were used to stratify patient groups: renal stone position at URSL, pre-URSL ureteral stent placement period > 21 days, and operation time > 75 min. Patients with a higher number of risk factors showed a significantly increased incidence of post-URSL fUTI (Fig. 3).

Discussion

Risk factors for fUTI after URSL have been reported as the presence of pre-URSL pyuria, a history of pre-URSL pyelonephritis, pre-URSL ureteral stent placement, and operation duration of 90 min or more [5, 9–11]. Youssef et al. reported that URSL in patients with a history of pre-URSL pyelonephritis with sepsis resulted in an increase in complications, including post-URSL fUTI, prolonged hospital stays, and prolonged post-URSL antibiotic administration [6]. A ureteral stent is often used for urinary drainage in stone-associated pyelonephritis, but there are no studies examining the relationship between the ureteral stenting period and post-URSL fUTI.

In this study, a risk factor for the development of fUTI following treatment of obstructive pyelonephritis and URSL was identified as > 21 days of ureteral stenting (Fig. 1a). Pre-stenting can improve the passive dilation of the ureter and increase the stone-free rate during URSL [12, 13]. It has been reported that bacteriuria and bacterial colonization of the stent occurs over time after stent placement [14]. Bacterial colonization of the stent was not observed within 2 weeks but was observed in 23.5–33% of patients after less than 4 weeks, 33.3–50% after 4–6 weeks, and 71.4% after more than 6 weeks [15]. Therefore, the optimal timing of URSL appears to be 7–21 days following stent placement.

An increased duration of operation was correlated with higher the risk of fUTI. Some studies have indicated that the risk of fUTI increases after an operation > 90 min [5, 11], but in this study the risk increased after operations of 75 min (Fig. 2). The reason for this may be that URSL performed after pyelonephritis poses a higher risk of bacterial exposure, so shorter operation times would reduce the incidence of fUTI. Furthermore, this study also showed that post-URSL sepsis complications increased with an operation time of > 90 min. These results indicate that the optimal duration of URSL after pyelonephritis should be 75 min or less, and operations longer than 90 min should be avoided in order to prevent severe fUTI.

Regarding the stone position, renal stones were considered to increase the intrapelvic pressure during URSL and cause fUTI regardless of the use of UAS [16]. However, in this study, there was no significant difference in the incidence of fUTI depending on the diameters of the access sheath. The reason for the high fUTI in patients with renal stones is considered to be that they are older than patients with ureteral stones, have many comorbidities such as DM, and have a large stone size and a long operation time, as shown in Table 2.

It has been previously reported that administration of prophylactic antibiotics reduced the rate of post-URSL bacteriuria, but the post-URSL fUTI incidence rate was not significantly different to the control group [17]. In a recent systematic review, it was reported that prophylactic antibiotics showed a certain effect [18]. In this study, no effect of prophylactic antibiotics on fUTI onset was observed, with similar results seen in selective cases of pre-URSL pyelonephritis with sepsis. However, the criteria for prophylactic antibiotic administration were not constant in this study, It is considered that prophylactic antibiotics should be more aggressively administered in the future to prevent the fUTI development, especially in patients with ureteral stent for > 21 days and renal stones with large stones. The Infectious Diseases Society of America guidelines state that replacing long-term indwelling catheters immediately before surgery is more effective than administering antibiotics [19]. Therefore, when URSL is performed on a patient with a ureteral stent that has been indwelling for > 21 days, it is recommended that the stent be replaced before URSL. However, the replacement procedure itself is mildly invasive, and there is a slight risk of fUTI, so indication needs to be considered.

This study has limitations, which must be considered. First, our retrospective analysis of data is from a single institution and of a small sample size, which are associated with a high risk of selection bias. Second, the types and duration of antibiotics administered during pyelonephritis and the prophylactic antibiotics before URSL were dependent on each attending physician and were not standardized. However, these factors would not increase the risk of post-URSL fUTI and were considered to have little effect on the results of the study.

Conclusions

It is suggested that fUTI following URSL could be avoided by compliance with a ureteral stent placement period of 21 days or less and operation time of 75 min or less in patients with obstructive pyelonephritis, especially in renal stone cases.

Abbreviations

BMI: Body mass index; CT: Computed tomography; fUTI: Febrile urinary tract infection; HU: Hounsfield unit; SIRS: Systemic inflammatory response syndrome; UAS: Ureteral access sheath; URSL: Ureteroscopic lithotripsy.

Authors' contributions

YI, SH contributed to study conception and design. TO, TI, DG contributed to data acquisition. MM, HM contributed to analysis and interpretation data. YI, MM contributed to drafting the manuscript. YI, MM, KF were involved in revising the manuscript. All authors have read and approved the manuscript.

Competing interests

The authors declare that they have no competing interests.

Author details

[1] Department of Urology, Hirao Hospital, 6-28 Hyobu-cho, Kashihara, Nara 634-0076, Japan. [2] Department of Urology, Nara Medical University, 840 Shijo-cho, Kashihara, Nara 634-8522, Japan.

References

1. Ramsey S, Robertson A, Ablett MJ, et al. Evidence-based drainage of infected hydronephrosis secondary to ureteric calculi. J Endourol. 2010;24:185–9.
2. Turk C, Knoll T, Petrik A, Sarica K, Straub M, Seitz C. Guidelines on Urolithiasis. 2010:1–106.
3. Yoshimura K, Utsunomiya N, Ichioka K, et al. Emergency drainage for urosepsis associated with upper urinary tract calculi. J Urol. 2005;173:458–62.
4. Members of the American College of Chest Physicians Society of Critical Care Medicine Consensus Conference Committee, American College of Chest Physicians Society of Critical Care Medicine Consensus Conference. Definition of sepsis and organ failure and guidelines for the use of innovative therapies in sepsis. Crit Care Med 1992; 20: 864–874.
5. Sugihara T, Yasunaga H, Horiguchi H, et al. A nomogram predicting severe adverse events after ureteroscopic lithotripsy: 12372 patients in a Japanese national series. BJU int. 2013;111:459–66.
6. Youssef RF, Neisius A, Goldsmith ZG, et al. Clinical outcomes after ureteroscopic lithotripsy in patients who initially presented with urosepsis: matched pair comparison with elective ureteroscopy. J Endourol. 2014;28:1439–43.
7. Erdil T, Bostanci Y, Ozden E, et al. Risk factors for systemic inflammatory response syndrome following percutaneous nephrolithotomy. Urolithiasis. 2013;41:395–401.
8. Singer M, Deutchman CS, Seymour CW, et al. The third international consensus definitions for sepsis and septic shock. JAMA. 2016;315:801–10.
9. Mitsuzuka K, Nakano O, Takahashi N, et al. Identification of factors associated with postoperative febrile urinary tract infection after ureteroscopy for urinary stones. Urolithiasis. 2016;44:257–62.
10. Uchida Y, Takazawa R, Kitayama S, et al. Predictive risk factors for systemic inflammatory response syndrome following ureteroscopic laser lithotripsy. Urolithiasis. 2018;46:375–81.
11. Fan S, Gong B, Hao Z, et al. Risk factors of infectious complications following flexible ureteroscope with a holmium laser: a retrospective study. Int J Clin Exp Med. 2015;8:11252–9.
12. Yang Y, Tang Y, Bai Y, et al. Preoperative double-J stent placement can improve the stone-free rate for patients undergoing ureteroscopic lithotripsy: a systematic review and meta-analysis. Urolithiasis. 2018;46:493–9.
13. Kawahara T, Ito H, Terao H, et al. Preoperative stenting for ureteroscopic lithotripsy for a large renal stone. Int J Urol. 2012;19:881–5.
14. Kehinde EO, Rotimi VO, Al-Awadi KA, et al. Factors predisposing to urinary tract infection after J ureteral stent insertion. J Urol. 2002;167:1334–7.
15. Lojanapiwat B. Colonization of internal ureteral stent and bacteriuria. World J Urol. 2006;24:681–3.
16. Zhong W, Leto G, Wang L, et al. Systemic inflammatory response syndrome after flexible ureteroscopic lithotripsy: a study of risk factors. J Endourol. 2015;29:25–8.
17. Knopf HJ, Graff HJ, Schulze H. Perioperative antibiotic prophylaxis in ureteroscopic stone removal. Eur Urol. 2003;44:115–8.
18. Chugh S, Pietropaolo A, Montanari E, et al. Predictors of urinary infections and urosepsis after ureteroscopy for stone disease: a systematic review from EAU section of urolithiasis (EULIS). Curr Urol Rep. 2020;21:16.
19. Nicolle LE, Bradley S, Colgan R, et al. Infectious Diseases Society of America guidelines for the diagnosis and treatment of asymptomatic bacteriuria in adults. Clin Infect Dis. 2005;40:643–54.

24

Case report of ureter obturator hernia and literature review analysis

Yongqiang Hong[1], Siyu Zhang[2], Xiuying Kong[3], Yuxin Zhang[1], Shaokun Hong[2] and Yuedong Chen[1,4*]

Abstract

Background: Ureteral obturator hernia is a rare condition, usually found accidentally during imaging examinations, or found during surgery. Ureteral hernia can easily lead to ureteral obstruction and hydronephrosis. Long-term hydronephrosis may lead to kidney damage and infection, and eventually cause kidney failure. As of December 31, 2020, there are only 2 literature reports.

Case presentation: This article reports a 67-year-old female patient with no symptoms. The computed tomography (CT) scan of the urinary system to show the left kidney and ureter had hydrops. The CTU imaging of the urinary tract revealed the left ureter pelvis herniated into the parietal pelvic fascia was accompanied by tortuosity and left hydronephrosis. She underwent laparoscopic abdominal wall hernia repair on April 29, 2020, and she recovered well.

Conclusions: Ureteral obturator hernia is an uncommon condition. The clinical symptoms are non-specific, including unclear abdominal pain, until the appearance of obstructive diseases of the urinary tract, such as renal insufficiency, urinary tract infection, kidney stones, and uremia. A comprehensive review of the literature shows that it is difficult to make an accurate diagnosis based on physical examination alone.Early urography can improve the possibility of accurate diagnosis. When a patient suffers from impaired renal function, timely surgical treatment can avoid deterioration of renal function.

Keywords: Ureteral obturator hernia, Ureteral stent implantation, Hernia repair, Hydronephrosis, Case report

Background

Ureteral obturator hernia a rare occurrence, usually found accidentally during imaging examinations or during surgery [1, 2]. Ureteral obturator hernia belongs to a category of ureteral hernia. Ureteral hernia can occur in the groin, femoral ring, ischial foramen, obturator and chest [3]. Among them, ureteral hernia is extremely rare in the obturator position. The obturator is composed of the pubic bone and ischial branch. Most of the holes are occupied by a layer of membrane, with small holes on the caudal side to allow the passage of obturator veins, arteries and nerves [4]. When the abdominal organs protrude through the obturator foramen of the hip to the femoral triangle (composed of the inguinal ligament, the inner edge of the adductor longus muscle, and the inner edge of the sartorius muscle), it is called an obturator hernia. Obturator hernia is a rare type of abdominal wall hernia with an incidence rate of 1% [5]. Once the ureter protrudes through the defect of the obturator foramen and cannot exit after entering the obturator tube, the ureteral hernia will occur into the obturator fora. We call it a "Ureteral obturator hernia". Through searching historical documents, we found that there are only 2 reported cases of obturator hernia with ureteral compression. Here, we provide an interesting case of an elderly woman with obturator hernia and left ureteral compression.

*Correspondence: chenyuedong8@126.com
[1] Department of Clinical Medicine, Fujian Medical University, Fuzhou 350000, China
Full list of author information is available at the end of the article

Case presentation

A 67-year-old female patient was admitted to another hospital for "rheumatic heart disease combined with mitral stenosis and regurgitation" and underwent "mitral valve replacement" surgery. During the hospitalization, a computerized tomography (CT) scan of the chest and abdomen was performed and it was found that the left kidney and ureter had hydrops. Three months later, in order to treat left kidney and ureteral hydrops, she was admitted to the Urology Department of our hospital. She has no symptoms such as frequent urination, urgency, abdominal pain, hematuria, and dysuria. She had no history of prior abdominal surgery, trauma, or congenital defects. Local examination showed no bulge or percussion pain in both kidney area and bilateral ureters. Laboratory examinations revealed a decrease in the glomerular filtration rate on both sides (70.15ml/min) and an increase in urine bacteria (7682.5/μL). After the physical examination, in order to further understand the degree of renal and ureteral hydrops, we recommended that she perform a computed tomography (CT) scan of the urinary tract. The results suggested that her left kidney and ureter were still present (Fig. 1). In order to clarify the cause of her kidney and ureteral hydrops, CTU imaging of the urinary tract was performed, and it was found that the left ureter pelvis herniated into the parietal pelvic fascia was accompanied by tortuosity and left hydronephrosis. In order to assess the function of the kidneys, she underwent nephro-dynamic imaging. The results suggest that the blood perfusion and function of the left kidney are slightly impaired, the excretion is significantly delayed, and the filtration rate of the left glomerulus is reduced (27.50ml/min); the glomerular filtration rate of the right kidney (38.60ml/min). The initial diagnosis was that the left ureter and hydronephrosis caused by pelvic perineal hernia, and general surgery consultation was invited, and laparoscopic exploration + tension-free repair of the left pelvic floor hernia was planned. We placed the patient in a lithotomy position, and placed trocars 1 cm above the navel, 5 cm on both sides of the navel, McBurney point and anti-McBurney point, and no hernias were found in the pelvic cavity through laparoscopy. Cut the left peritoneum during the operation and open the left side Toldt space.Toldt's space is the fusion fascia space, which is formed by the fusion of the mesangium and the following tissues (mesenia or parietal peritoneum) after the midgut volvulus during embryonic development. It is called Toldt's fascia, and the potential gap is called Toldt's gap. Next, look for the left ureter, cut the peritoneum along the surface of the ureter to the pelvic floor. Later, observation of the pelvic cavity revealed that the left obturator space became larger, the ureter passed through the obturator area, and the upper ureter was significantly dilated (Fig. 2). Therefore, we changed the diagnosis to left obturator hernia with left ureteral hydrops and left hydronephrosis, and decided to perform left obturator hernia repair. And implemented the left ureterolysis, see the expansion of the ureter has returned to normal. The incised pelvic peritoneum was continuously sealed with a 3-0 Barbed thread behind the ureter. Pelvic part of the ureter was moved into the abdominal cavity. No obvious bleeding was seen after flushing the abdominal cavity, and the incision was sutured layer by layer. The result of the operation was very successful. One week after the operation, she had a follow-up visit. Color Doppler ultrasound of the urinary system showed that the upper dilatation of the left ureter was better than before. And the patient is very satisfied with the treatment.

Discussion

Ureteral obturator hernia is very rare in clinical practice. We only found 2 reports by searching and reviewing relevant literature (as of December 31, 2020, Pubmed, Embase and Cochrane, as well as CNKI and Wanfang electronic journals full-text database search).At present, the main cause of the disease is not clear. Some scholars believe that the main susceptibility factors may be piriformis atrophy, congenital or acquired defects of pelvic wall fascia [6]. Generally speaking, the clinical symptoms of ureteral obturator hernia are non-specific, including unclear abdominal pain, until the appearance of urinary obstructive diseases, such as renal insufficiency, urinary tract infection, kidney stones and uremia [7]. Weingarten, KE and others found a case of ureteral obturator hernia after kidney transplantation. This patient developed intermittent, dullness, and left lower abdominal discomfort within a few years after kidney transplantation. The serum creatinine level rose from 133 to 293 μmol/L. L (1.5 mg/dL to 3.3 mg/dL). In the next 2 weeks, the patient's renal function deteriorated, and the serum creatinine level showed an irregular upward trend, with a peak value of 506 μmol/L (5.7 mg/dL). Ultrasound examination of the transplanted kidney showed moderate hydronephrosis, and antegrade pyelography showed a long and tortuous ureter, accompanied by distal ureteral obstruction. So they first placed a percutaneous nephrostomy tube for drainage, and manually reset the prolapsed ureter through gentle palpation and groin manipulation. Subsequently, obturator hernia repair was performed [8]. Izzo, M. et al. reported a case of obturator hernia with ureteral compression. This patient suddenly developed vomiting, weakness, constipation and left lower abdominal pain and came to see a doctor. After hospitalization, he found C-reactive protein and creatinine levels. High; Urine examination showed leukopenia and hematuria,

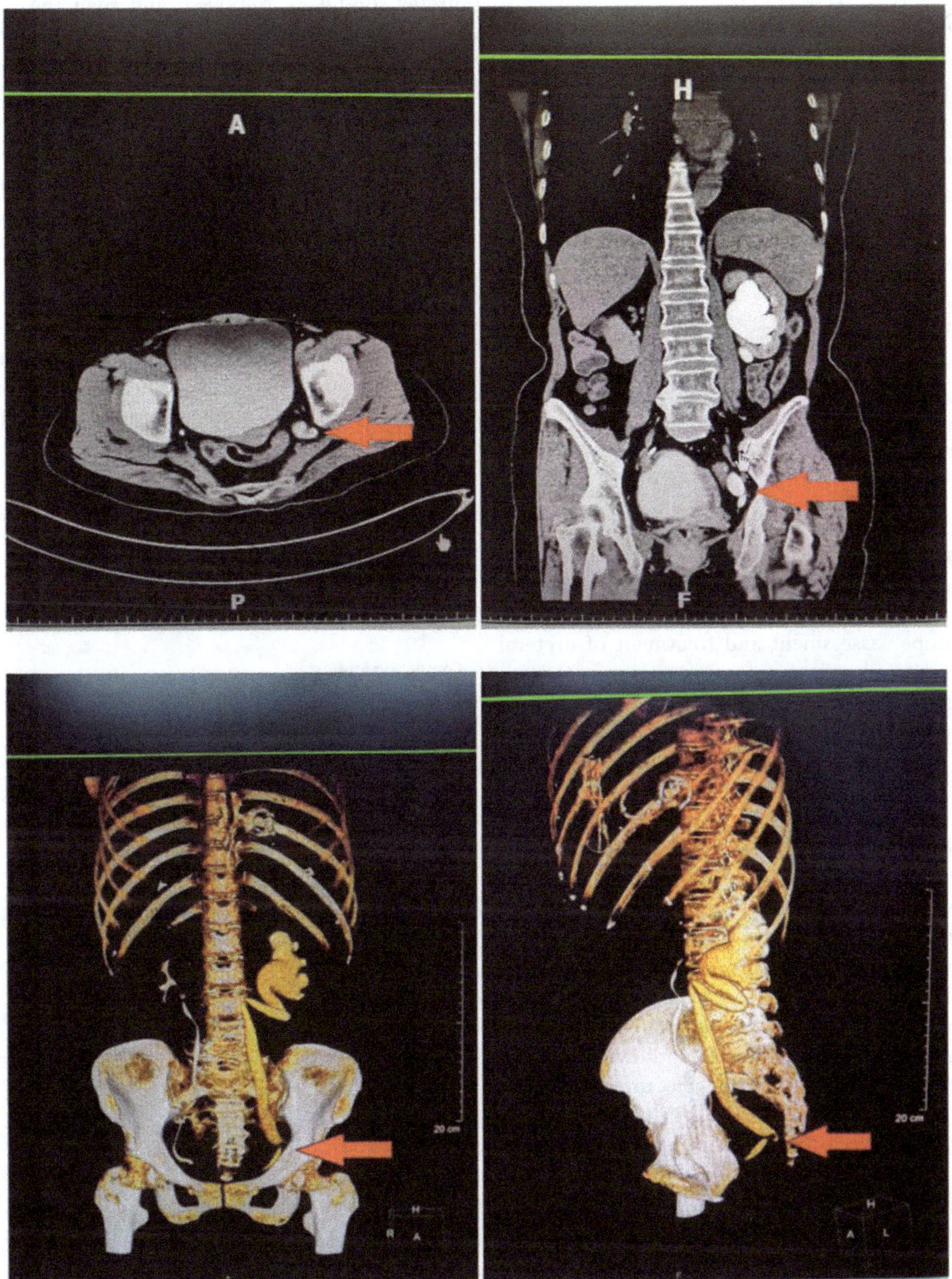

Fig. 1 Urinary system CTU and three-dimensional reconstruction, suggesting tortuous hydronephrosis on the left ureter and hydronephrosis on the left

ultrasound examination showed hydronephrosis in the left kidney, and computed tomography showed that the left obturator foramen and ipsilateral ureter were compressed, and the small intestinal ring was completely prominent. Because the patient's renal function was damaged, they considered elective surgery after the renal function was restored [9].

The clinical symptoms of ureteral obturator hernia are non-specific. In rare cases, just like our case, there are no symptoms, only the preoperative CT suggests that

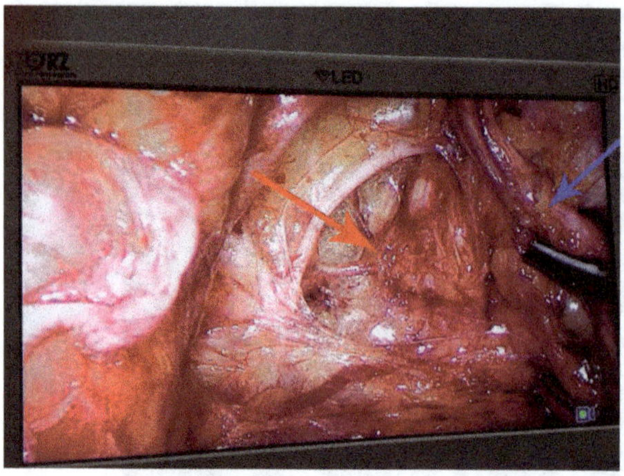

Fig. 2 Intraoperative exploration revealed enlarged obturator. The red arrow refers to the enlarged obturator and the blue arrow refers to the twisted ureter

the lower part of the ureter is obstructed. It is difficult to diagnose ureteral obturator hernia by physical examination alone. In essence, it is idiopathic ureteral stenosis. Therefore, proper assessment and treatment of ureteral stenosis is of great significance for protecting renal function and eliminating malignant tumors. The causes of ureteral stenosis include: (A) Malignant diseases, such as transitional cell carcinoma and cervical tumors. In addition, ureteral stenosis can also occur in the in situ metastasis of cancers such as cervical cancer, prostate cancer, and ovarian cancer. (B) Ureteral stones. (C) Radiation injury. (D) Ischemia and trauma caused by surgery. (E) Injury caused by ureteroscopy. (F) Infection, such as urinary tuberculosis. Therefore, urography (i.e., intravenous urography, retrograde pyelography and CT) can assist in the diagnosis [10]. Urography can identify the location of the obstruction. The main imaging manifestations are ureteral dilatation, hydronephrosis, and even ureteral cyst. Frank C. Lin et al. suggested that ureteral hernia should be treated conservatively unless there is emergency treatment (such as obstruction, uremia, or intractable lumbar pain). And conduct long-term laboratory and imaging follow-up to monitor progress [3].

We believe that when ureteral hernia leads to ureteral obstruction and impaired renal function, intervention should be made as soon as possible. Especially in this type of patient, long-term hydronephrosis may lead to kidney damage and infection, and even eventually Will cause the kidneys to fail [11]. When renal function is severely impaired, percutaneous nephrostomy for external drainage and ureteral stent implantation for internal drainage will help reduce obstructive symptoms and protect renal function. When the protruding ureter appears obvious dilation, atresia, inflammation or necrosis, the ureter should be removed, and then the ureterocystoscope should be performed [7]. There are many surgical approaches, including inguinal approach, retropubic approach, and transperitoneal approach. Generally, the abdominal approach via a low median incision is the most popular because it can fully expose the obturator ring and identify and remove any adhesions. This method allows the surgeon to establish a diagnosis, avoid any obturator vessels, and better expose the obturator ring [9].

Once unexplained hydronephrosis or ureteral obstruction is found, you need to be alert to the possibility of ureteral hernia. Early urography can improve the possibility of accurate diagnosis. When a patient has impaired renal function, early surgical intervention is effective.

Authors' contributions

YQH participated in the surgery, participated in the follow up care, performed literature review, and drafted the manuscript. XYK performed literature review, and drafted the manuscript. YXZ performed literature review. SKH participated in the surgery. SYZ carried out the surgery, participated in the follow up care, edited the manuscript. YDC carried out the surgery, participated in the follow up care, and edited the manuscript. All authors read and approved the final manuscript.

Competing interest

The authors declare that they have no competing interests.

Author details

[1]Department of Clinical Medicine, Fujian Medical University, Fuzhou 350000, China. [2]Department of General Surgery, The First Affiliated Hospital of Xiamen niversity, Xiamen 361001, China. [3]Xiamen University School of Medicine, Xiamen 361001, China. [4]Department of Urology, The First Affiliated Hospital of Xiamen University, Xiamen 361001, China.

References

1. Pollack H, Popky G, Blumberg M. Hernias of the ureter. An anatomic-roentgenographic study. Radiology. 1975;117(2):275–81.
2. Orlando CA, Nunziata BC, Alfredo S. Retrocrural loop of the ureter: CT findings. Am J Roentgenol. 1998;170:1293–4.
3. Lin FC, Lin JS, Kim S, Walker JR. A rare diaphragmatic ureteral herniation case report: endoscopic and open reconstructive management. BMC Urol. 2017;17(1).
4. Herath M, Kanhere H. Loin to groin pain-a case report of an intermittent obturator hernia mimicking ureteric colic. Int J Surg Case Rep. 2020;66:356–9.
5. Kulkarni SR, Punamiya AR, Naniwadekar RG, Janugade HB, Chotai TD, Vimal Singh T, Natchair A. Obturator hernia: a diagnostic challenge. Int J Surg Case Rep. 2013;4(7):606–8.
6. Loffroy R, Bry J, Guiu B, Dubruille T, Michel F, Cercueil JP, Krause D. Uretero-sciatic hernia: a rare cause of ureteral obstruction visualized by multislice helical computed tomography. Urology. 2007;69(2):385 e381–3.
7. Bertolaccini L, Giacomelli G, Bozzo RE, Gastaldi L, Moroni M. Inguino-scrotal hernia of a double district ureter: case report and literature review. Hernia. 2005;9(3):291–3.
8. Weingarten KE, D'Agostino HB, Dunn J, Steiner RW. Obturator herniation of the ureter in a renal transplant recipient causing hydronephrosis: perioperative percutaneous management. J Vasc Interv Radiol. 1996;7(6):939–41.
9. Izzo M, Regusci L, Fasolini F. Obturator hernia with ureteral entrapment. Case Rep Gastroenterol. 2014;8(2):156–61.
10. Yanagi K, Kan A, Sejima T, Takenaka A. Treatment of ureterosciatic hernia with a ureteral stent. Case Rep Nephrol Dial. 2015;5(1):83–6.
11. Allam ES, Johnson ES, Grewal SG, Johnson FE. Inguinoscrotal herniation of the ureter: description of five cases. Int J Surg Case Rep. 2015;14:160–3.

25

Photodynamic diagnostic ureteroscopy using the VISERA ELITE video system for diagnosis of upper-urinary tract urothelial carcinoma

Koichiro Wada[1,4], Motoo Araki[1,4*], Ryuta Tanimoto[2,4], Takuya Sadahira[1,4], Shogo Watari[1,4], Yuki Maruyama[1,4], Yosuke Mitsui[1,4], Hirochika Nakajima[3,4], Herik Acosta[1], Satoshi Katayama[1,4], Takehiro Iwata[1,4], Shingo Nishimura[1,4], Atsushi Takamoto[1,4], Tomoko Sako[1,4], Kohei Edamura[1,4], Yasuyuki Kobayashi[1,4], Masami Watanabe[1,4], Toyohiko Watanabe[1,4] and Yasutomo Nasu[1,4]

Abstract

Background: The advantages of photodynamic diagnostic technology using 5-aminolevulinic acid (ALA-PDD) have been established. The aim of this prospective cohort study was to evaluate the usefulness of ALA-PDD to diagnose upper tract urothelial carcinoma (UT-UC) using the Olympus VISERA ELITE video system.

Methods: We carried out a prospective, interventional, non-randomized, non-contrast and open label cohort pilot study that involved patients who underwent ureterorenoscopy (URS) to detect UT-UC. 5-aminolevulinic acid hydrochloride was orally administered before URS. The observational results and pathological diagnosis with ALA-PDD and traditional white light methods were compared, and the proportion of positive subjects and specimens were calculated.

Results: A total of 20 patients were enrolled and one patient who had multiple bladder tumors did not undergo URS. Fifteen of 19 patients were pathologically diagnosed with UT-UC and of these 11 (73.3%) were ALA-PDD positive. Fourteen of 19 patients were ALA-PDD positive and of these 11 were pathologically diagnosed with UC. For the 92 biopsy specimens that were malignant or benign, the sensitivity for both traditional white light observation and ALA-PDD was the same at 62.5%, whereas the specificities were 73.1% and 67.3%, respectively. Of the 38 specimens that were randomly biopsied without any abnormality under examination by both white light and ALA-PDD, 11 specimens (28.9%) from 5 patients were diagnosed with high grade UC. In contrast, four specimens from 4 patients, which were negative in traditional white light observation but positive in ALA-PDD, were diagnosed with carcinoma in situ (CIS).

Conclusions: Our results suggest that ALA-PDD using VISERA ELITE is not sufficiently applicable for UT-UC. Nevertheless, it might be better particularly for CIS than white light and superior results would be obtained using VISERA ELITE II video system.

*Correspondence: motoosh@md.okayama-u.ac.jp
[1] Department of Urology, Okayama University Graduate School of Medicine, Dentistry and Pharmaceutical Sciences, 2-5-1, Shikata-cho, Kita-ku, Okayama 700-8558, Japan
Full list of author information is available at the end of the article

Keywords: Photodynamic diagnosis, 5-Aminolevulinic acid, ALA-PDD, Upper urinary tract urothelial carcinoma, VISERA ELITE video system

Background

Photodynamic diagnostic (PDD) technology using 5-aminolevulinic acid (ALA-PDD) is currently being used for the diagnosis of brain tumors in Japan. For patients with bladder cancer, the sensitivity and specificity of ALA-PDD using scopes and video systems produced by Karl Storz SE & Co. KG (Tuttlingen, Germany) can be as high as 75.8% and 68.2%, respectively [1]. Thus, in 2017 Japanese national health insurance approved ALA-PDD for visualization of non-muscle-invasive bladder cancer at the time of transurethral resection of bladder tumors (TURBT). ALA is an amino acid that is naturally present in living animals and plants, as well as in commonly consumed foods and beverages, and protoporphyrin IX (PpIX), which is also present in the human body. Neither compound shows toxicity and the safety of both has been confirmed in healthy individuals [2]. The premise for ALA-PDD is that orally ingested ALA accumulates as PpIX in tumor cells to a greater degree than in normal cells. Upon excitation with visible blue light (375–445 nm), PpIX emits red light (600–740 nm).

Upper tract urothelial carcinoma (UT-UC) includes renal pelvic and ureteral cancer, which are the same as bladder cancer from a pathological perspective. Although standard treatment for UT-UC is total nephroureterectomy and partial cystectomy, techniques involving endoscopic diagnosis and resection with URS have been developed [3, 4]. However, small satellite tumors, flat tumors and carcinoma in situ (CIS) in the upper urinary tract are difficult to diagnose and treat endoscopically [5, 6]. ALA-PDD allows visualization of lesions that cannot be diagnosed by conventional observation using white light, thus increasing the likelihood of accurate diagnosis and effective treatment in patients with UT-UC [7, 8]. ALA-PDD performed for UT-UC patients using a ureteroscope and a video system produced by Karl Storz SE & Co. KG. has been described [9, 10], but no similar study has been carried out using a video system manufactured by Olympus Co., Ltd. (Tokyo, Japan).

The aim of this prospective cohort study was to evaluate the usefulness of ALA-PDD for diagnosis of UT-UC using the VISERA ELITE video system produced by Olympus Co., Ltd.

Methods

All methods were carried out in accordance with relevant guidelines and regulations.

Study design

We carried out a pilot, prospective interventional, non-randomized, non-contrast and open label cohort study. Enrollment began following approval by the review board. Patients who were suspected of having UT-UC and were undergoing ureterorenoscopy (URS) were enrolled. Since this study was a pilot study, 20 cases were considered based on the annual number of cases treated at our institution. The primary endpoint was the proportion of positive subjects and secondary endpoints were sensitivity, specificity, positive predictive value (PPV), negative predictive value (NPV) and adverse events for ALA-PDD.

Patients

Patients that were enrolled in the study were adults who were suspected of having UT-UC and were undergoing URS. All patients were aware of the conditions associated with the disease, and provided informed consent to participate. All enrolled patients agreed to use contraception until 1 month after the administration of 5-ALA. Exclusion criteria were patients with porphyria, allergy to porphyrin or 5-ALA, hepatic dysfunction, use of drugs that induced photosensitivity, pregnancy, or severe underlying diseases such as cardiovascular diseases or infection.

Protocols

On the day of the URS, 20 mg/kg of 5-aminolevulinic acid hydrochloride (5-ALA HCl) was orally administered over 180 min (range: 120–240 min) before the scheduled insertion time for the ureteroscope. After oral administration of 5-ALA HCl, patients drank 250 mL of an L-arginine-intensive drink and 500 mL of fruit juice to maintain blood pressure. At the time of examination, normal observations using white light and ALA-PDD using visible blue light were carried out using a two-color LED light source (ALADUCK LS-DLED, SBI Pharmaceuticals, Tokyo, Japan). All endoscopic images were recorded.

After the procedures, patients had proper shading to prevent photosensitivity for up to 48 h after ingesting

5-ALA HCl and light exposure of less than 500 lx was maintained. Hematologic and biochemical examinations were performed on postoperative days (POD) 1 and 3 and the occurrence of adverse events was noted.

5-ALA (5-aminolevulinic acid)

5-ALA HCl was supplied as a white powder similar to that for ALAGLIO by SBI Pharmaceuticals (SBI Pharmaceuticals, Tokyo, Japan). The chemical compound was stored according to strict quality control guidelines and detailed usage records were maintained by the Division of Clinical Research of New Drugs and Therapeutics in the Center for Innovative Clinical Medicine, Okayama University Hospital.

Endourological techniques

The endourological techniques and URS procedures performed at our institution for observation of the upper urinary tract and ablation of tumors were previously described [11, 12]. All the patients underwent URS using "no-touch" technique, which is without any insertion of guidewire or ureteral catheter prior to ureteroscope, under general anesthesia in a lithotomy position. Before the procedures, 10 μM PpIX in a glass vial was observed using blue light and the ureteroscopes were confirmed to glow red. After cystoscopy, a 6/7.5 Fr semi-rigid ureteroscope (E-line, Richard Wolf, Knittlingen, Germany) was inserted with or without a guidewire as high as possible, and then changed to an 8.4 or 7.95 Fr flexible ureteroscope (URF-P5 or P6, Olympus Co. Ltd., Tokyo, Japan). At observation, white light and blue light, switched with a foot pedal, were alternately used. When abnormalities, such as a tumor or red fluorescence, were observed, cold cup biopsies were performed using 3.3 Fr Forceps™ (Cook Medical, Bloomington, IN, USA) without any hemostatic technique. Among patients who had preoperative positive urine cytology and had no abnormality, cold cup biopsies from the renal pelvis and ureter were randomly performed. All endourological procedures were performed using the VISERA ELITE video system and camera head produced by Olympus Co., Ltd.

Data analysis

The observational results and pathological diagnoses, the proportion of positive subjects, positive specimens, sensitivity, and specificity were calculated. Adverse events were also investigated and severity was categorized using the Clavien-Dindo classification.

Results

Characteristics of the 20 patients enrolled in this study are shown in Table 1. A total of 5 patients (25%) had positive preoperative urine cytology and no abnormalities on CT urography. Another 5 patients (25%) had abnormalities on CT urography but negative urine cytology.

Table 1 Patient characteristics before URS using ALA-PDD

	Number of patients	(%)
Median age (IQR)	71	(67–79)
Gender		
Male	16	(80)
Female	4	(20)
Co-morbidities		
Malignancy	2	(10)
Urothelial carcinoma	1	(5)
UT-UC	0	
Bladder cancer	1	(5)
Other	0	
Cardiovascular diseases	5	(25)
Diabetes mellitus	6	(30)
Other	4	(20)
None	7	(35)
Laterality		
Right	8	(40)
Left	9	(45)
Bilateral	2	(10)
Unknown	1	(5)
Disease site		
Renal pelvis	6	(30)
Clinical stage		
$<$cT2	3	(15)
$\geq$cT2	3	(15)
Ureter	7	(35)
Clinical stage		
$<$cT2	4	(20)
$\geq$cT2	3	(15)
Unknown (no lesion on CT or MRI)	7	(35)
Urine cytology		
Positive	13	(65)
Negative	7	(35)

The median (IQR) time from oral administration of 5-ALA HCl to biopsy was 246 (227–269) minutes. One patient had multiple tumors in the bladder and URS was aborted. Among the 19 remaining patients, biopsy was not performed because of absence of any abnormality in one patient, for whom URS was performed as follow-up. Fifteen patients were pathologically diagnosed with UT-UC and of these, 11 (73.3%) were ALA-PDD positive. Fourteen of 19 patients were ALA-PDD positive and of these, 11 were pathologically diagnosed with UC. Among the 50 specimens that are ALA-PDD positive, 25 (50%) were pathologically diagnosed with UC, 17 (34%)

were not malignant, and the status for 8 (16%) could not be determined because the specimens were too small. Among the 7 patients that were ALA-PDD positive and white light negative (Fig. 1), 4 were diagnosed with CIS. Of the 38 specimens from 12 patients that showed no abnormalities under examination by both white light and ALA-PDD, 11 specimens (28.9%) from 5 patients were diagnosed with high grade UC. Comparing white light and ALA-PDD, 4 specimens taken from definite tumors in 2 patients were ALA-PDD negative but diagnosed with UC. On the other hand, 4 specimens which were white light negative and ALA-PDD positive taken from 4 patients were diagnosed with CIS. Of the 31 specimens diagnosed with high grade UC, 18 and 13 (58% and 42%) were ALA-PDD positive and negative, respectively. For specimens from patients with low grade UC, 7 (78%) of 9 were ALA-PDD positive, but 2 (22%) specimens were ALA-PDD negative.

For observational accuracy calculations, 2 patients who had pathological diagnoses were excluded and 18 patients were enrolled. Based on the results for these 18 patients, the sensitivity and specificity of ALA-PDD were calculated to be 80.0% and 33.3%, respectively, whereas for white light observation the respective values were 86.7% and 66.7% (Table 2). Considering biopsy specimens that could be diagnosed as malignant or benign (n = 92), the sensitivity of white light observation and ALA-PDD was the same at 62.5%, whereas the specificities were 73.1% for white light and 67.3% for ALA-PDD, respectively. The PPV and NPV of ALA-PDD were 59.5% and 70.0%, respectively. The combined observation had the highest sensitivity at 72.5%, but the lowest specificity at 51.9%.

For adverse events, all patients took the first 50 mL of drug solution including 5-ALA HCl; however, two patients complained of nausea and one vomited 2 h after taking 5-ALA HCl. Other symptoms included elevated serum aminotransferase that required no additional treatment (Clavien-Dindo Grade I) in 6 patients and hypotension requiring vasopressors (Grade II) in one patient. No allergic episodes, cardiovascular complications or photosensitivity were observed in our study.

Discussion

In this prospective cohort study to evaluate the effectiveness of ALA-PDD for UT-UC diagnosis using the VISERA ELITE video system, the sensitivity and specificity were 62.5% and 67.3%, respectively. Of the 38 specimens that were randomly biopsied without any abnormality under examination by both white light and ALA-PDD, 11 specimens (28.9%) from 5 patients were diagnosed with high grade UC. On the other hand, four biopsy specimens that had abnormal findings with ALA-PDD but not with normal white light observation were diagnosed with CIS.

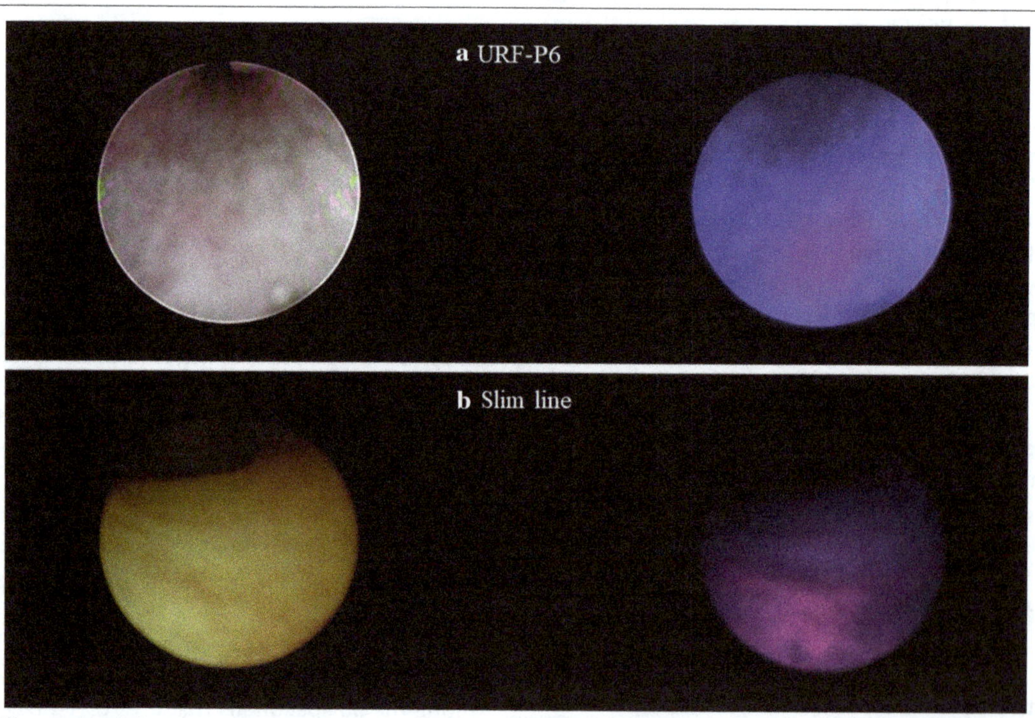

Fig. 1 Two different white light negative and ALA-PDD positive lesions using flexible URS (URS-P6, **a**) and semi-rigid ureteroscopy (Slim line, **b**) followed by diagnosis with carcinoma in situ

Table 2 Diagnostic accuracy of normal white light observation, ALA-PDD and combined observation

	White light			ALA-PDD			Combined observation		
	Positive	Negative	Total	Positive	Negative	Total	Positive	Negative	Total
A. Analysis by participant (n = 18)									
Pathological diagnosis									
UC	13	2	15	12	3	15	15	0	15
Non-UC	1	2	3	2	1	3	2	1	3
Total	14	4	18	14	4	18	17	1	18
Accuracy of each observational method	Sensitivity		86.7%	Sensitivity		80.0%	Sensitivity		100.0%
	Specificity		66.7%	Specificity		33.3%	Specificity		33.3%
	PLR[a]		2.6	PLR		1.2	PLR		1.5
	NLR[b]		0.2	NLR		0.6	NLR		-
	FPR[c]		13.3%	FPR		20.0%	FPR		0.0%
	FNR[d]		33.3%	FNR		66.7%	FNR		66.7%
	PPVe		92.9%	PPV		85.7%	PPV		88.2%
	NPV[f]		50.0%	NPV		25.0%	NPV		100.0%
	Normal observation			ALA-PDD			Combined observation		
	Positive	Negative	Total	Positive	Negative	Total	Positive	Negative	Total
B. Analysis by biopsy specimen (n = 92)									
Pathological diagnosis									
Urothelial carcinoma	25	15	40	25	15	40	29	11	40
Non-urothelial carcinoma	14	38	52	17	35	52	25	27	52
Total	39	53	92	42	50	92	54	38	92
Accuracy of each observational method	Sensitivity		62.5%	Sensitivity		62.5%	Sensitivity		72.5%
	Specificity		73.1%	Specificity		67.3%	Specificity		51.9%
	PLR		2.3	PLR		1.9	PLR		1.5
	NLR		0.5	NLR		0.4	NLR		0.5
	FPR		37.5%	FPR		37.5%	FPR		27.5%
	FNR		26.9%	FNR		32.7%	FNR		48.1%
	PPV		64.1%	PPV		59.5%	PPV		53.7%
	NPV		71.7%	NPV		70.0%	NPV		71.1%

[a] PLR: positive likelihood ratio
[b] NLR: negative likelihood ratio
[c] FPR: false positive ratio
[d] FNR: false negative ratio
[e] PPV: positive predictive value
[f] NPV: negative predictive value

ALA-PDD was approved only for bladder cancer by Japanese national health insurance in 2017. This approach is expected to have value not only for bladder cancer diagnosis but also for treatment, namely complete resection at TURBT [1, 13–16]. On the other hand, studies describing photodynamic treatment using ALA (ALA-PDT) [17] and some pilot studies [18, 19] involving ALA-PDD for UT-UC reported that ALA-PDT and ALA-PDD could be effective and useful even for UT-UC (Table 3). Among studies concerning ALA-PDT and -PDD conducted since 2012, most used ureteroscopes with a video system produced by Karl Storz SE & Co. KG (Tuttlingen, Germany) to diagnose ALA-PDD and this technique was shown to have higher accuracy for UT-UC diagnosis than methods involving white light [10, 20–22] and CT urography [22]. Thus, before carrying out the present study, we confirmed that PpIX fluorescence could be observed using a ureteroscope with the VISERA ELITE video system [23]. Our present study revealed that sensitivity and specificity values for ALA-PDD for UT-UC were lower than other studies for UT-UC and slightly lower than those for bladder cancer. These outcomes could be due to differences in: (1) cystoscopes and ureteroscopes; (2) image quality; and (3) video system

Table 3 Previous studies describing use of ALA-PDT/PDD to diagnose UT-UC

References	Country	Study design	Objective	Sample size	Video system supplier	Sensitivity (%)	Specificity (%)
Waidelich [17]	Germany	Pilot study	PDT[a]	4	Not stated	–	–
Somani et al. [18]	UK	Pilot study	PDD[b]	4	Karl Storz	–	–
Audenet et al. [19]	France	Review	–	–	–	–	–
Ahmad et al. [20]	UK	Prospective cohort	PDD	26	Karl Storz	100	62.5
Aboumarzouk et al. [21]	UK	Prospective cohort	PDD	32	Karl Storz	96	100
Aboumarzouk et al. [22]	UK	Prospective cohort	PDD	30	Karl Storz	94	100
Bondad et al. [25]	UK	Retrospective	Unknown	24	–	–	–
Kata et al. [9]	UK	Review	PDD	–	Karl Storz	–	–
Kata et al. [10]	UK	Prospective cohort	PDD	54	Karl Storz	95.8	96.6
Osman et al. [7]	Bahrain	Review	–	–	–	–	–
This study (2019)	Japan	Prospective cohort	PDD	20	VISERA ELITE, Olympus	62.5	67.3%

[a] *PDT* photodynamic therapy

[b] *PDD* photodynamic diagnosis

quality. First, images obtained using ureteroscopy are dark and small because ureteroscopes are longer and thinner than cystoscopes. Second, image processing software that optimizes gradations of collected images has not been available yet. Third, neither the VISERA ELITE nor camera head are designated for ALA-PDD, and thus surgeons must insert a special filter between the camera head and the endoscope. Use of the newest video system such as the VISERA ELITE II could produce a higher sensitivity and specificity since we did perform additional ex vivo experiments to evaluate which video system was better for ALA-PDD using ureteroscopy, and found that images produced by the VISERA ELITE II were superior to those obtained using VISERA ELITE (Fig. 2).

Interestingly, 11 of the 38 (28.9%) specimens that exhibited no abnormalities in either white light or ALA-PDD examinations were pathologically diagnosed with high grade UC. The reasons for this result are unclear, but some abovementioned factors may have contributed to this outcome. To our knowledge there are no studies that examined random biopsy samples taken from the upper urinary tract, and additional investigations are needed.

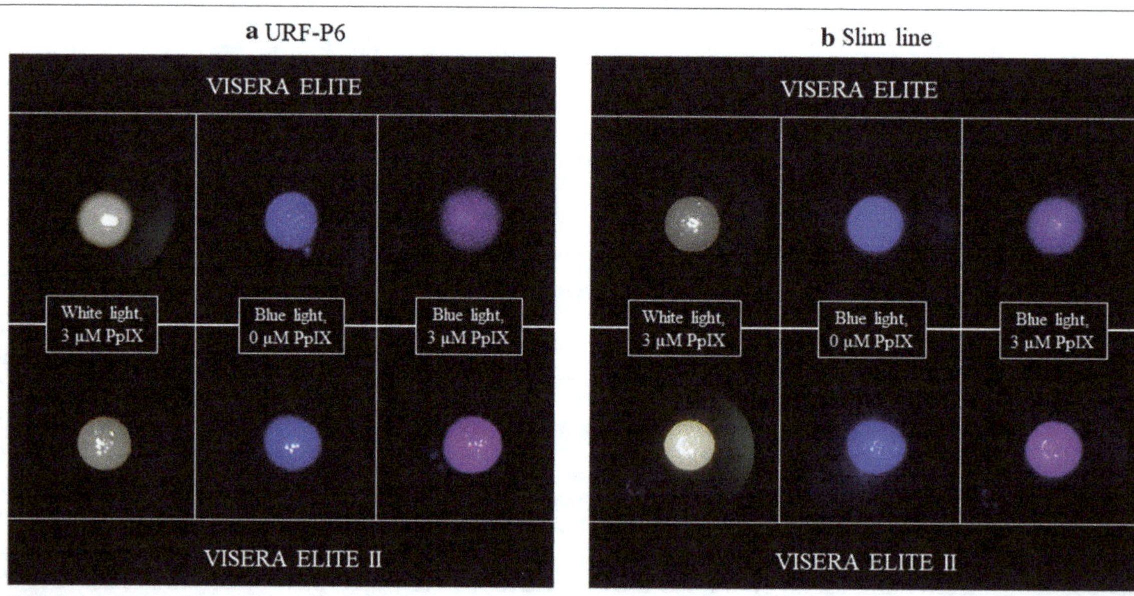

Fig. 2 Ex vivo experiments for evaluation of ELITE and ELITE II. Cotton swabs containing 0 or 3 μM PpIX are observed using the same flexible URS (URS-P6, **a**) and semi-rigid ureteroscopy (Slim line, **b**) by white light or blue light (ALA-PDD) at a distance of 5 mm. In both case of flexible URS and semi-rigid ureteroscopy, a higher fluorescent intensity with ELITE II (white arrows) compared to ELITE (black arrows) is seen observing the cotton swabs containing 3 μM PpIX by blue light

According to European guidelines [24], diagnostic ureteroscopy is strongly recommended to diagnose UT-UC tumor type and tumor grade. Furthermore, endoscopic management for UT-UC is the primary treatment option as a kidney-sparing surgery for patients with low-risk tumors (unifocal tumor; tumor size < 2 cm; low-grade cytology; low-grade URS biopsy; no invasive aspect on CT urography). Although in our study 2 specimens from one patient with low grade UC were ALA-PDD negative, low grade UC can be positive even in normal white light observation. In addition, 4 specimens diagnosed with CIS were negative in normal observation but positive in ALA-PDD. Hence, our results indicate that ALA-PDD might be an effective method for detection of CIS in the upper urinary tract.

Adverse events of ALA-PDD have been reported as liver toxicity, allergic episode, cardiovascular complications, photosensitivity, hypotension, nausea and vomiting [9, 25]. In our study, no severe adverse events were observed outside of hypotension in one patient because of some preventative measures such as oral intake before the procedure, shading for 48 h to avoid photosensitivity, and other factors. However, one patient who had vomited 2 h after administration of 5-ALA was diagnosed with high grade UC while any abnormality could not be observed under examination by both white light and PDD. The fact suggests the possibility that vomiting had some effect on ALA-PDD.

The present study has several limitations. Although this pilot study was prospective, it was performed at a single center, was non-randomized and included small number of patients (n = 20). Second, there were 2 patients who underwent protocol URS after endoscopic laser ablation and cognitive bias could be associated with the previous procedure. Third, we evaluated the usefulness of ALA-PDD only in the diagnostic process and not the treatment process. Fourth, we did not compare endoscopic devices including semirigid/flexible ureteroscopes, light cables, and video systems, and did not evaluate their compatibility with ALA-PDD. Despite these limitation, the ureteroscopy with ALA-PDD might be more useful for diagnosis in patients with UT-UC, particularly with CIS.

Conclusions

Our results of this pilot study suggest that ALA-PDD using VISERA ELITE is not sufficiently applicable for UT-UC. Nevertheless, it might be better particularly for CIS than white light and superior results would be obtained using VISERA ELITE II video system. Further studies on patient selection, endoscopic equipment and image processing methods are needed for the broad application of ALA-PDD for UT-UC diagnosis.

Acknowledgements

The authors thank the clinical laboratory technicians of Okayama University Hospital for their technical support.

Authors' contributions

K.W.: Research conception and design, obtaining funding, data acquisition, data analysis and interpretation, drafting and editing the manuscript; M.A.: Research conception and design, data analysis and interpretation, drafting and editing the manuscript, approval of the final manuscript; R.T.: Data acquisition; T.S.: Obtaining funding, data acquisition, data analysis and interpretation, drafting the manuscript; S.W.: Data analysis; Y.M.: Data analysis; Y.M.: Data analysis and interpretation; H.N.: Revision of the manuscript; H.A.: Data analysis and interpretation, revision of the manuscript; S.K.: Data acquisition; T.I.: Data analysis and interpretation; S.N.: Data acquisition; A.T.: Data acquisition; T.S.: Data acquisition; K.E.: Data acquisition, revision of the manuscript; Y.K.: Data acquisition; M.W.: Critical revision of the manuscript; T.W.: Critical revision of the manuscript; Y.N: Supervision of this study. All authors read and approved the final manuscript.

Competing interests

All the authors have no conflicts of interest to be disclosed.

Author details

[1] Department of Urology, Okayama University Graduate School of Medicine, Dentistry and Pharmaceutical Sciences, 2-5-1, Shikata-cho, Kita-ku, Okayama 700-8558, Japan. [2] Department of Urology, Kagawa Prefectural Central Hospital, 1-2-1, Asahi-machi, Takamatsu 760-8557, Japan. [3] Department of Urology, Fukuyama City Hospital, 5-23-1, Zao-cho, Fukuyama 721-8511, Japan. [4] Okayama Urological Research Group: OURG, 2-2-7-1, Ima-cho, Kita-ku, Okayama 700-0975, Japan.

References

1. Inoue K, Anai S, Fujimoto K, Hirao Y, Furuse H, Kai F, et al. Oral 5-aminolevulinic acid mediated photodynamic diagnosis using fluorescencecystoscopy for non-muscle-invasive bladder cancer: a randomized, double-blind, multicentre phase II/III study. Photodiagnosis Photodyn Ther. 2015;12:193–200.
2. Mustajoki P, Timonen K, Gorchein A, Seppäläinenet AM, Matikainen E, Tenhunen R. Sustained high plasma 5-aminolaevulinic acid concentration in a volunteer: no porphyric symptoms. Eur J Clin Invest. 1992;22:407–11.
3. Fiuk JV, Schwartz BF. Upper tract urothelial carcinoma: paradigm shift towards nephron sparing management. World J Nephrol. 2016;5:158–65.
4. Raman JD, Park R. Endoscopic management of upper-tract urothelial carcinoma. Expert Rev Anticancer Ther. 2017;17:545–54.
5. Sasaki K, Wada K, Araki M, Kobayashi Y, Sugimoto M, Ebara S, et al. Diagnostic ureteroscopy for cases clinically suspected of carcinoma in situ of the upper urinary tract. Acta Med Okayama. 2017;71:227–32.
6. Gillan A, El-Mokadem I, Rai B, Lang S, Alcorn J, Shams Ud Din A, et al. Carcinoma in situ is significantly underdetected by prenephroureterectomy ureteroscopy in the management of uppertracturothelial cancers. Biomed Res Int. 2015;2015:547586.
7. Osman E, Alnaib Z, Kumar N. Photodynamic diagnosis in upper urinary tract urothelial carcinoma: a systematic review. Arab J Urol. 2017;15:100–9.
8. Soria F, Shariat SF, Lerner SP, Fritsche HM, Rink M, Kassouf W, et al. Epidemiology, diagnosis, preoperative evaluation and prognostic assessment of upper-tract urothelial carcinoma (UTUC). World J Urol. 2017;35:379–87.
9. Kata SG, Nabi G, Eljamel S, Chlosta P, Moseley H, Aboumarzouk OM. Photodynamic diagnostic ureterorenoscopy with orally administered 5-aminolaevulinic acid as photosensitiser: how I do it. Urol Int. 2014;93:384–8.
10. Kata SG, Aboumarzouk OM, Zreik A, Somani B, Ahmad S, Nabi G, et al. Photodynamic diagnostic ureterorenoscopy: a valuable tool in the detection of upper urinary tract tumour. Photodiagnosis Photodyn Ther. 2016;13:255–60.
11. Takao A, Saika T, Uehara S, Monden K, Abarzua F, Nasu Y, et al. Indications for ureteropyeloscopy based on radiographic findings and urine cytology in detection of upper urinary tract carcinoma. Jpn J Clin Oncol. 2010;40:1087–91.
12. Araki M, Uehara S, Sasaki K, Monden K, Tsugawa M, Watanabe T, et al. Ureteroscopic management of chronic unilateral hematuria: a single-center experience over 22 years. PLoS ONE. 2012;7:e36729.

13. O'Brien T, Ray E, Chatterton K, Khan MS, Chandra A, Thomas K. Prospective randomized trial of hexylaminolevulinate photodynamic-assisted transurethral resection of bladder tumour (TURBT) plus single-shot intravesical mitomycin C vs conventional white-light TURBT plus mitomycin C in newly presenting non-muscle-invasive bladder cancer. BJU Int. 2013;112:1096–104.
14. Tandogdu Z, Lewis R, Duncan A, Penegar S, McDonald A, Vale L, PHOTO Trial Management Group, et al. PHOTO Trial Management Group Photodynamic versus white light-guided treatment of non-muscle invasive bladder cancer: a study protocol for a randomised trial of clinical and cost-effectiveness. BMJ Open. 2019;9:e022268.
15. Nakai Y, Inoue K, Tsuzuki T, Shimamoto T, Shuin T, Nagao K, et al. Oral 5-aminolevulinic acid-mediated photodynamic diagnosis using fluorescence cystoscopy for non-muscle-invasive bladder cancer: a multicenter phase III study. Int J Urol. 2018;25:723–9.
16. Stenzl A, Penkoff H, Dajc-Sommerer E, Zumbraegel A, Hoeltl L, Scholz M, et al. Detection and clinical outcome of urinary bladder cancer with 5-aminolevulinic acid-induced fluorescence cystoscopy: a multicenter randomized, double-blind, placebo-controlled trial. Cancer. 2011;117:938–47.
17. Waidelich R, Hofstetter A, Stepp H, Baumgartner R, Weninger E, Kriegmair M. Early clinical experience with 5-aminolevulinic acid for the photodynamic therapy of upper tract urothelial tumors. J Urol. 1998;159:401–4.
18. Somani BK, Moseley H, Eljamel MS, Nabi G, Kata SG. Photodynamic diagnosis (PDD) for upper urinary tract transitional cell carcinoma (UT-TCC): evolution of a new technique. Photodiagnosis Photodyn Ther. 2010;7:39–43.
19. Audenet F, Traxer O, Yates DR, Cussenot O, Rouprêt M. Potential role of photodynamic techniques combined with new generation flexible ureterorenoscopes and molecular markers for the management of urothelial carcinoma of the upper urinary tract. BJU Int. 2012;109:608–14.
20. Ahmad S, Aboumarzouk O, Somani B, Nabi G, Kata SG. Oral 5-aminolevulinic acid in simultaneous photodynamic diagnosis of upper and lower urinary tract transitional cell carcinoma—a prospective audit. BJU Int. 2012;110(11 Pt B):E596-600.
21. Aboumarzouk OM, Ahmad S, Moseley H, Kata SG. Accuracy of photodynamic diagnosis in the detection and follow-up of patients with upper urinary tract lesions: Initial 3-year experience. Arab J Urol. 2012;10:138–42.
22. Aboumarzouk OM, Mains E, Moseley H, Kata SG. Diagnosis of upper urinary tract tumours: is photodynamic diagnosis assisted ureterorenoscopy required as an addition to modern imaging and ureterorenoscopy? Photodiagnosis Photodyn Ther. 2013;10:127–33.
23. Tanimoto R, Wada K, Ishizuka M, Murakami K, Ishii T, Mitsui Y, et al. Preclinical *ex-vivo* experiment of photodynamic diagnosis using 5-aminolevulinic acid for upper urinary tract urothelial cancer. J Endourol. 2017;31(S2):A26.
24. Rouprêt M, Babjuk M, Burger M, Compérat E, Cowan NC, Gontero P, et al. European Association of Urology Guidelines on Upper Urinary Tract Urothelial Cell Carcinoma: 2020 Update. 2020. https://uroweb.org/wp-content/uploads/EAU-Guidelines-on-Upper-Urinary-Tract-Urothelial-Carcinoma-2020.pdf. Accessed 1st Oct 2020.
25. Bondad J, Aboumarzouk OM, Moseley H, Kata SG. Oral 5-aminolevulinic acid induced Photodynamic Diagnostic Ureterorenoscopy–does the blood pressure require monitoring? Photodiagnosis Photodyn Ther. 2013;10:39–41.

26

The use of mono- and combination drug therapy in men and women with lower urinary tract symptoms (LUTS) in the UK

Mahmood Ali[1,2*†], Margarita Landeira[2†], Patrick J. O. Covernton[2], Nurul Choudhury[2†], Ashley Jaggi[1,2†], Francis Fatoye[1] and Rob van Maanen[3†]

Abstract

Background: Combination drug therapy for lower urinary tract symptoms (LUTS) is beneficial to selected patients and recommended by guidelines. Patterns of real-world LUTS drug use, especially combination drug therapy, have not been studied extensively. Moreover, further understanding of the recent landscape is required following the introduction of the beta-3-adrenoceptor agonist mirabegron in the UK in 2013 for overactive bladder (OAB). The objective was to describe mono- and combination drug therapy use for LUTS in patients in UK clinical practice.

Methods: This was a retrospective, descriptive, observational database study using UK Clinical Practice Research Datalink GOLD and linked databases. Men and women ≥ 18 years with a first prescription for any LUTS drug from 2014 to 2016 with ≥ 12 months continuous enrollment pre- and post-index date were included. Primary endpoints were mono- or combination drug therapy use for LUTS in male and female cohorts. Secondary endpoints were description of treatment prescribed, treatment persistence and patient demographics. Data were analyzed descriptively. Subcohorts were defined by drugs prescribed at index date.

Results: 79,472 patients (61.3% male) were included, based on index treatments. Of all men, 82.5% received any benign prostatic obstruction (BPO) drug, 25.4% any OAB drug, and 7.9% any BPO drug plus any OAB drug. As either mono- or combination drug therapy, 77.1% received an alpha-blocker, 18.9% a 5-alpha reductase inhibitor, 23.9% an antimuscarinic agent, and 2.1% mirabegron. Of all women, 94.5% received any OAB drug, 6.0% duloxetine, and 0.5% any OAB drug plus duloxetine. As either mono- or combination drug therapy, 87.7% received an antimuscarinic, and 9.7% mirabegron. In men or women receiving OAB treatment, approximately 2.5% received combination drug therapy with an antimuscarinic agent and mirabegron. For OAB drug monotherapies, mirabegron had the highest persistence in both male and female cohorts.

Conclusions: This study provides a better understanding of the recent landscape of LUTS drug use in UK clinical practice. It highlights potential undertreatment of storage symptoms in men with LUTS and the low use of combination OAB treatments.

*Correspondence: mmd.ali01@gmail.com
†At the time of study or manuscript preparation
[1] Manchester Metropolitan University, Manchester, UK
Full list of author information is available at the end of the article

Keywords: Benign prostatic obstruction (BPO), Overactive bladder (OAB), Lower urinary tract symptoms (LUTS), Persistence, Stress urinary incontinence (SUI)

Background

Lower urinary tract symptoms (LUTS) is an overarching term for symptoms in men and women, comprising storage, voiding and post-voiding components [1, 2]. In both men and women, storage LUTS are commonly attributed to overactive bladder (OAB) syndrome [1–3], which is defined as urinary urgency, usually with increased daytime frequency and/or nocturia, with/without urinary incontinence, and with no urinary tract infection or other detectable disease [1, 2, 4]. Stress urinary incontinence (SUI) is another common cause of LUTS, especially in women, and involves involuntary urine leakage associated with physical activity (e.g., coughing, sneezing), often as a consequence of childbirth [1, 3, 5]. Voiding LUTS in men are commonly attributed to benign prostatic obstruction (BPO: bladder outlet obstruction [BOO] due to benign prostatic enlargement) [1, 6].

Although conservative treatment, including lifestyle intervention and behavioral therapies (such as bladder training), remains the foundation of LUTS management, several pharmacological treatments are available [6–8]. If conservative treatment fails, pharmacological therapy for OAB/urgency urinary incontinence (UUI) includes antimuscarinic agents or the beta-3 agonist, mirabegron [7]. Combination of an antimuscarinic agent plus mirabegron has also been shown to be effective [9] and is recommended as an option if patients respond inadequately to monotherapy [7, 8]. In patients with SUI where surgery is not indicated, duloxetine is the only recommended pharmacotherapy [7]; it is unknown to what extent duloxetine is used in combination with OAB drugs. Women with LUTS can experience symptoms of both OAB and SUI [10], but there are no recommendations regarding combination therapy with OAB/UUI drugs for such patients.

In men with LUTS suggestive of BPO, the main treatment options include alpha-blockers for rapid symptomatic relief [11, 12] and 5-alpha reductase inhibitors (5-ARIs) to delay progression of BPO and help manage symptoms over the long term in men at risk of disease progression [6, 12]. Alpha-blockers are usually used as first-line treatment [6], but the European Association of Urology (EAU) guidelines recommend combined alpha-blocker and 5-ARI treatment in men with moderate-to-severe LUTS and an increased risk of disease progression [6]. However, many men with LUTS (approximately 50%) experience mixed symptoms suggestive of both OAB and BPO [13]. Only one-third of these men with mixed symptoms will achieve adequate symptom control with an alpha-blocker alone, with the remainder requiring additional pharmacotherapy to manage residual storage LUTS [14]. Clinical trials in men on alpha-blocker monotherapy who still have bothersome storage LUTS have shown that adding an OAB drug can significantly reduce storage symptoms and improve quality of life [15–18]. The addition of an antimuscarinic agent or beta-3-agonist if storage symptoms are not relieved by alpha-blocker monotherapy is a recommended treatment strategy in clinical guidelines [6].

Patterns of real-world LUTS drug use, especially combination drug therapy, have not been studied extensively in the UK. Our study investigated the recent landscape of pharmacotherapy for men and women with LUTS in UK clinical practice, including the types and extent of combination therapies used, and persistence with treatment.

Methods

Study design

This was a retrospective, descriptive, observational database study of LUTS treatment in the UK primary care setting. Data were extracted from the UK Clinical Practice Research Datalink (CPRD) GOLD, a national longitudinal primary care database, which contains anonymized electronic health records of over 15.6 million patients (September 2018 version) [19]. Only de-identified data were obtained, and patients could opt out if they did not wish to have their data used for research purposes. CPRD GOLD was linked to the Hospital Episode Statistic database in England for the exploration of resource use, and the Index of Multiple Deprivation (IMD). The IMD provides an indication of patients' socio-economic status measured at the GP surgery level. All methods were carried out in accordance with relevant guidelines and regulations.

Population

The study included adults (≥ 18 years of age) identified with LUTS (evidenced by prescription of drugs used to treat LUTS) between 1 January 2014 and 31 December 2016, with ≥ 12 months continuous enrollment pre- and post-index date (index date was the date on which patients were prescribed a new index pharmacotherapy [one pharmacotherapy or combination of two or more pharmacotherapies] for the first time between 1 January 2014 and 31 December 2016). Patients prescribed the same index drug in the 12-month pre-index period were excluded. Male and female cohorts were considered separately. Sub-cohorts were defined by the drugs received at index date (Additional file 1: Table S1), and combination therapy was categorized by index drug with patients placed into one sub-cohort only. If > 1 drug was prescribed at index date and this indicated assignment to different sub-cohorts, the order of preference was as follows: LUTS (including OAB) had priority over BPO in the male cohort and LUTS (including OAB) over SUI in the female cohort. Patients were classified as being on combination therapy if the additional drug(s) was prescribed within the prescription duration of the first drug (prescription duration was calculated by total tablets prescribed divided by total daily dose) and the index date was the first prescription of the most recently prescribed drug.

The LUTS (including OAB) cohort were patients receiving an OAB drug (antimuscarinic agent and/or mirabegron), with or without a BPO drug (alpha-blocker and/or 5-ARI) in the male cohort and with or without a SUI drug (duloxetine) in the female cohort. BPO patients were those receiving an alpha-blocker and/or 5-ARI without an OAB drug. SUI patients were those receiving duloxetine without an OAB drug (Additional file 1: Table S1).

Endpoints

Primary endpoints were use of mono- or combination drug therapy for LUTS in a) male or b) female cohorts. Secondary endpoints were socio-demographic and clinical characteristics, and description of monotherapy/combination drugs. Exploratory variables included treatment persistence and presence of a LUTS diagnostic Read code in the pre-index period.

Data analyses

Socio-demographic characteristics were recorded by age, sex and IMD; clinical characteristics were recorded by comorbidity (number of chronic diseases from the Quality and Outcomes Framework [QOF]), polypharmacy (number of distinct British National Formulary headers from CPRD GOLD), and antimuscarinic treatment experience (≥ 1 antimuscarinic agent prescription, other than index treatment, in CPRD GOLD), within the 12-month pre-index period.

Statistical analyses

Data were analyzed descriptively for the overall population and by cohort and sub-cohort. Analyses were conducted using SAS Studio version 3.5.

Persistence was analyzed by median time (from index date) to first discontinuation (TTD, during the 12-month post-index period), and persistence rate at 12 months, calculated using the Kaplan–Meier method. Discontinuation was defined as exceeding the maximum allowable gap duration (MAGD) between prescriptions. For the base-case, the MAGD was defined as 1.5 times the estimated duration of the most recent prescription. Combination treatment was classed as discontinued upon discontinuation of any one of the component drugs. Data were classed as Not Observable when the number of patients still at risk was below the 20% of the initial sample threshold required to allow for persistence to be calculated or, the median was not reached.

Sensitivity analyses

Sensitivity analyses (SA1-7) varied the combination drug therapy definition, MAGD definition and presence of LUTS diagnostic code. The combination drug therapy definition was changed to: a second drug of interest is prescribed within 1.5 times the estimated prescription interval of the first drug (SA1); two drugs of interest are prescribed on the same day (SA2); both drugs continue to be prescribed for ≥ 90 days from index date (SA3). MAGD definition was changed to: equivalent to (SA4) or double (SA5) the length of most recent prescription. To be considered a patient with LUTS, patients required a LUTS diagnosis code (Additional file 1: Tables S2a–c) registered any time before the index date (SA6). In the final sensitivity analysis, patients diagnosed with hypertension were excluded (SA7).

Results

Patients

Of 223,831 patients with one or more LUTS drug prescription between 1 January 2014 and 31 December 2016, 79,472 were included in the study (61.3% [$n = 48,690$] in the male and 38.7% [$n = 30,782$] in the female cohort) (Fig. 1) (Additional file 1: Table S3a and b).

At index date, the mean age was 65.5 years. In the 12-month pre-index period, patients had a mean of 0.2 new diagnoses of QOF chronic diseases and were prescribed a mean of 9.6 drugs; 5.1% of patients had received an antimuscarinic agent (Tables 1, 2). Approximately one in five patients (16.3%) had a LUTS diagnostic code, the notable exceptions being for doxazosin and duloxetine monotherapy (3% each).

Extent of monotherapy and combination drug use

Of all men ($n = 48,690$), 82.5% received any BPO drug (alpha-blocker and/or 5-ARI), 74.6% received any (one or more) BPO drug without an OAB drug, 25.4% received any OAB drug (antimuscarinic agent and/or mirabegron) (17.5% received any [one or more] OAB drug without a BPO drug, and 7.9% received any BPO drug plus any OAB drug). As either mono- or combination therapy, 77.1% were receiving an alpha-blocker, 18.9% received a

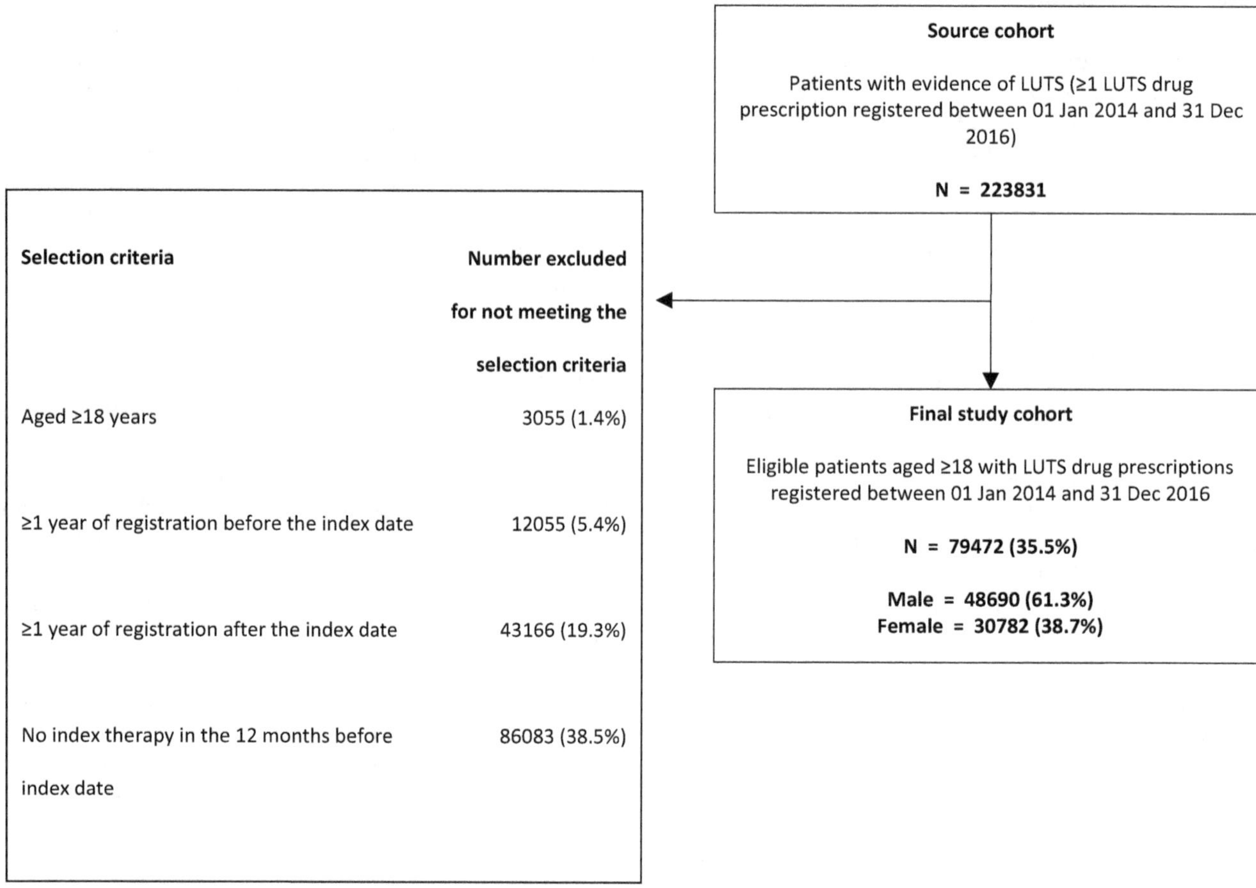

Fig. 1 Selection criteria and study cohorts

5-ARI, 23.9% an antimuscarinic agent and 2.1% mirabegron. The most common drug received either as mono- or combination therapy was tamsulosin (61.2% of all men) and the most common combination was finasteride plus tamsulosin (8.6%, with or without additional drugs). Of all women ($n = 30{,}782$), 94.5% received any OAB drug, 6.0% received a SUI drug, and 0.5% received any OAB drug plus a SUI drug (Additional file 1: Table S3b). As either mono- or combination therapy, 87.7% were receiving an antimuscarinic agent and 9.7% mirabegron. The extent of drug class use is summarized in Tables 3, 4 and 5, and in Additional file 1: Tables S3b and 4.

Male LUTS (including OAB) sub-cohort

In this sub-cohort of 12,383 men treated with any OAB drug, 64.2% received monotherapy with an OAB drug and 35.8% received combinations (31.2% with any OAB drug plus any BPO drug and 7.8% with two or more OAB drugs [3.2% with and 4.6% without a BPO drug]) (Table 3). In addition, 94.1% received any antimuscarinic agent, 8.4% received mirabegron, 2.5% received any antimuscarinic agent plus mirabegron and 5.4% received two or more antimuscarinic agents (Table 3). In this sub-cohort 26.9% of patients received combination therapy including any alpha-blocker and any antimuscarinic agent and 2.6% received any alpha-blocker plus mirabegron. Furthermore, 7.7% of this sub-cohort received triple therapy with any alpha-blocker plus any 5-ARI plus any OAB drug (Table 3).

The most frequently prescribed OAB monotherapies in this sub-cohort were solifenacin (22.3%), oxybutynin (21.1%), tolterodine (11.7%) and mirabegron (4.1%) (Table 3; Additional file 1: Table S5).

The most common OAB drug either alone or in combination was solifenacin (40.6% of the OAB sub-cohort). The most frequently prescribed combination was solifenacin plus tamsulosin (7.3% of sub-cohort for this two-drug combination alone; 11.7% when also including additional drugs), followed by oxybutynin plus tamsulosin and then tolterodine plus tamsulosin, with 2.9% and 2.0% of sub-cohort, respectively. A total of 0.8% of this sub-cohort received mirabegron plus solifenacin alone (1.4% when also including additional drugs).

Table 1 Population demographic and clinical characteristics for male sub-cohorts

		LUTS (including OAB) N = 12,383	BPO only N = 36,307
Age at index date	n	12,383	36,307
	Mean (SD)	65.54 (15.73)	67.98 (12.47)
	18–24	192 (1.6%)	119 (0.3%)
	25–34	434 (3.5%)	356 (1.0%)
	35–44	736 (5.9%)	997 (2.7%)
	45–54	1438 (11.6%)	3586 (9.9%)
	55–64	2188 (17.7%)	7746 (21.3%)
	65–74	3379 (27.3%)	11,905 (32.8%)
	≥75	4016 (32.4%)	11,598 (31.9%)
Index of multiple deprivation at index prescription (GP surgery level)	n	5112	16,534
	1 = least deprived	633 (12.4%)	2770 (16.8%)
	2	1124 (22.0%)	3654 (22.1%)
	3	968 (18.9%)	3175 (19.2%)
	4	963 (18.8%)	2926 (17.7%)
	5 = most deprived	1424 (27.9%)	4009 (24.2%)
New comorbidities	n	12,383	36,307
Count of newly diagnosed chronic diseases from the QOF within the 12-month pre-index period	Mean (SD)	0.21 (0.50)	0.22 (0.51)
	0	10,228 (82.6%)	29,480 (81.2%)
	1	1790 (14.5%)	5700 (15.7%)
	2	313 (2.5%)	978 (2.7%)
	3+	52 (0.4%)	149 (0.4%)
Polypharmacy	n	12,383	36,307
Number of distinct BNF headers within the 12-month pre-index period	Mean (SD)	9.81 (7.27)	8.52 (6.45)
	0	576 (4.7%)	1757 (4.8%)
	[1; 3]	1931 (15.6%)	6668 (18.4%)
	[4; 7]	2936 (23.7%)	10,342 (28.5%)
	[8; 19]	5707 (46.1%)	15,220 (41.9%)
	20+	1233 (10.0%)	2320 (6.4%)
Antimuscarinic treatment experience within the 12-month pre-index period	n	12,383	36,307
	Yes	908 (7.3%)	397 (1.1%)
	No	11,475 (92.7%)	35,910 (98.9%)

Male LUTS (including OAB) sub-cohort patients were those receiving an OAB drug (antimuscarinic and/or mirabegron) with or without a BPO drug (either an alpha-blocker and/or 5-ARI). Male BPO sub-cohort patients were those receiving an alpha-blocker and/or 5-ARI without an OAB drug. Percentages may not total exactly 100 due to rounding

BNF: British National Formulary; *BPO*: benign prostatic obstruction; *GP*: general practitioner; *LUTS*: lower urinary tract symptoms; *OAB*: overactive bladder; *QOF*: Quality and Outcomes Framework; *SD*: standard deviation

Male BPO sub-cohort

In this sub-cohort of 36,307 men, 81.9% received monotherapy (75.6% with any alpha-blocker; 6.3% with any 5-ARI) and 18.1% received combination therapy (15.3% with any alpha-blocker plus any 5-ARI). Tamsulosin monotherapy was the most commonly prescribed (58.3% of sub-cohort patients), followed by doxazosin (15.0%) (Table 4; Additional file 1: Table S6). For combination therapy, 49.7% of combination therapy patients were prescribed finasteride plus tamsulosin (9.0% of this sub-cohort for these two drugs alone; 10.0% when also including additional drugs), followed by dutasteride plus tamsulosin and doxazosin plus tamsulosin. In addition, 93.6% of patients in this sub-cohort overall received an alpha-blocker and 21.7% a 5-ARI.

Female LUTS (including OAB) sub-cohort

In this sub-cohort of 29,094 women, 90.5% of patients received monotherapy (83.4% any antimuscarinic, 7.1% mirabegron) and 9.5% combination therapy (9.0% with two or more OAB drugs). In addition, 0.5% of women in this sub-cohort received any OAB drug plus duloxetine

Table 2 Population demographic and clinical characteristics for female sub-cohorts

		LUTS (including OAB) N = 29,094	SUI N = 1688
Age at index date	n	29,094	1688
	Mean (SD)	62.92 (16.77)	54.24 (16.29)
	18–24	604 (2.1%)	32 (1.9%)
	25–34	1121 (3.9%)	159 (9.4%)
	35–44	2536 (8.7%)	315 (18.7%)
	45–54	4835 (16.6%)	399 (23.6%)
	55–64	5264 (18.1%)	315 (18.7%)
	65–74	6446 (22.2%)	248 (14.7%)
	≥75	8288 (28.5%)	220 (13.0%)
Index of multiple deprivation at index prescription (GP surgery level)	n	11,999	665
	1 = least deprived	1534 (12.8%)	86 (12.9%)
	2	2418 (20.2%)	148 (22.3%)
	3	2292 (19.1%)	137 (20.6%)
	4	2285 (19.0%)	105 (15.8%)
	5 = most deprived	3470 (28.9%)	189 (28.4%)
New comorbidities	n	29,094	1688
Count of newly diagnosed chronic diseases from the QOF within the 12-month pre-index period	Mean (SD)	0.20 (0.48)	0.23 (0.53)
	0	24,327 (83.6%)	1374 (81.4%)
	1	3950 (13.6%)	248 (14.7%)
	2	712 (2.4%)	56 (3.3%)
	3+	105 (0.4%)	10 (0.6%)
Polypharmacy	n	29,094	1688
Number of distinct BNF headers within the 12-month pre-index period	Mean (SD)	10.77 (7.49)	11.55 (7.42)
	0	681 (2.3%)	29 (1.7%)
	[1; 3]	3766 (12.9%)	165 (9.8%)
	[4; 7]	6944 (23.9%)	384 (22.7%)
	[8; 19]	14,178 (48.7%)	873 (51.7%)
	20+	3525 (12.1%)	237 (14.0%)
Antimuscarinic treatment experience within the 12-month pre-index period	n	29,094	1688
	Yes	2681 (9.2%)	56 (3.3%)
	No	26,413 (90.8%)	1632 (96.7%)

Female LUTS (including OAB) sub-cohort patients were those receiving an OAB drug (antimuscarinic and/or mirabegron) with or without a SUI drug (duloxetine). Female SUI sub-cohort patients were those receiving duloxetine without an OAB drug. Percentages may not total exactly 100 due to rounding

BNF: British National Formulary; *GP*: general practitioner; *LUTS*: lower urinary tract symptoms; *OAB*: overactive bladder; *QOF*: Quality and Outcomes Framework; *SD*: standard deviation; *SUI*: stress urinary incontinence

(Table 5). Mirabegron plus duloxetine was prescribed to 0.04% of patients in this sub-cohort. A combination of any two or more antimuscarinic agents (± mirabegron) was used by 6.3% of sub-cohort patients and any antimuscarinic agent plus mirabegron by 2.7%. The most common OAB drug either alone or in combination was solifenacin (41.0% of the OAB sub-cohort) and 10.2% of this sub-cohort overall received mirabegron.

Solifenacin was the most frequently prescribed monotherapy (34.7% of this sub-cohort), followed by oxybutynin and tolterodine (Table 5; Additional file 1: Table S7); 92.8% of sub-cohort patients were prescribed any antimuscarinic agent. The most frequently prescribed combinations were solifenacin plus tolterodine, oxybutynin plus solifenacin and mirabegron plus solifenacin.

Female SUI sub-cohort

Duloxetine was prescribed to all ($n = 1688$) sub-cohort patients and was the only drug used in women with SUI, as defined in the base-case.

Persistence

Kaplan Meier curves of TTD by mono- and combination drug therapy for the male BPO sub-cohort, and for

Table 3 Extent of mono- and combination drug therapy use in the male LUTS (including OAB) sub-cohort

Monotherapy	N	% of monotherapy patients	% of all patients in male OAB sub-cohort	% of all male patients
Any OAB drug monotherapy	7946	100.0	64.2	16.3
Any antimuscarinic monotherapy	7443	93.7	60.1	15.3
Solifenacin	2759	34.7	22.3	5.7
Oxybutynin	2613	32.9	21.1	5.4
Tolterodine	1445	18.2	11.7	3.0
Mirabegron	503	6.3	4.1	1.0
Fesoterodine	285	3.6	2.3	0.6
Trospium	227	2.9	1.8	0.5
Flavoxate	49	0.6	0.4	0.1
Darifenacin	47	0.6	0.4	0.1
Propiverine	18	0.2	0.1	0.04
Combination drug therapy	**N**	**% of combination drug therapy patients**	**% of all patients in male OAB sub-cohort**	**% of all male patients**
Any combination drug therapy	4437	100.0	35.8	9.1
Any BPO drug + any OAB drug	3863	87.1	31.2	7.9
Any BPO drug + any antimuscarinic	3643	82.1	29.4	7.5
Any BPO drug + mirabegron	347	7.8	2.8	0.7
Any alpha-blocker + any OAB drug (±5-ARI)	3538	79.7	28.6	7.3
Any alpha-blocker + any antimuscarinic (± mirabegron and/or 5-ARI)	3330	75.1	26.9	6.8
Any alpha-blocker + mirabegron (± antimuscarinic and/or 5-ARI)	326	7.3	2.6	0.7
Triple drug therapy (any alpha-blocker + any 5-ARI + any OAB drug)	958	21.6	7.7	2.0
Any OAB drug + any 5-ARI (± alpha-blocker)	1284	28.9	10.4	2.6
Any OAB drug + any 5-ARI (excl. alpha-blocker)	325	7.3	2.6	0.7
Mirabegron + any antimuscarinic (± BPO drug)	307	6.9	2.5	0.6
Any ≥ 2 OAB (± BPO drug)	964	21.7	7.8	2.0
Any ≥ 2 OAB (no BPO drug)	574	12.9	4.6	1.2
Any ≥ 2 antimuscarinics (± BPO drug and/or mirabegron)	666	15.0	5.4	1.4
Solifenacin + tamsulosin	902	20.3	7.3	1.9
Oxybutynin + tamsulosin	364	8.2	2.9	0.7
Tamsulosin + tolterodine	248	5.6	2.0	0.5
Finasteride + solifenacin + tamsulosin	233	5.3	1.9	0.5
Doxazosin + solifenacin	114	2.6	0.9	0.2
Solifenacin + tolterodine	114	2.6	0.9	0.2
Finasteride + oxybutynin + tamsulosin	111	2.5	0.9	0.2
Oxybutynin + solifenacin	102	2.3	0.8	0.2
Finasteride + solifenacin	96	2.2	0.8	0.2
Mirabegron + tamsulosin	96	2.2	0.8	0.2
Doxazosin + oxybutynin	95	2.1	0.8	0.2
Mirabegron + solifenacin	95	2.1	0.8	0.2
Fesoterodine + tamsulosin	83	1.9	0.7	0.2
Dutasteride + solifenacin + tamsulosin	79	1.8	0.6	0.2
Doxazosin + tolterodine	69	1.6	0.6	0.1
Other combinations	1636	36.9	13.2	3.4
Drug class	**N**		**% of all patients in male OAB sub-cohort**	**% of all male patients**
Any OAB drug	12,383		100	25.4

Table 3 (continued)

Drug class	N	% of all patients in male OAB sub-cohort	% of all male patients
Any OAB drug (no BPO drug)	8520	68.8	17.5
Any antimuscarinic	11,653	94.1	23.9
Total mirabegron	1039	8.4	2.1
Any alpha-blocker	3538	28.6	7.3
Any 5-ARI	1284	10.4	2.6

5-ARI: 5-alpha reductase inhibitor; *BPO*: benign prostatic obstruction; *LUTS*: lower urinary tract symptoms; *OAB*: overactive bladder

Table 4 Extent of mono- and combination drug therapy use in the male BPO sub-cohort

Monotherapy	N	% of monotherapy patients	% of all patients in BPO sub-cohort	% of all male patients
Any BPO drug monotherapy	29,739	100.0	81.9	61.1
Any alpha-blocker monotherapy	27,462	92.3	75.6	56.4
Any 5-ARI monotherapy	2277	7.7	6.3	4.7
Tamsulosin	21,158	71.1	58.3	43.5
Doxazosin	5456	18.3	15.0	11.2
Finasteride	2131	7.2	5.9	4.4
Alfuzosin	665	2.2	1.8	1.4
Dutasteride	146	0.5	0.4	0.3
Prazosin	101	0.3	0.3	0.2
Terazosin	44	0.1	0.1	0.1
Indoramin	38	0.1	0.1	0.1
Combination drug therapy	**N**	**% of combination drug therapy patients**	**% of all patients in BPO sub-cohort**	**% of all male patients**
Any combination drug therapy	6568	100.0	18.1	13.5
Any alpha-blocker + any 5-ARI	5573	84.9	15.3	11.4
Finasteride + tamsulosin	3262	49.7	9.0	6.7
Dutasteride + tamsulosin	1189	18.1	3.3	2.4
Doxazosin + tamsulosin	614	9.3	1.7	1.3
Doxazosin + finasteride	289	4.4	0.8	0.6
Alfuzosin + finasteride	233	3.5	0.6	0.5
Alfuzosin + tamsulosin	208	3.2	0.6	0.4
Doxazosin + finasteride + tamsulosin	167	2.5	0.5	0.3
Dutasteride + finasteride + tamsulosin	125	1.9	0.3	0.3
Other combinations	481	7.3	1.3	1.0
Drug class	**N**		**% of all patients in BPO sub-cohort**	**% of all male patients**
Any BPO drug	36,307		100	74.6
Any alpha-blocker	33,984		93.6	69.8
Any 5-ARI	7896		21.7	16.2

5-ARI: 5-alpha reductase inhibitor; *BPO*: benign prostatic obstruction

Table 5 Extent of mono- and combination drug therapy use in the female LUTS (including OAB) sub-cohort

Monotherapy	N	% of monotherapy patients	% of all patients in female OAB sub-cohort	% of all female patients
Any OAB drug monotherapy	26,338	100.0	90.5	85.6
Any antimuscarinic monotherapy	24,263	92.1	83.4	78.8
Solifenacin	10,083	38.3	34.7	32.8
Oxybutynin	7852	29.8	27.0	25.5
Tolterodine	4020	15.3	13.8	13.1
Mirabegron	2075	7.9	7.1	6.7
Fesoterodine	1173	4.5	4.0	3.8
Trospium	754	2.9	2.6	2.4
Darifenacin	209	0.8	0.7	0.7
Flavoxate	96	0.4	0.3	0.3
Propiverine	76	0.3	0.3	0.2
Combination drug therapy	**N**	**% of combination drug therapy patients**	**% of all patients in female OAB sub-cohort**	**% of all female patients**
All combination drug therapy	2756	100.0	9.5	9.0
Any ≥ 2 OAB drugs	2621	95.1	9.0	8.5
Mirabegron + any antimuscarinic	788	28.6	2.7	2.6
Any ≥ 2 antimuscarinics (± mirabegron)	1847	67.0	6.3	6.0
Duloxetine + any OAB drug	144	5.2	0.5	0.5
Solifenacin + tolterodine	507	18.4	1.7	1.6
Oxybutynin + solifenacin	458	16.6	1.6	1.5
Mirabegron + solifenacin	417	15.1	1.4	1.4
Fesoterodine + solifenacin	174	6.3	0.6	0.6
Oxybutynin + tolterodine	174	6.3	0.6	0.6
Other combinations	1026	37.2	3.5	3.3
Drug class	**N**		**% of all patient in OAB sub-cohort**	**% of all female patients**
Any OAB drug	29,094		100	94.5
Any antimuscarinic	27,010		92.8	87.7
Total mirabegron	2972		10.2	9.7

LUTS: lower urinary tract symptoms; *OAB*: overactive bladder

duloxetine in the female SUI sub-cohort, are included in Additional file 1: Figures S1–S3.

Male LUTS (including OAB) sub-cohort

For monotherapy, mirabegron had the longest median TTD (205 days), followed by fesoterodine (115 days), trospium (102 days) and solifenacin (97 days) (Fig. 2a; Table 6). These drugs also displayed the highest 12-month persistence rates (Table 7). For combination therapies, tamsulosin plus trospium had the longest median TTD (144 days); however, the sample size was small ($n = 65$). The longest median TTD for combination therapy with a sample size > 100 was 121 days for finasteride plus solifenacin plus tamsulosin (Fig. 2b). The highest 12-month persistence was with finasteride plus solifenacin (32.3%) (Table 7).

Male BPO sub-cohort

For monotherapy, median TTD was longest for doxazosin and finasteride (> 365 days each [median not reached]), followed by tamsulosin (329 days) and dutasteride (305 days) (however, see sensitivity analyses below). Doxazosin had the highest 12-month persistence (67.8%) followed by finasteride (53.3%) and tamsulosin (48.4%). For combination therapies, the highest 12-month persistence was for dutasteride plus tamsulosin (56.3%) followed by doxazosin plus dutasteride (55.6%) (Additional file 1: Tables S8 and S9).

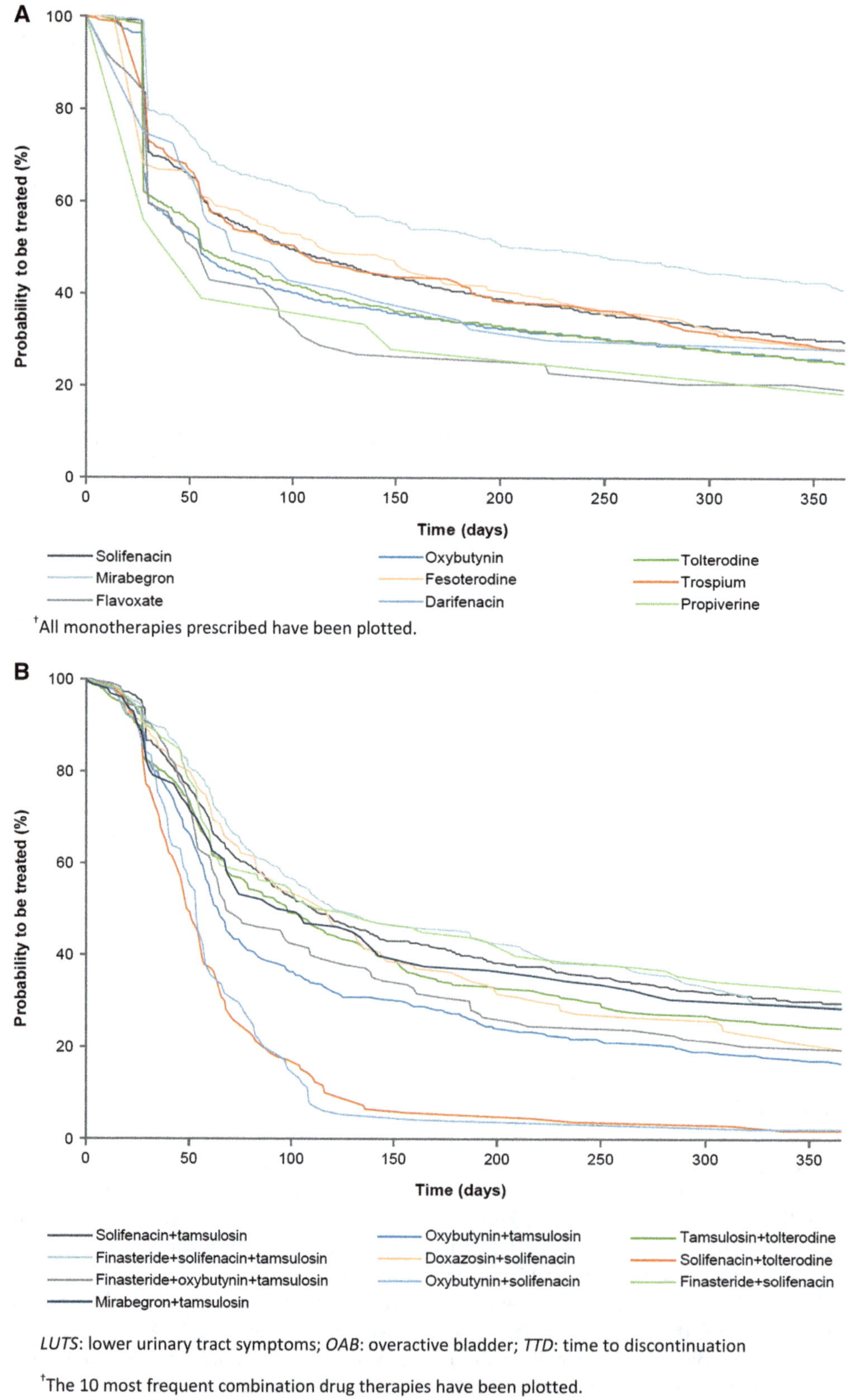

Fig. 2 TTD in male LUTS (including OAB) sub-cohort (Kaplan–Meier estimates)† for **A** monotherapies. †All monotherapies prescribed have been plotted. **B** Combination drug therapies. *LUTS*: lower urinary tract symptoms; *OAB*: overactive bladder; *TTD*: time to discontinuation. †The 10 most frequent combination drug therapies have been plotted

Table 6 Persistence in post-index period in the male LUTS (including OAB) sub-cohort

Index drug	N	Persistence days Median (Q1–Q3)
Monotherapy		
Solifenacin	2759	97 (30–365[a])
Oxybutynin	2613	56 (28–363)
Tolterodine	1445	56 (28–359)
Mirabegron	503	205 (50–365[a])
Fesoterodine	285	115 (28–365[a])
Trospium	227	102 (30–365[a])
Flavoxate	49	54 (30–222)
Darifenacin	47	71 (28–365[a])
Propiverine	18	42 (28–273)
Combination drug therapy		
Solifenacin + tamsulosin	902	111 (53–365[a])
Oxybutynin + tamsulosin	364	65 (42–195)
Tamsulosin + tolterodine	248	99 (48–335.5)
Finasteride + solifenacin + tamsulosin	233	121 (61–365[a])
Doxazosin + solifenacin	114	117 (59–308)
Solifenacin + tolterodine	114	50 (34–75)
Finasteride + oxybutynin + tamsulosin	111	69 (49–215)
Oxybutynin + solifenacin	102	54 (38–82)
Finasteride + solifenacin	96	120 (55–365[a])
Mirabegron + tamsulosin	96	98 (47–365[a])
Doxazosin + oxybutynin	95	60 (44–128)
Mirabegron + solifenacin	95	61 (42–95)
Fesoterodine + tamsulosin	83	80 (50–221)
Dutasteride + solifenacin + tamsulosin	79	74 (51–235)
Doxazosin + tolterodine	69	95 (50–365[a])
Tamsulosin + trospium	65	144 (61–365[a])
Finasteride + oxybutynin	62	77 (42–240)
Finasteride + tamsulosin + tolterodine	57	119 (62–365[a])
Alfuzosin + solifenacin	47	124 (42–365[a])
Other combinations	1405	63 (41–151)

LUTS: lower urinary tract symptoms; *OAB*: overactive bladder; *Q1*: lower quartile; *Q3*: upper quartile

[a] Q3 not reached by 365 days

Female LUTS (including OAB) sub-cohort

For monotherapy, median TTD (244 days) and 12-month persistence (43.5%) was longest for mirabegron (Fig. 3a). Among combination therapies, persistence rates at 12 months were often not observable; however, the longest median TTD was 69 days for duloxetine plus tolterodine and 70 days for fesoterodine plus mirabegron (Fig. 3b, and Additional file 1: Tables S10 and S11).

Female SUI sub-cohort

For duloxetine, median TTD was 55 days and 12-month persistence rate was 22.0%.

Sensitivity analyses

Results of sensitivity analyses were consistent with the main analyses, with one notable exception. In the male BPO sub-cohort, patients with a confirmed LUTS diagnosis had a lower median TTD on doxazosin (144 versus > 365 days) and finasteride (170 versus > 365 days) versus the main analysis (Additional file 1: Figures S4a and b). There were no notable findings in the other sensitivity analyses performed (Additional file 1: Table S12).

Discussion

This retrospective analysis in a UK GP primary care database complements previous UK studies of LUTS/OAB and LUTS/BPO [20–22]. The study highlights the relatively low use of combination treatments that target OAB. Only a small proportion of LUTS (including OAB) patients were prescribed mirabegron with an antimuscarinic agent. However, use of this combination may have increased since the publication of studies such as BESIDE in 2016, SYNERGY in 2017 and SYNERGY II in 2018, which showed benefits of combination versus an antimuscarinic alone [9, 23, 24]. It was also notable that around 5% each of men and women receiving OAB drugs were on a combination of two or more antimuscarinic agents (Tables 3 and 4), despite a lack of evidence supporting any benefit of this approach.

Our study also highlights the relatively low treatment rates for storage symptoms in men, despite the fact that these symptoms can be highly bothersome in men, even more so than voiding symptoms [25]. In the EPIC study, of all men identified with LUTS, over 80% had storage LUTS [10]. In the EpiLUTS study [13], storage symptoms were experienced by around two-thirds of men, with approximately 50% of men reporting mixed storage and voiding symptoms [13]. Alpha-blockers are the usual first-line treatment for men with LUTS suggestive of BPO [6, 26] and while they have been shown to relieve both voiding and storage symptoms [27], evidence suggests that up to two-thirds will not respond adequately to alpha-blocker monotherapy [14]. In these cases, the EAU guidelines recommend adding an OAB drug [6]. Therefore, it would be expected that the percentage of men who required OAB treatment would be similar to the percentage of those with storage symptoms. This percentage is around 45% when calculated using data from the EpiLUTS study [13]—the percentage of LUTS patients with storage symptoms alone combined with around two thirds of LUTS patients with mixed symptoms (i.e., those who do not respond to first-line alpha-blocker therapy). However, in our study only around a quarter of all men being treated for LUTS received treatment specifically targeting storage symptoms (i.e., an antimuscarinic and/or mirabegron alone or combined with a BPO drug),

Table 7 Persistence at 1 month, 6 months and 1 year in male LUTS (including OAB) sub-cohort

	N	1 month % [95% CI]	6 months % [95% CI]	1 year % [95% CI]	Median (months) [95% CI]
All	12,383	72.9	34.8	25.2	2.5
		[72.1, 73.6]	[33.9, 35.6]	[24.4, 26.0]	[2.4, 2.7]
Number of patients still at risk[a]		9024	4304	3105	
Monotherapy	7946	65.6	37.6	27.7	2.5
		[64.5, 66.6]	[36.5, 38.6]	[26.8, 28.7]	[2.3, 2.7]
Number of patients still at risk[a]		5211	2986	2193	
Combination drug therapy	4437	85.9	29.7	20.6	2.5
		[84.9, 86.9]	[28.4, 31.1]	[19.4, 21.8]	[2.4, 2.7]
Number of patients still at risk[a]		3813	1318	912	
Monotherapy					
Darifenacin	47	74.5	34.0	27.7	2.3
		[59.4, 84.6]	[21.0, 47.5]	[15.9, 40.8]	[1.7, 5.4]
Number of patients still at risk[a]		35	16	13	
Fesoterodine	285	67.4	41.8	28.1	3.8
		[61.6, 72.5]	[36.0, 47.4]	[23.0, 33.4]	[2.7, 5.2]
Number of patients still at risk[a]		192	119	80	
Flavoxate	49	59.2	26.5	20.4	1.8
		[44.2, 71.4]	[15.2, 39.3]	[10.5, 32.6]	[1.0, 3.1]
Number of patients still at risk[a]		29	13	9	
Mirabegron	503	79.5	53.1	40.9	6.7
		[75.7, 82.8]	[48.6, 57.3]	[36.6, 45.2]	[5.2, 9.5]
Number of patients still at risk[a]		400	267	204	
Oxybutynin	2613	59.6	33.5	25.1	1.8
		[57.7, 61.4]	[31.7, 35.3]	[23.5, 26.8]	[1.7, 1.9]
Number of patients still at risk[a]		1557	875	653	
Propiverine	18	55.6	27.8	22.2	1.4
		[30.5, 74.8]	[10.1, 48.9]	[6.9, 42.9]	[0.9, 4.9]
Number of patients still at risk[a]		10	5	4	
Solifenacin	2759	70.2	40.2	29.5	3.2
		[68.5, 71.9]	[38.4, 42.1]	[27.8, 31.2]	[2.9, 3.6]
Number of patients still at risk[a]		1938	1110	812	
Tolterodine	1445	61.2	33.7	24.8	1.8
		[58.6, 63.6]	[31.3, 36.1]	[22.6, 27.1]	[1.8, 2.2]
Number of patients still at risk[a]		884	487	355	
Trospium	227	73.1	41.4	27.8	3.4
		[66.9, 78.4]	[35.0, 47.7]	[22.1, 33.7]	[2.2, 4.9]
Number of patients still at risk[a]		166	94	63	
Combination drug therapy					
Alfuzosin + solifenacin	47	87.2	40.4	29.8	4.1
		[73.8, 94.1]	[26.5, 53.9]	[17.6, 43.0]	[2.1, 6.9]
Number of patients still at risk[a]		41	19	14	
Doxazosin + oxybutynin	95	87.4	18.9	NO	2
		[78.8, 92.6]	[11.8, 27.4]	–	[1.8, 2.3]
Number of patients still at risk[a]		83	18	13	
Doxazosin + solifenacin	114	89.5	36.0	20.2	3.8
		[82.2, 93.9]	[27.3, 44.7]	[13.4, 28.0]	[2.8, 4.7]
Number of patients still at risk[a]		102	41	23	
Doxazosin + tolterodine	69	87.0	39.1	29.0	3.1

Table 7 (continued)

	N	1 month % [95% CI]	6 months % [95% CI]	1 year % [95% CI]	Median (months) [95% CI]
		[76.4, 93.0]	[27.7, 50.4]	[18.8, 39.9]	[2.1, 6.4]
Number of patients still at risk[a]		60	27	20	
Dutasteride + solifenacin + tamsulosin	79	89.9	27.8	21.5	2.4
		[80.8, 94.8]	[18.5, 38.0]	[13.3, 31.1]	[2.1, 3.6]
Number of patients still at risk[a]		71	22	17	
Fesoterodine + tamsulosin	83	85.5	28.9	NO	2.6
		[75.9, 91.5]	[19.6, 38.9]	–	[2.1, 3.3]
Number of patients still at risk[a]		71	24	12	
Finasteride + oxybutynin	62	88.7	32.3	17.7	2.5
		[77.8, 94.5]	[21.1, 43.9]	[9.5, 28.1]	[1.8, 3.6]
Number of patients still at risk[a]		55	20	11	
Finasteride + oxybutynin + tamsulosin	111	91.0	30.6	19.8	2.3
		[83.9, 95.0]	[22.3, 39.3]	[13.0, 27.7]	[2.0, 3.6]
Number of patients still at risk[a]		101	34	22	
Finasteride + solifenacin	96	90.6	44.8	32.3	3.9
		[82.8, 95.0]	[34.7, 54.4]	[23.2, 41.7]	[2.1, 6.9]
Number of patients still at risk[a]		87	43	31	
Finasteride + solifenacin + tamsulosin	233	91.0	45.1	28.8	4
		[86.5, 94.0]	[38.6, 51.3]	[23.1, 34.7]	[3.4, 6.2]
Number of patients still at risk[a]		212	105	67	
Finasteride + tamsulosin + tolterodine	57	96.5	40.4	28.1	3.9
		[86.7, 99.1]	[27.7, 52.7]	[17.2, 40.0]	[2.8, 6.7]
Number of patients still at risk[a]		55	23	15	
Finasteride + tolterodine	41	85.4	29.3	22.0	1.7
		[70.3, 93.1]	[16.4, 43.4]	[10.9, 35.5]	[1.5, 3.9]
Number of patients still at risk[a]		35	12	9	
Mirabegron + solifenacin	95	85.3	NO	NO	2
		[76.4, 91.0]	–	–	[1.7, 2.5]
Number of patients still at risk[a]		81	11	6	
Mirabegron + tamsulosin	96	82.3	37.5	29.2	3.2
		[73.1, 88.6]	[27.9, 47.1]	[20.5, 38.4]	[2.2, 4.7]
Number of patients still at risk[a]		79	36	28	
Oxybutynin + solifenacin	102	84.3	NO	NO	1.8
		[75.7, 90.1]	–	–	[1.6, 1.9]
Number of patients still at risk[a]		86	4	2	
Oxybutynin + tamsulosin	364	82.4	26.9	16.5	2.1
		[78.1, 86.0]	[22.5, 31.6]	[12.9, 20.5]	[2.0, 2.3]
Number of patients still at risk[a]		300	98	60	
Solifenacin + tamsulosin	902	86.7	39.9	29.4	3.6
		[84.3, 88.7]	[36.7, 43.1]	[26.4, 32.4]	[3.2, 4.1]
Number of patients still at risk[a]		782	360	264	
Solifenacin + tolterodine	114	77.2	NO	NO	1.6
		[68.3, 83.9]	–	–	[1.5, 1.8]
Number of patients still at risk[a]		88	6	2	
Tamsulosin + tolterodine	248	82.3	33.5	24.2	3.3
		[76.9, 86.5]	[27.7, 39.4]	[19.1, 29.7]	[2.6, 4.0]
Number of patients still at risk[a]		204	83	60	
Tamsulosin + trospium	65	90.8	41.5	29.2	4.7

Table 7 (continued)

	N	1 month % [95% CI]	6 months % [95% CI]	1 year % [95% CI]	Median (months) [95% CI]
		[80.6, 95.7]	[29.5, 53.1]	[18.8, 40.5]	[2.9, 7.1]
Number of patients still at risk[a]		59	27	19	
Other combinations	1364	85.1	22.4	15.9	2.1
		[83.1, 86.9]	[20.2, 24.6]	[14.0, 17.9]	[2.0, 2.2]
Number of patients still at risk[a]		1161	305	217	

Not Observable indicates that the number of patients still at risk was below the 20% of the initial sample threshold required to calculate persistence, or the median was not reached

CI: confidence interval; *LUTS*: lower urinary tract symptoms; *NO*: not observable; *OAB*: overactive bladder [a]Number of patients still observable at a given time and for whom no events occurred

although this figure refers only to men with treated LUTS, in contrast to the other studies which were based on the general population. Thus, some men with storage symptoms may be receiving inadequate treatment in clinical practice, despite storage symptoms often being the most bothersome component of LUTS [28].

We might also expect to see OAB/BPO drug combination therapy in up to one-third of all men being treated for LUTS (i.e., two-thirds of those with mixed symptoms) [13, 14]. However, in the current study, only 7% were receiving alpha-blocker plus antimuscarinic combination treatment therapy (and only 8% were on any OAB/BPO drug combination), which is consistent with another UK study in which 15% of men with mixed LUTS were reported to be receiving an alpha-blocker combined with an antimuscarinic agent [20].

As well as alpha-blockers and 5-ARIs, the EAU guidelines recommend the use of phosphodiesterase type 5 inhibitors (PDE5Is) for the treatment of men with moderate-to-severe LUTS with or without erectile dysfunction [6]. Tadalafil, the only currently licensed PDE5I for male LUTS [6], has been shown to relieve both voiding and storage symptoms [29], although additional therapy may be required for patients with severe LUTS related to BOO [30]. However, this study did not look at tadalafil use due to potential misclassification of patients receiving the drug for erectile dysfunction.

The reasons for the low treatment of storage symptoms in men may be historical, reflecting overemphasis on the prostate-related component of LUTS rather than bladder-related issues. Furthermore, there may be a perceived risk of precipitating urinary retention when using bladder antimuscarinic agents in men with evidence of obstruction, although the available evidence suggests that this risk is low [31]. There is already good evidence supporting the use of alpha-blocker/antimuscarinic combination therapy in men with mixed symptoms [16, 17]. More recently, two randomized, placebo-controlled trials have also demonstrated that mirabegron add-on therapy in men who have residual OAB symptoms while being treated with tamsulosin for LUTS is both effective and well-tolerated [18, 32]. It is hoped that this new evidence will help to improve the overall management of men with mixed symptoms.

Antimuscarinic agents and beta-3 agonists are recommended first-line pharmacological treatments for both men and women with OAB [7, 8] and men with moderate-to-severe LUTS with predominant bladder storage symptoms [6]. However, with antimuscarinics, long-term persistence is often poor due to unmet treatment expectations or adverse events [33]. In our study, mirabegron monotherapy had the highest persistence (both in men and women). Several observational studies also reported higher persistence with mirabegron vs antimuscarinics [22, 34]. Persistence was greater with drug monotherapy than in combination drug therapy, and was particularly poor with combinations of two antimuscarinics in both men and women.

For monotherapy targeting BPO and voiding symptoms (e.g. alpha-blockers and 5-ARIs), persistence was highest for doxazosin and finasteride, but this was not evident in sensitivity analyses based on confirmed LUTS diagnosis. This suggests that the higher persistence with these agents in the main sub-cohorts may be driven by their use in other disorders (e.g., doxazosin for hypertension) and it is notable that only 3% of patients on doxazosin had a LUTS diagnostic code.

A limitation of our study is that in CPRD GOLD, GPs do not systematically report prescriptions issued in secondary care, and reasons for discontinuation were not available in CPRD, which limits interpretation of persistence results. In addition, some treatments are prescribed for conditions other than OAB, LUTS, BPO or SUI (e.g., doxazosin, finasteride and duloxetine), which may influence some of the treatment pattern and/or persistence estimates. The inclusion of fixed-dose combinations may

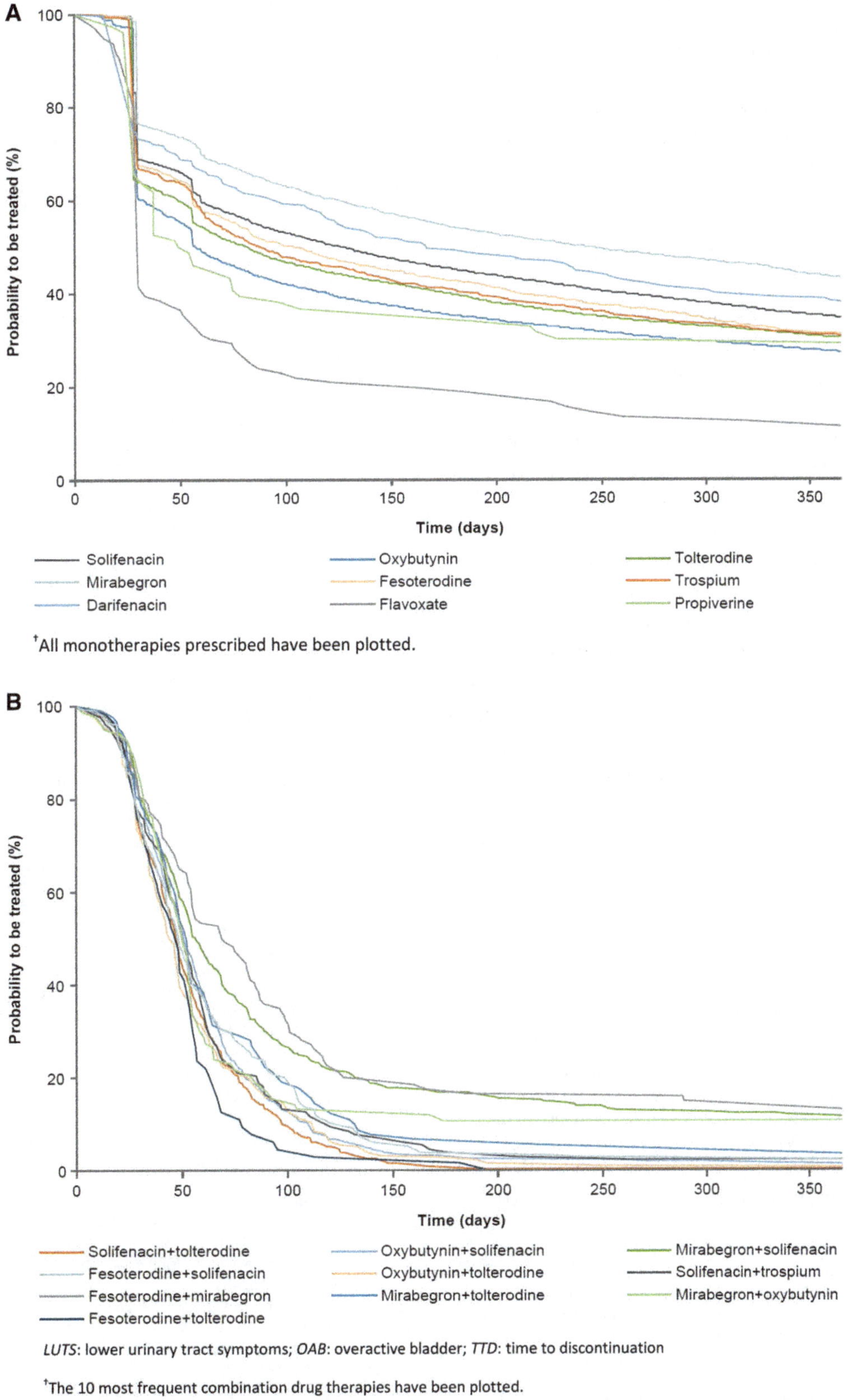

Fig. 3 TTD in female LUTS (including OAB) sub-cohort (Kaplan–Meier estimates)[†]for **A** monotherapies. [†]All monotherapies prescribed have been plotted. **B** Combination drug therapies. *LUTS*: lower urinary tract symptoms; *OAB*: overactive bladder; *TTD*: time to discontinuation. [†]The 10 most frequent combination drug therapies have been plotted

increase the overall persistence with tamsulosin/solifenacin combination therapy [35]; for tamsulosin/dutasteride fixed-dose combination, the available evidence suggests it may have no impact on persistence [36]. Finally, as this study was performed using a UK general practice database, it is unclear to what extent the results would be generalizable to other healthcare systems.

Conclusions

This study provides new real-world evidence suggesting that men with LUTS may be under-treated with pharmacotherapies that specifically target storage symptoms. Only around a quarter of the men being treated for any LUTS received treatment specifically targeting storage symptoms and around 8% of men received a combination of BPO/OAB drugs for mixed symptoms. In addition, use of combination OAB treatment was low in both men and women, which may reflect the lack of evidence for this approach at the time these patients were being treated. Of all OAB medications, numerically the highest rates of monotherapy persistence were seen with mirabegron in both men and women. Persistence was worse when using combination drug therapy and particularly poor when using two antimuscarinic agents. By highlighting the possible under-treatment of men with treatments that target storage symptoms and the low use of combination OAB treatment (especially with mirabegron plus an antimuscarinic agent), this may help clinicians in the UK to reassess their approach to pharmacotherapy for patients with bothersome LUTS.

Abbreviations

5-ARI: 5-Alpha reductase inhibitor; BNF: British National Formulary; BOO: Bladder outlet obstruction; BPO: Benign prostatic obstruction; CI: Confidence interval; CPRD: Clinical Practice Research Datalink; EAU: European Association of Urology; GP: General practitioner; IMD: Index of Multiple Deprivation; LUTS: Lower urinary tract symptoms; MAGD: Maximum allowable gap duration; NO: Not observable; NRES: National Research Ethics Service Committee; OAB: Overactive bladder; PDE5I: Phosphodiesterase type 5 inhibitor; Q1: Lower quartile; Q3: Upper quartile; QOF: Quality and Outcomes Framework; SA: Sensitivity analysis; SD: Standard deviation; SUI: Stress urinary incontinence; TTD: Time to discontinuation.

Acknowledgements

Medical writing support was provided by Hayley Owen and Tom Lavelle (Bioscript Medical Ltd, Macclesfield, UK).

Authors' contributions

Conception and design of study: MA, ML, PJOC, NC, AJ, FF and RvM. Data acquisition: MA and ML. Data analysis and interpretation: MA, ML, PJOC, NC, AJ, FF and RvM. Statistical analysis: MA and ML. Obtaining funding: MA, ML, NC, AJ and FF. Administrative, technical or material support: MA, ML, AJ and FF. Supervision: MA, ML and FF. Study report preparation, review and finalization process: MA and ML. Critical revision of the publication for intellectual content: MA, ML, PJOC, AJ, FF and RvM. All authors read and approved the final manuscript.

Competing interests

MA, ML and PJOC are employees of Astellas Pharma Europe Ltd.; NC was an employee of Astellas Pharma Europe Ltd. when the manuscript was written; MA and AJ were working as associates as part of the Knowledge Transfer Partnership (KTP) between Astellas and Manchester Metropolitan University during the time this research was carried out; FF received grant funding from Astellas Pharma during the conduct of the study; RvM was an employee of Astellas Global Development, Leiden at the time of this work.

Author details

[1]Manchester Metropolitan University, Manchester, UK. [2]Present Address: Astellas Pharma Europe Ltd, Addlestone, UK. [3]Astellas Global Development, Leiden, The Netherlands.

References

1. Abrams P, Cardozo L, Fall M, Griffiths D, Rosier P, Ulmsten U, van Kerrebroeck P, Victor A, Wein A. The standardisation of terminology of lower urinary tract function: report from the Standardisation Subcommittee of the International Continence Society. Neurourol Urodyn. 2002;21(2):167–78.
2. D'Ancona C, Haylen B, Oelke M, Abranches-Monteiro L, Arnold E, Goldman H, Hamid R, Homma Y, Marcelissen T, Rademakers K, et al. The International Continence Society (ICS) report on the terminology for adult male lower urinary tract and pelvic floor symptoms and dysfunction. Neurourol Urodyn. 2019;38(2):433–77.
3. Haylen BT, de Ridder D, Freeman RM, Swift SE, Berghmans B, Lee J, Monga A, Petri E, Rizk DE, Sand PK, et al. An International Urogynecological Association (IUGA)/International Continence Society (ICS) joint report on the terminology for female pelvic floor dysfunction. Neurourol Urodyn. 2010;29(1):4–20.
4. International Continence Society: ICS Glossary - Overactive bladder (OAB, urgency) syndrome. https://www.ics.org/glossary/symptom/overactive bladderoaburgencysyndrome. Accessed June 2021.
5. DeMaagd GA, Davenport TC. Management of urinary incontinence. P T. 2012;37(6):345-361H.
6. Gravas S, Cornu JN, Gacci M, Gratzke C, Herrmann TRW, Mamoulakis C, Rieken M, Speakman MJ, Tikkinen KAO, Guidelines Associates et al. EAU guidelines on management of non-neurogenic male lower urinary tract symptoms (LUTS), incl. benign prostatic obstruction (BPO). https://uroweb.org/guideline/treatment-of-non-neurogenic-male-luts/. Accessed May 2021.
7. Burkhard FC, Bosch JLHR, Cruz F, Lemack GE, Nambiar AK, Thiruchelvam N, Tubaro A, Associates: G, Ambühl D, Bedretdinova DA et al. EAU guidelines on urinary incontinence. https://uroweb.org/guideline/urinary-incontinence/. Accessed December 2019.
8. Gormley EA, Lightner DJ, Burgio KL, Chai TC, Clemens JQ, Culkin DJ, Das AK, Foster HE, Jr., Scarpero HM, Tessier CD et al. Diagnosis and treatment of non-neurogenic overactive bladder (OAB) in adults: an AUA/SUFU guideline (2019). https://www.auanet.org/guidelines/overactive-bladder-(oab)-guideline#x2903. Accessed October 2019.
9. Gratzke C, van Maanen R, Chapple C, Abrams P, Herschorn S, Robinson D, Ridder A, Stoelzel M, Paireddy A, Yoon SJ, et al. Long-term safety and efficacy of mirabegron and solifenacin in combination compared with monotherapy in patients with overactive bladder: a randomised, multicentre phase 3 study (SYNERGY II). Eur Urol. 2018;74(4):501–9.
10. Irwin DE, Milsom I, Hunskaar S, Reilly K, Kopp Z, Herschorn S, Coyne K, Kelleher C, Hampel C, Artibani W, et al. Population-based survey of urinary incontinence, overactive bladder, and other lower urinary tract symptoms in five countries: results of the EPIC study. Eur Urol. 2006;50(6):1306–14 (**discussion 1314–1315**).
11. de Mey C. alpha(1)-blockers for BPH: are there differences? Eur Urol. 1999;36(Suppl 3):52–63.
12. McVary KT, Roehrborn CG, Avins AL, Barry MJ, Bruskewitz RC, Donnell RF, Foster HE Jr, Gonzalez CM, Kaplan SA, Penson DF, et al. Update on AUA guideline on the management of benign prostatic hyperplasia. J Urol. 2011;185(5):1793–803.
13. Sexton CC, Coyne KS, Kopp ZS, Irwin DE, Milsom I, Aiyer LP, Tubaro A, Chapple CR, Wein AJ. EpiLUTS Team: The overlap of storage, voiding and postmicturition symptoms and implications for treatment seeking in the USA, UK and Sweden: EpiLUTS. BJU Int. 2009;103(Suppl 3):12–23.

14. Lee HN, Lee KS, Kim JC, Chung BH, Kim CS, Lee JG, Kim DK, Park CH, Park JK, Hong SJ. Rate and associated factors of solifenacin add-on after tamsulosin monotherapy in men with voiding and storage lower urinary tract symptoms. Int J Clin Pract. 2015;69(4):444–53.
15. Filson CP, Hollingsworth JM, Clemens JQ, Wei JT. The efficacy and safety of combined therapy with alpha-blockers and anticholinergics for men with benign prostatic hyperplasia: a meta-analysis. J Urol. 2013;190(6):2153–60.
16. van Kerrebroeck P, Chapple C, Drogendijk T, Klaver M, Sokol R, Speakman M, Traudtner K, Drake MJ, Group NS. Combination therapy with solifenacin and tamsulosin oral controlled absorption system in a single tablet for lower urinary tract symptoms in men: efficacy and safety results from the randomised controlled NEPTUNE trial. Eur Urol. 2013;64(6):1003–12.
17. Rees J, Foley S, Huang M, Rosa Arias J, Skoumal R, Walters C, Yavuz Y, De Wachter S. Vesomni improves the quality of life in men with lower urinary tract symptoms in routine clinical practice in Europe. Neurourol Urodyn. 2019;38(3):981–9.
18. Kaplan SA, Herschorn S, McVary KT, Staskin D, Chapple C, Foley S, Cambronero Santos J, Kristy RM, Choudhury N, Hairston J, et al. Efficacy and safety of mirabegron versus placebo add-on therapy in men with overactive bladder symptoms receiving tamsulosin for underlying benign prostatic hyperplasia: a randomized, phase 4 study (PLUS). J Urol. 2020;203(6):1163–71.
19. Herrett E, Gallagher AM, Bhaskaran K, Forbes H, Mathur R, van Staa T, Smeeth L. Data resource profile: Clinical Practice Research Datalink (CPRD). Int J Epidemiol. 2015;44(3):827–36.
20. Hakimi Z, Johnson M, Nazir J, Blak B, Odeyemi IA. Drug treatment patterns for the management of men with lower urinary tract symptoms associated with benign prostatic hyperplasia who have both storage and voiding symptoms: a study using the health improvement network UK primary care data. Curr Med Res Opin. 2015;31(1):43–50.
21. Wagg A, Compion G, Fahey A, Siddiqui E. Persistence with prescribed antimuscarinic therapy for overactive bladder: a UK experience. BJU Int. 2012;110(11):1767–74.
22. Chapple CR, Nazir J, Hakimi Z, Bowditch S, Fatoye F, Guelfucci F, Khemiri A, Siddiqui E, Wagg A. Persistence and adherence with mirabegron versus antimuscarinic agents in patients with overactive bladder: a retrospective observational study in UK clinical practice. Eur Urol. 2017;72(3):389–99.
23. Drake MJ, Chapple C, Esen AA, Athanasiou S, Cambronero J, Mitcheson D, Herschorn S, Saleem T, Huang M, Siddiqui E, et al. Efficacy and safety of mirabegron add-on therapy to solifenacin in incontinent overactive bladder patients with an inadequate response to initial 4-week solifenacin monotherapy: a randomised double-blind multicentre phase 3B study (BESIDE). Eur Urol. 2016;70(1):136–45.
24. Herschorn S, Chapple CR, Abrams P, Arlandis S, Mitcheson D, Lee KS, Ridder A, Stoelzel M, Paireddy A, van Maanen R, et al. Efficacy and safety of combinations of mirabegron and solifenacin compared with monotherapy and placebo in patients with overactive bladder (SYNERGY study). BJU Int. 2017;120(4):562–75.
25. Agarwal A, Eryuzlu LN, Cartwright R, Thorlund K, Tammela TL, Guyatt GH, Auvinen A, Tikkinen KA. What is the most bothersome lower urinary tract symptom? Individual- and population-level perspectives for both men and women. Eur Urol. 2014;65(6):1211–7.
26. Rees J, Bultitude M, Challacombe B. The management of lower urinary tract symptoms in men. BMJ. 2014;348:e3861.
27. Chapple CR, Wyndaele JJ, Nordling J, Boeminghaus F, Ypma AF, Abrams P, on behalf of the European Tamsulosin Study Group. Tamsulosin, the first prostate-selective α1A-adrenoceptor antagonist. A meta-analysis of two randomized, placebo-controlled, multicentre studies in patients with benign prostatic obstruction (symptomatic BPH). Eur Urol. 1996;29(2):155–67.
28. Peters TJ, Donovan JL, Kay HE, Abrams P, de la Rosette JJ, Porru D, Thuroff JW. The International Continence Society "Benign Prostatic Hyperplasia" Study: the botherosomeness of urinary symptoms. J Urol. 1997;157(3):885–9.
29. Matsukawa Y, Majima T, Matsuo K, Funahashi Y, Kato M, Yamamoto T, Gotoh M. Effects of tadalafil on storage and voiding function in patients with male lower urinary tract symptoms suggestive of benign prostatic hyperplasia: a urodynamic-based study. Int J Urol. 2018;25(3):246–50.
30. Sebastianelli A, Spatafora P, Morselli S, Vignozzi L, Serni S, McVary KT, Kaplan S, Gravas S, Chapple C, Gacci M. Tadalafil alone or in combination with tamsulosin for the management for LUTS/BPH and ED. Curr Urol Rep. 2020;21(12):56.
31. Oelke M, Speakman MJ, Desgrandchamps F, Mamoulakis C. Acute urinary retention rates in the general male population and in adult men with lower urinary tract symptoms participating in pharmacotherapy trials: a literature review. Urology. 2015;86(4):654–65.
32. Kakizaki H, Lee KS, Yamamoto O, Jong JJ, Katou D, Sumarsono B, Uno S, Yamaguchi O. Mirabegron add-on therapy to tamsulosin for the treatment of overactive bladder in men with lower urinary tract symptoms: a randomized, placebo-controlled study (MATCH). Eur Urol Focus. 2020;6(4):729–37.
33. Benner JS, Nichol MB, Rovner ES, Jumadilova Z, Alvir J, Hussein M, Fanning K, Trocio JN, Brubaker L. Patient-reported reasons for discontinuing overactive bladder medication. BJU Int. 2010;105(9):1276–82.
34. Yeowell G, Smith P, Nazir J, Hakimi Z, Siddiqui E, Fatoye F. Real-world persistence and adherence to oral antimuscarinics and mirabegron in patients with overactive bladder (OAB): a systematic literature review. BMJ Open. 2018;8(11):e021889.
35. Drake MJ, Bowditch S, Arbe E, Hakimi Z, Guelfucci F, Amri I, Nazir J. A retrospective study of treatment persistence and adherence to alpha-blocker plus antimuscarinic combination therapies, in men with LUTS/BPH in the Netherlands. BMC Urol. 2017;17(1):36.
36. Eisen C, Lulic Z, Palacios-Moreno JM, Adalig B, Hennig M, Cortes V, Gilg F, Kostev K. Persistence and adherence to dutasteride/tamsulosin fixed-dose versus free-combination alpha blocker/5ARI therapy in patients with benign prostate hyperplasia in Germany. Int J Clin Pharmacol Ther. 2020;58(1):37–49.

The effect of screening and treatment of *Ureaplasma urealyticum* infection on semen parameters in asymptomatic leukocytospermia

Qi-Feng Zhang[1*], Yu-Ji Zhang[2], Sheng Wang[3], Yu Wei[3], Feng Li[3] and Ke-Jian Feng[3]

Abstract

Background: *Ureaplasma urealyticum* (UU) infection, as well as asymptomatic leukocytospermia, whether it has effect on semen parameters and whether it needs screening and treatment is still a confusing and controversial topic for clinicians.

Methods: Among 1530 adult males who visited Guilin People's Hospital due to infertility, 295 were diagnosed with asymptomatic leukocytospermia, and 95 were further screened for UU-positive. 81 UU-positive asymptomatic leukocytospermia patients received 7-day or 14-day treatment plan with doxycycline, and 70 cases were cured. The semen parameters of non-leukocytospermia, leukocytospermia, UU-positive leukocytospermia and UU-negative leukocytospermia groups were compared, and the differences between the two treatment plans and the semen parameters before UU treatment and 1 month after UU-cured were compared.

Results: Compared with non-leukocytospermia patients, the sperm concentration, progressive motility (PR), and normal morphology of patients with leukocytospermia decreased, while those with UU-positive leukocytospermia performed more significantly. The PR, total motility, and normal morphology of UU-positive leukocytospermia patients were significantly lower than those of UU-negative leukocytospermia patients (all $p < 0.001$). The UU cure rates of the 7-day and 14-day treatment plan with doxycycline was 84.62% and 89.66% ($p = 0.738$), respectively, and the sperm concentration, PR, total motility, and normal morphology of the cured UU-positive leukocytospermia patients were all increased after 1 month ($p = 0.001$, $p = 0.022$, $p = 0.004$ and $p = 0.008$, respectively).

Conclusions: It is significant to screen and treat UU infection in asymptomatic leukocytospermia for improving sperm quality. Where appropriate, the 7-day treatment plan with doxycycline may be a good choice.

Keywords: Leukocytospermia, *Ureaplasma urealyticum*, Semen parameters, Doxycycline

Background

Leukocytospermia is an abnormal laboratory finding defined by the World Health Organization as the presence of 1×10^6 seminal leukocytes per mL in human ejaculate [1], It is generally accepted that leukocytospermia may indicate infection or inflammation of the male urogenital and sex glands tract [2, 3], and it is a poor marker for either bacteriospermia or impaired semen quality [4], which has a negative impact on spermatogenesis or maturation, and is related to the decrease of semen parameters such as sperm concentration, motility, normal morphology and DNA fragmentation index [5, 6]. A prospective, controlled, blinded study suggests that leukocytospermia has a significant effect on sperm

*Correspondence: lanwind@163.com
[1] Department of Andrology, Guilin People's Hospital, Guilin 541002, China
Full list of author information is available at the end of the article

dynamic motility patterns, DNA and chromosome integrity in infertile men, and the pregnancy rate of patients cured with antibiotics is significantly higher than that of patients with persistent leukocytospermia [7]. Studies showed that antibiotics might improve the rate of resolution of leukocytospermia, the bacteriologic cure rate, and even improve sperm parameters to increase pregnancy rate [8]. A meta-analysis of 12 studies showed that using broad spectrum antibiotics in the treatment of patients with leukocytospermia might be useful in improving sperm concentration, motility, and morphology [9]. But a number of studies have shown that there is no correlation between elevated levels of semen leukocytes and bacteriospermia [10], and evidence from an RCT study also suggests that antibiotic therapy is not beneficial for the treatment of asymptomatic leucocytospermia [11], even in infertile men, leukocytospermia does not affect the success rate of IVF or ICSI [12]. Although a large number of studies have proved the relationship between semen leukocytosis and bacterial infection, sperm quality, and even the effectiveness of antibiotic treatment, the conflicting results are not convincing, the association of leukocytospermia with semen quality or male fertility and the significance of antibiotic therapy are still under debate.

Similarly, asymptomatic carrying of *Ureaplasma urealyticum* (UU) and *Mycoplasma hominis* (MH) is common, most people will not develop into diseases, and there is not enough evidence to prove that it is beneficial to detect and treat these infections, so it is not recommended to carry out routine detection and treatment for asymptomatic or symptomatic men and women [13, 14]. On the other hand, some studies suggest that the presence of UU and MH is related to the abnormal sperm parameters [15], sperm vitality and Progressive motility of UU infected men were significantly lower than those of uninfected men [16], and the mean sperm concentration was also lower [17]. The relationship between UU infection and sperm quality or male fertility is also debated.

Therefore, we designed this study to find more evidence of the effect of asymptomatic leukocytospermia and UU infection on sperm quality and whether antibiotic therapy is beneficial.

Methods

We retrospectively analyzed adult males who visited Guilin People's Hospital due to infertility and performed routine semen analysis and UU screening and treatment for patients with leukocytospermia from April 2017 to December 2019. After excluded patients with systemic diseases, cryptorchidism, chromosome abnormalities, varicocele, male azoospermia, bacteriospermia, as well as patients who drank excessively, smoked heavily, had symptoms of genitourinary tract infection or a history of antibiotic use in recent 4 weeks, 1530 patients and medical records were finally collected. Among them, 295 cases were diagnosed with leukocytospermia, 95 cases were further screened for UU-positive, 81 cases were treated with doxycycline, and 14 cases were treated with other sensitive antibiotics due to antibiotic sensitivity tests showing doxycycline resistance or intermediate sensitivity, or for other reasons. The semen parameters of non-leukocytospermia, leukocytospermia, UU-positive leukocytospermia and UU-negative leukocytospermia groups were compared, and the differences between two treatment plans with doxycycline and the semen parameters before UU treatment and 1 month after UU-cured were compared. The study was approved by the ethical review committee.

Semen samples were collected in sterile containers by masturbation after 2–7 days of abstinence. Sperm Quality Analyzer (SQA-V, Medical Electronic Systems Co., Ltd.) was used for the semen analysis within 60 min after ejaculation and liquefaction, and the semen volume, pH value, sperm concentration, progressive motility (PR), total motion (PR + NP) (NP, Non-progressive motility) and normal morphology were measured by the World Health Organization (WHO, 5th Edition). The seminal leukocytes was detected using the peroxidase method and leukocytospermia was diagnosed by seminal peroxidase-positive leukocyte concentration not less than 1×10^6 per mL. Culture appraisal of UU/MH was carried out with urethral swab samples by the modified broth dilution testing methods (Kit provided by Zhuhai Langfeng Biotech Co., Ltd.), and reexamined by the same method at least one week after treatment. Antibiotic sensitivity test results were obtained at high and low concentrations for 12 antibiotics: Cyclolipoerythromycin, Doxycycline, Josamycin, Thiamphenicol, Clarithromycin, Erythromycin, Ciprofloxacin, Roxithromycin, Levofloxacin, Minocycline, Azithromycin and Gatifloxacin. The susceptibility of bacteria to each antibiotic was graded as either susceptible, intermediate or resistant. For UU-positive leukocytospermia patients with doxycycline susceptible, no history of allergies, and contraindications, doxycycline was preferred, and 7-day or 14-day treatment plan (doxycycline 100 mg twice daily for 7 days or 14 days, double the first dose) options were selected according to the patient's wishes.

Data analysis was performed using IBM SPSS Statistics for Windows, Version 24 (IBM Corp., Armonk, New York, United States). Compliance of variables with a normal distribution was analyzed with the Kolmogorov–Smirnov test. Continuous variables were presented as means with standard deviations (mean ± SD) or medians (25–75%). Categorical variables were represented as numbers with percentages. Continuous data were analyzed by Independent-samples t-test or Paired-samples t-test for normally distributed variables and Mann–Whitney U test or Wilcoxon Signed-Ranks Test for non-normally distributed variables. Categorical data were analyzed using Pearson's chi-square test or Fisher's exact test. Statistical significance was defined as $p < 0.05$.

Results

According to the detection of seminal leukocytes, 1235 of 1530 infertile patients were diagnosed with non-leukocytospermia and 295 with leukocytospermia. The sperm concentration, PR and normal morphology of patients with leukocytospermia were lower than those of the patients with Non-leukocytospermia ($p < 0.001$, $p = 0.017$ and $p = 0.019$, respectively). According to the culture appraisal, 95 patients with leukocytospermia were positive for UU (8 cases of them were UU and MH positive at the same time, there was no single MH positive), while 200 patients were negative. Compared with Non-leukocytospermia patients, the sperm concentration and total motility of UU-negative leukocytospermia patients decreased significantly ($p < 0.001$ and $p = 0.022$, respectively), while the sperm concentration, PR, total motility and normal morphology of UU-positive leukocytospermia patients decreased significantly (all $p < 0.001$). Compared with UU-negative and UU-positive leukocytospermia group, The PR, total motility and normal morphology of UU-positive leukocytospermia patients were significantly lower than those of UU-negative leukocytospermia patients (all $p < 0.001$). (Table 1).

Antibiotic sensitivity test showed that the susceptible rate of Cyclolipoerythromycin was 94.74%, Minocycline was 93.68%, and doxycycline was 92.63% (Fig. 1), As doxycycline is inexpensive and easily available, we usually recommend doxycycline for patients who are susceptible to doxycycline and have no history of allergies or contraindications, and choose 7-day or 14-day treatment plan according to the patient's wishes. As a result, 14 UU-positive patients were treated with other sensitive antibiotics due to antibiotic sensitivity tests showing doxycycline resistance or intermediate sensitivity, or for other reasons, and 81 UU-positive patients received doxycycline treatment. We collected 52 patients with a 7-day treatment plan and 29 patients with a 14 day treatment plan with doxycycline, the cure rates were 84.62% and 89.66% respectively, and there was no significant difference between the two treatment plans ($p = 0.738$). (Table 2). At the same time, we also found that the two treatment plans have no significant difference in semen volume, PH, sperm concentration, PR, total motility and normal morphology for UU cured patients ($p = 0.490$,

Table 1 General information and comparison of Non-leukocytospermia group, leukocytospermia group, UU-negative leukocytospermia group and UU-positive leukocytospermia group

	Non-leukocytospermia group	Leukocytospermia group	UU-negative leukocytospermia group	UU-positive leukocytospermia group	^1p value^a	^2p value^a	^3p value^a	^4p value^a
n	1235	295	200	95				
Age (years)	33.32 (29.00–37.00)	33.20 (29.00–37.00)	33.39 (29.00–37.00)	32.80 (29.00–36.00)	0.530	0.408	0.952	0.543
BMI (kg/m^2)	21.24 (19.94–22.39)	21.29 (20.17–22.38)	21.32 (20.34–22.38)	21.22 (19.66–22.39)	0.544	0.930	0.201	0.277
Semen volume (mL)	3.52 (2.50–4.50)	3.42 (2.50–4.50)	3.47 (2.50–4.50)	3.31 (2.50–4.50)	0.275	0.658	0.163	0.326
PH	7.66 (7.30–8.00)	7.69 (7.30–8.10)	7.71 (7.40–8.00)	7.63 ± 0.63	0.253	0.121	0.859	0.330
Sperm concentration (× 10^6/mL)	82.13 (43.00–113.8.80)	65.55 (33.60–83.30)	66.29 (38.88–82.45)	63.99 (24.4–92.00)	< 0.001	< 0.001	< 0.001	0.228
PR (%)	36.02 (27.00–47.00)	31.80 (9.00–49.00)	35.23 (19.25–53.00)	24.58 (0–39.00)	0.017	0.514	< 0.001	< 0.001
Total motility, PR + NP (%)	47.55 (40.00–59.00)	43.35 (24.00–64.00)	47.64 (34.50–66.00)	34.33 (4.00–55.00)	0.510	0.022	< 0.001	< 0.001
Normal morphology (%)	8.57 (5.00–11.00)	7.81 (3.00–8.00)	8.70 (4.00–13.00)	5.93 (0–9.00)	0.019	0.492	< 0.001	< 0.001

UU Ureaplasma urealyticum, BMI body mass index, *PR* progressive motility, *NP* non-progressive motility

[a] Mann–Whitney U-test

[1] *p* value (Comparison between non-leukocytospermia group and leukocytospermia group)

[2] *p* value (Comparison between non-leukocytospermia group and UU-negative leukocytospermia group)

[3] *p* value (Comparison between non-leukocytospermia group and UU-positive leukocytospermia group)

[4] *p* value (Comparison between UU-negative leukocytospermia group and UU-positive leukocytospermia group)

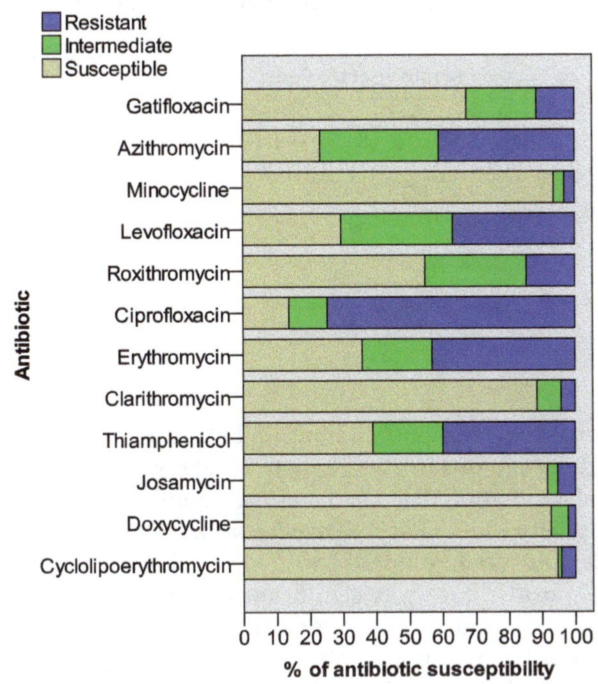

Fig. 1 Susceptibility of *Ureaplasma urealyticum* to 12 different antibiotics

Table 2 Comparison of UU cure rates between the two treatment plans

	n	UU cured case (%)	UU uncured case (%)	*p* value[a]
7-day treatment plan	52	44 (84.62)	8 (15.38)	0.738
14-day treatment plan	29	26 (89.66)	3 (10.34)	

UU Ureaplasma urealyticum

[a] Fisher's exact test

$p=0.529$, $p=0.995$, $p=0.592$, $p=0.486$ and $p=0.293$, respectively). (Table 3).

A further study of 70 UU-positive leukocytospermia patients before and after treatment showed that the sperm concentration, PR, total motility, and normal morphology of the UU cured patients were all increased after 1 month after UU-cured ($p=0.001$, $p=0.022$, $p=0.004$ and $p=0.008$, respectively), but there was no significant difference in semen volume and pH value ($p=0.324$ and $p=0.663$, respectively). (Table 4).

Discussion

Leukocytospermia or pyospermia is still a confusing and controversial topic for clinicians. Although it has been proposed by the World Health Organization as an indicator of reproductive tract infection and inflammation, the evidence is not convincing. The frequency of leukocytospermia among infertile males is quite wide, and the reliable incidence is about 30% [18, 19]. Some pathophysiological views recognize that bacteria and infiltrating leukocytes, two major inflammatory mediators, directly or indirectly affect human sperm function [20], However, most leukocytospermia is not caused by bacterial infection or bacteriospermia, or there is no evidence of microbial infection, this may be because the invasion of male reproductive tract by microorganisms may be divided into three different stages. In the first stage, bacterial infection can be induced by microorganisms, and pathological bacterial strains can be observed in semen, without attracting a large number of white blood cells; in the second stage, activated white blood cells appear in ejaculation; in the third stage, bacteria are removed, usually with isolated leukocytospermia as the representative [21]. Bacteria are mainly involved in the intrinsic and mitochondrial dependent

Table 3 Comparison of semen parameters of UU-positive leukocytospermia patients before treatment and 1 month after UU Cured

	Before treatment		*p* value	1 month after UU Cured		*p* value
	7-day treatment plan	14-day treatment plan		7-day treatment plan	14-day treatment plan	
n	44	26		44	26	
Semen volume (mL)	3.12 (2.13–4.00)	3.34 ± 1.67	0.659[a]	3.15 (2.50–3.38)	3.44 (2.50–4.13)	0.490[a]
PH	7.60 ± 0.66	7.67 ± 0.61	0.693[b]	7.62 ± 0.65	7.72 ± 0.49	0.529[b]
Sperm concentration (× 10^6/mL)	65.13 (28.40–99.38)	59.96 ± 45.44	0.738[a]	70.25 (34.60–87.28)	68.04 ± 44.94	0.995[a]
PR (%)	23.20 (0.25–35.75)	25.23 (2.5–40.75)	0.359[a]	25.43 ± 18.07	27.82 ± 17.85	0.592[b]
Total motility, PR + NP (%)	32.91 (5.00–50.75)	36.42 (12.5–59.00)	0.274[a]	36.72 ± 20.27	40.21 ± 19.82	0.486[b]
Normal morphology (%)	5.52 (0.50–8.00)	5.96 (1.50–9.25)	0.401[a]	6.09 (2.25–9.00)	7.31 ± 4.41	0.293[a]

UU Ureaplasma urealyticum, *PR* progressive motility, *NP* non-progressive motility

[a] Mann–Whitney U-test

[b] Independent-samples t-test

Table 4 Comparison of semen parameters of UU-positive leukocytospermia patients before treatment and 1 month after UU cured

	Before treatment	1 month after UU Cured	*p* value[a]
Semen volume (mL)	3.20 (2.08–4.00)	3.26 (2.50–4.00)	0.324
PH	7.63 (7.15–8.20)	7.66 ± 0.59	0.663
Sperm concentration ($\times 10^6$/mL)	63.21 (24.00–95.88)	69.43 (35.03–88.73)	0.001
PR(%)	23.96 (1.00–39.00)	26.32 (9.75–41.25)	0.022
Total motility, PR + NP (%)	34.21 (7.25–53.25)	38.02 ± 20.03	0.004
Normal morphology (%)	5.69 (1.5–9.00)	6.54 (3.00–10.00)	0.008

UU Ureaplasma urealyticum, *PR* progressive motility, *NP* non-progressive motility

[a] Wilcoxon signed-ranks test

apoptosis cell death, while oxidative stress may play a role in reducing the conventional sperm parameters in leukocytospermia, and the combined effect of bacteria and leukocytes accelerated the apoptosis and necrosis of sperm [22]. The increased seminal leukocytes may mediate reactive oxygen species (ROS) production by direct cell–cell contact or soluble products released by leukocytes [23]. A Systematic Review and Meta-Analysis of Case–Control Studies indicated that patients with leukocytospermia showed lower sperm concentration and lower progressive motility compared to men without leukocytospermia, however, the significant differences disappeared, along with the large inter-study heterogeneity, when analyses were restricted to studies clearly reporting the inclusion of men without clinical evidence of seminal tract infection [24]. It seems that the clinical evidence of seminal tract infection is the key to sperm quality decline, and clinical studies have also found that compared with some pathogenic bacterial strains, the direct contact between conditioned pathogenic bacteria and sperm may play a greater role in promoting apoptosis [25].

Ureaplasma urealyticum (UU), usually considered as a conditional pathogen, belongs to the genus Ureaplasma and the family Mycoplasmataceae in the order Mycoplasmatales. A meta-analysis found that UU, but not undifferentiated Ureaplasma infections or U. parvum, has been shown to be the pathogen of nongonococcal urethritis (NGU) [26]. Moreover, UU is easy to be implanted in urethra, but not necessarily cause urethritis [27], quite a few patients with these infections are not aware of their infections because they may be asymptomatic, even whether it is pathogenic and the impact on fertility is still uncertain. The incidence of UU was reported inconsistently, a study of 19,098 infertile men and 3368 fertile men found that 10.22% and 3.65% of UU infertile and fertile men's urethra specimens, and 3.16% and 0.89% of MH specimens, UU infection will significantly affect sperm quality, and there is a significant relationship between UU infection and male infertility [28]. A systematic review and meta-analysis found that there was a significant relationship between UU and *Mycoplasma hominis* with male infertility, and compared with the global average, the UU-positive rate was significantly higher in both the infertility group and the control group in China, while the positive rate was significantly lower in *Mycoplasma hominis* [29]. Similarly, UU infection can directly affect sperm, cause leukocyte-mediated inflammatory response, and affect sperm by producing ROS [30].

Oxidative stress (OS) is considered to be the pathological molecular mechanism of most clinical, environmental and lifestyle factors that lead to male infertility. OS occurs when the physiological balance of oxidants and reducers in the system is reduced by excessive ROS or antioxidant levels [31], including some internal and external factors, such as inflammation and infection, varicocele, smoking, drinking, obesity, exposure to radiation and chemotherapy [32], and even male reproductive hormone disorders [33]. In the process of spermatogenesis, reactive oxygen species are very harmful, and the content of unsaturated fatty acids in sperm membrane is easily affected by oxidative stress, and these lipids can be oxidized through a series of chain reactions to release potential toxicity and mutagenic aldehydes and alkenals [34–36], finally, excessive ROS has a pathological impact on spermatogenesis, resulting in the decrease of sperm concentration, motility and fertilization rate [37]. A large number of clinical studies have shown that leukocytospermia-induced sperm damage may be due to high levels of leukocyte-derived ROS and inflammatory mediators, Such as toll-like receptors 2 and 4 (TLR-2/4), cyclooxygenase-2 (COX-2), nuclear factor erythryoid-2 related factor (Nrf-2), interleukin-6 (IL-6) and tumor necrosis factor-alpha (TNF-α), etc. [38, 39], even low levels of leukocytospermia have seminal oxidative stress [40]. It is not certain that the effect of leukocytospermia or UU infection on sperm exists, but it seems to be explainable from the current mechanism research.

However, on this issue, clinicians need more clinical evidence and feasible clinical solutions.

In our observation, there was no significant change in the semen volume and pH in all groups. Patients with leukocytospermia have lower sperm concentration, PR and normal morphology than patients with non-leukocytospermia. However, when we exclude UU-positive leukocytospermia patients and only consider UU-negative leukocytospermia patients, although there was a difference in the total motility, the difference between the PR and normal morphology disappeared, but only consider the UU-positive leukocytospermia patients, the sperm concentration, PR, total motility and normal morphology were significantly lower than the patients with non-leukocytospermia. At the same time, compared with UU-negative leukocytospermia patients, the PR, total motor ability and normal morphology of UU-positive leukocytospermia patients were significantly lower. These results seem to confirm that leukocytospermia has a definite effect on semen parameters, at least in terms of sperm concentration. Perhaps the leukocytes in semen itself is a factor that affects semen parameters, of course, these need more extensive research to confirm. However, the effect on PR and normal morphology, like many controversial studies on leukocytospermia, is not convincing. Our research showed that UU-negative leukocytospermia was not like leukocytospermia in terms of PR and normal morphology, which was no significantly different from non-leukocytospermia. Such results indicate that the effect of UU-negative leucospermia on sperm quality is rather limited. However, when patients with leukocytospermia are infected with UU at the same time, the effect on sperm quality is more obvious and serious, which can involve multiple aspects of semen parameters such as PR, total motor ability and normal morphological. This seems to suggest that infectious factors may be an important factor in the decline of sperm quality in asymptomatic leukocytospermia, and UU infection is a common infectious factor in asymptomatic leukocytospermia. Therefore, screening for UU infection in asymptomatic leukocytospermia is meaningful.

According to the antibiotic sensitivity test of UU, the top three susceptible antibiotics were Cyclolipoerythromycin, Minocycline and Doxycycline, and because doxycycline is inexpensive and easy to obtain, we prefer to choose doxycycline in clinic. According to the results of the 7-day and the 14-day treatment plan, there is no significant difference in cure rates, and there is no significant difference in the effect of the two plans on the sperm quality of UU cured leukocytospermia patients. If patients are susceptible to doxycycline and have no history of allergies and contraindications, we think that the doxycycline 7-day treatment plan is a good choice and this antibiotic treatment is meaningful. From our results, the semen parameters such as sperm concentration, PR, total motility, and normal morphology of UU-positive leukocytospermia patients were significantly improved 1 month after UU was cured. Unfortunately, some patients also received antioxidant and other treatments after our observation period, and no correct pregnancy rate was observed. However, our research shows that screening and treating UU in asymptomatic leukocytospermia is meaningful, not only can improve sperm quality but also save a lot of resources and costs, reduce the use of antibiotics, which seems to be an efficient diagnosis and treatment program.

This study has some limitations. Since more pathogens such as chlamydia or mycoplasma have been tested only in symptomatic leukocytespermia rather than asymptomatic leukocytospermia, this may miss some pathogens. In addition, some patients received additional treatments later, and we were unable to follow up with the UU-cured patients for longer periods to obtain more data.

Conclusion

Asymptomatic leukocytospermia may have some effect on sperm parameters, which seem to be mainly manifested in sperm concentration. When patients with asymptomatic leukocytospermia are infected with UU at the same time, the effect on sperm quality is more obvious and serious, which can involve multiple aspects of semen parameters such as PR, total motor ability and normal morphological. It is significant to screen and treat UU infection in asymptomatic leukocytospermia for improving sperm quality. Where appropriate, we recommend the 7-day treatment plan with doxycycline.

Abbreviations

UU: *Ureaplasma urealyticum*; MH: *Mycoplasma hominis*; BMI: Body mass index; PR: Progressive motility; NP: Non-progressive motility.

Authors' contributions

QFZ and YJZ designed this study; QFZ, SW, YW, FL and KJF participated in data collection; QFZ and YJZ carried out data analysis and interpretation. QFZ drafted the manuscript; SW and YW revised the manuscript. All authors read and approved the final manuscript.

Competing interests

The authors declare that they have no competing interests.

Author details

[1] Department of Andrology, Guilin People's Hospital, Guilin 541002, China. [2] Department of Medical Record Management, The First Affiliated Hospital of Hainan Medical University, Haikou 571137, China. [3] Department of Urology, Guilin People's Hospital, Guilin 541002, China.

References

1. World Health Organization. WHO laboratory manual for the examination and processing of human semen. Geneva: World Health Organization; 2010.

2. Pentyala S, Lee J, Annam S, Alvarez J, Veerraju A, Yadlapalli N, Khan SA. Current perspectives on pyospermia: a review. Asian J Androl. 2007;9(5):593–600.
3. Sandoval JS, Raburn D, Muasher S. Leukocytospermia: Overview of diagnosis, implications, and management of a controversial finding. Middle East Fertil Soc J. 2013;18(3):129–34.
4. Rodin DM, Larone D, Goldstein M. Relationship between semen cultures, leukospermia, and semen analysis in men undergoing fertility evaluation. Fertil Steril. 2003;79:1555–8.
5. Domes T, Lo KC, Grober ED, Mullen JBM, Mazzulli T, Jarvi K. The incidence and effect of bacteriospermia and elevated seminal leukocytes on semen parameters. Fertil Steril. 2012;97(5):1050–5.
6. Pratap H, Hottigoudar SY, Nichanahalli KS, Rajendran S, Bheemanathi HS. Sperm DNA integrity in leukocytospermia and its association with seminal adenosine deaminase. J Hum Reprod Sci. 2019;12(3):182–8.
7. Moubasher A, Sayed H, Mosaad E, Mahmoud A, Farag F, Taha EA. Impact of leukocytospermia on sperm dynamic motility parameters, DNA and chromosomal integrity. Cent European J Urol. 2018;71(4):470–5.
8. Jung JH, Kim MH, Kim J, Baik SK, Koh SB, Park HJ, Seo JT. Treatment of leukocytospermia in male infertility: a systematic review. World J Mens Health. 2016;34(3):165–72.
9. Skau PA, Folstad I. Do bacterial infections cause reduced ejaculate quality? A meta-analysis of antibiotic treatment of male infertility. Behav Ecol. 2003;14(1):40–7.
10. Bachir BG, Jarvi K. Infectious, inflammatory, and immunologic conditions resulting in male infertility. Urol Clin North Am. 2014;41(1):67–81.
11. Krisp A, Hörster S, Skrzypek J, Krause W. Treatment with levofloxacin does not resolve asymptomatic leucocytospermia–a randomized controlled study. Andrologia. 2003;35(4):244–7.
12. Ricci G, Granzotto M, Luppi S, Giolo E, Martinelli M, Zito G, Borelli M. Effect of seminal leukocytes on in vitro fertilization and intracytoplasmic sperm injection outcomes. Fertil Steril. 2015;104(1):87–93.
13. Horner P, Donders G, Cusini M, Gomberg M, Jensen JS, Unemo M. Should we be testing for urogenital *Mycoplasma hominis*, *Ureaplasma parvum* and *Ureaplasma urealyticum* in men and women?—a position statement from the European STI Guidelines Editorial Board. J Eur Acad Dermatol Venereol. 2018;32(11):1845–51.
14. Andrade-Rocha FT. *Ureaplasma urealyticum* and *Mycoplasma hominis* in men attending for routine semen analysis. Prevalence, incidence by age and clinical settings, influence on sperm characteristics, relationship with the leukocyte count and clinical value. Urol Int. 2003;71(4):377–81.
15. Salmeri M, Valenti D, La Vignera S, Bellanca S, Morello A, Toscano MA, Mastrojeni S, Calogero AE. Prevalence of *Ureaplasma urealyticum* and *Mycoplasma hominis* infection in unselected infertile men. J Chemother. 2012;24(2):81–6.
16. Lee JS, Kim KT, Lee HS, Yang KM, Seo JT, Choe JH. Concordance of *Ureaplasma urealyticum* and *Mycoplasma hominis* in infertile couples: impact on semen parameters. Urology. 2013;81(6):1219–24.
17. Liu J, Wang Q, Ji X, Guo S, Dai Y, Zhang Z, Jia L, Shi Y, Tai S, Lee Y. Prevalence of *Ureaplasma urealyticum*, *Mycoplasma hominis*, *Chlamydia trachomatis* infections, and semen quality in infertile and fertile men in China. Urology. 2014;83(4):795–9.
18. Gambera L, Serafini F, Morgante G, Focarelli R, De Leo V, Piomboni P. Sperm quality and pregnancy rate after COX-2 inhibitor therapy of infertile males with abacterial leukocytospermia. Hum Reprod. 2007;22(4):1047–51.
19. Henkel R, Maass G, Jung A, Haidl G, Schill W-B, Schuppe H-C. Age-related changes in seminal polymorphonuclear elastase in men with asymptomatic inflammation of the genital tract. Asian J Androl. 2007;9(3):299–304.
20. Fraczek M, Kurpisz M. Mechanisms of the harmful effects of bacterial semen infection on ejaculated human spermatozoa: potential inflammatory markers in semen. Folia Histochem Cytobiol. 2015;53(3):201–17.
21. Sanocka D, Fraczek M, Jedrzejczak P, Szumała-Kakol A, Kurpisz M. Male genital tract infection: an influence of leukocytes and bacteria on semen. J Reprod Immunol. 2004;62(1–2):111–24.
22. Fraczek M, Hryhorowicz M, Gill K, Zarzycka M, Gaczarzewicz D, Jedrzejczak P, Bilinska B, Piasecka M, Kurpisz M. The effect of bacteriospermia and leukocytospermia on conventional and nonconventional semen parameters in healthy young normozoospermic males. J Reprod Immunol. 2016;118:18–27.
23. Saleh RA, Agarwal A, Kandirali E, Sharma RK, Thomas AJ, Nada EA, Evenson DP, Alvarez JG. Leukocytospermia is associated with increased reactive oxygen species production by human spermatozoa. Fertil Steril. 2002;78(6):1215–24.
24. Castellini C, D'Andrea S, Martorella A, Minaldi E, Necozione S, Francavilla F, Francavilla S, Barbonetti A. Relationship between leukocytospermia, reproductive potential after assisted reproductive technology, and sperm parameters: a systematic review and meta-analysis of case–control studies. Andrology. 2020;8(1):125–35.
25. Fraczek M, Hryhorowicz M, Gaczarzewicz D, Szumala-Kakol A, Kolanowski TJ, Beutin L, Kurpisz M. Can apoptosis and necrosis coexist in ejaculated human spermatozoa during in vitro semen bacterial infection? J Assist Reprod Genet. 2015;32(5):771–9.
26. Zhang N, Wang R, Li X, Liu X, Tang Z, Liu Y. Are Ureaplasma spp a cause of nongonococcal urethritis? A systematic review and meta-analysis. PLoS ONE. 2014;9(12):e113771.
27. Jordan SJ, Toh E, Williams JA, Fortenberry L, LaPradd ML, Katz BP, Batteiger BE, Nelson DE, Batteiger TA. Aetiology and prevalence of mixed-infections and mono-infections in non-gonococcal urethritis in men: a case–control study. Sex Transm Infect. 2020;96:306–11.
28. Huang C, Long X, Jing S, Fan L, Xu K, Wang S, Zhu W. *Ureaplasma urealyticum* and *Mycoplasma hominis* infections and semen quality in 19,098 infertile men in China. World J Urol. 2016;34(7):1039–44.
29. Huang C, Zhu HL, Xu KR, Wang SY, Fan LQ, Zhu WB. Mycoplasma and ureaplasma infection and male infertility: a systematic review and meta-analysis. Andrology. 2015;3(5):809–16.
30. Zhang ZH, Zhang HG, Dong Y, Han RR, Dai RL, Liu RZ. *Ureaplasma urealyticum* in male infertility in Jilin Province, North-east China, and its relationship with sperm morphology. J Int Med Res. 2011;39(1):33–40.
31. Bisht S, Dada R. Oxidative stress: major executioner in disease pathology, role in sperm DNA damage and preventive strategies. Front Biosci (Schol Ed). 2017;9:420–47.
32. Wagner H, Cheng JW, Ko EY. Role of reactive oxygen species in male infertility: an updated review of literature. Arab J Urol. 2018;16(1):35–43.
33. Darbandi M, Darbandi S, Agarwal A, Sengupta P, Durairajanayagam D, Henkel R, Sadeghi MR. Reactive oxygen species and male reproductive hormones. Reprod Biol Endocrinol. 2018;16(1):87.
34. Moazamian R, Polhemus A, Connaughton H, Fraser B, Whiting S, Gharagozloo P, Aitken RJ. Oxidative stress and human spermatozoa: diagnostic and functional significance of aldehydes generated as a result of lipid peroxidation. Mol Hum Reprod. 2015;21(6):502–15.
35. Aitken RJ, Gibb Z, Baker MA, Drevet J, Gharagozloo P. Causes and consequences of oxidative stress in spermatozoa. Reprod Fertil Dev. 2016;28(1–2):1–10.
36. Aitken RJ. Reactive oxygen species as mediators of sperm capacitation and pathological damage. Mol Reprod Dev. 2017;84(10):1039–52.
37. Du Plessis SS, Agarwal A, Halabi J, Tvrda E. Contemporary evidence on the physiological role of reactive oxygen species in human sperm function. J Assist Reprod Genet. 2015;32(4):509–20.
38. Hagan S, Khurana N, Chandra S, Abdel-Mageed AB, Mondal D, Hellstrom WJG, Sikka SC. Differential expression of novel biomarkers (TLR-2, TLR-4, COX-2, and Nrf-2) of inflammation and oxidative stress in semen of leukocytospermia patients. Andrology. 2015;3(5):848–55.
39. Eldamnhoury EM, Elatrash GA, Rashwan HM, El-Sakka AI. Association between leukocytospermia and semen interleukin-6 and tumor necrosis factor-alpha in infertile men. Andrology. 2018;6(5):775–80.
40. Agarwal A, Mulgund A, Alshahrani S, Assidi M, Abuzenadah AM, Sharma R, Sabanegh E. Reactive oxygen species and sperm DNA damage in infertile men presenting with low level leukocytospermia. Reprod Biol Endocrinol. 2014;12:126.

28

Assessment and treatment of recurrent urinary tract infections in women: Development of a questionnaire based on a qualitative study of patient expectations in secondary care

J. J. Pat[2*], T. v. d. Aart[2], M. G. Steffens[1], L. P. W. Witte[1] and M. H. Blanker[2]

Abstract

Background: To develop a questionnaire to facilitate the inventorying of women's expectations for the assessment and treatment of recurrent urinary tract infection (UTI) in secondary care.

Methods: Semi-structured interviews were conducted among women with recurrent UTI referred to our urology department. The interviews were conducted by one interviewer, recorded, transcribed verbatim, and analyzed thematically by two researchers. We first developed 35 questions to identify potential themes, and we then tested them among women with and without recurrent UTI. Changes were made according to the feedback received.

Results: Six interviews were conducted before saturation was reached. Thematic analysis identified three themes: patient pathway, personal knowledge, and social implications. All respondents had received multiple antibiotic courses but no prophylactic antibiotic therapy, and although all were aware of some preventive measures, they wanted more information about their disease. However, some women were afraid to access information for fear of what they might learn. Recurrent UTI also significantly affected the daily lives all respondents. Some women expressed fears over frequent antibiotic use, and others felt that there must be something wrong with their body to have so many UTIs. Women expected the urologist to provide an explanation and to start adequate therapy for their recurrent UTI. We created a 32-item questionnaire based on these themes

Conclusion: This study not only developed a questionnaire for use when assessing patient expectations of recurrent UTI management in secondary care but also provided novel insights into the thoughts, opinions, and expectations of women who are referred.

Keywords: Female, Urinary tract infections, Questionnaire, Interview

Background

Urinary tract infections (UTIs) are among the most common bacterial infections worldwide [1], with estimates indicating that over 30% of all women will experience at least one UTI in their lives. Studies have shown that 20–50% of these women will experience at least one recurrence, defined as at least two UTIs in 6 months or at least three UTIs in 12 months [2, 3].

Several guidelines are available for the assessment and treatment of recurrent UTI, but there is no agreement on the optimal diagnostic process [1, 4, 5]. The Dutch Association of Urology commissioned a specific guideline about bacterial UTI in which it advised using a voiding diary, urine sediment assessment, and uroflowmetry in

*Correspondence: j.j.pat@umcg.nl
[2] Department of General Practice, University of Groningen, University Medical Centre, Groningen, Hanzeplein 1, 9713 GZ Groningen, The Netherlands
Full list of author information is available at the end of the article

all patients with recurrent infection [1]. It only advocated additional diagnostic procedures, such as ultrasound or cystoscopy, in the presence of macroscopic hematuria or loin pain. The American Urology Association (AUA), Canadian Urology Association (CUA), and Society of Urodynamics, Female Pelvic Medicine and Urogenital Reconstruction (SUFU) recently published a guideline on recurrent UTI in which it was stated that cystoscopy and imaging should not be performed routinely [6]. Instead, assessments of women with recurrent UTI should focus on modifiable behaviors that are known to reduce the risk of recurrence, while excluding structural or functional abnormalities of the genitourinary tract.

Each year about 250 patients with recurrent UTI are referred to our outpatient clinic, and of these, approximately 20% have previously attended for this reason. It has been shown that patients often attend consultations in primary care with certain expectations for the outcomes [7]. However, these expectations have not been inventoried in secondary care for patients with recurrent UTI. Failure to consider these expectations is likely to affect consultation outcomes adversely. Using a questionnaire would help caregivers start important clinical conversations.

In this study, we aimed to assess patient expectations regarding the assessment and treatment of recurrent UTI in secondary care and to use the newly acquired information to develop a questionnaire on this topic.

Methods

We conducted a qualitative study based on semi-structured interviews of women referred to our urology department with recurrent UTI. The interview guide was first tested with two patients. Women were excluded from participation if at least one of the following criteria was met: referral for complicated UTI, known urological malignancy, intermittent or continuous catheterization, pregnancy, or insufficient proficiency with the Dutch language. Eligible patients were given an invitation letter and a written informed consent form. The study was approved by our local medical ethics committee under approval number 180319.

After patients signed the informed consent form, a single researcher held face-to-face or telephone interviews according to an interview guide (Additional file 1). To minimize interviewer bias, the researcher (TvdA) was a trained medical student who clarified to participants that she was not a medical doctor. All interviews were recorded and transcribed verbatim. The interviewer started with an open question about the patient's expectations of the visit to the urologist, and although open questions were used throughout the interview, the interviewer was free to seek elaboration on initial responses. Additional interviews were held until saturation was reached, which was defined as obtaining no new information from two consecutive interviews. The questionnaire was written in Dutch and translated to English by a native speaker. The English version was then translated back to Dutch to check if the English version matched the original questionnaire.

Analysis

We performed thematic analysis using Atlas.TI 8® (ATLAS.ti Scientific Software Development GmbH). Two researchers (TvdA and JJP) separately read and re-read the transcripts to become familiar with the data, then analyzed the text and added codes to the responses. Open coding was used, allowing the codes to be developed and adjusted as the interview transcripts were analyzed. After the initial coding, we evaluated the codes and organized them into themes, re-read the interviews with the themes in mind, and formulated questions that covered the content of those themes. We took care to ensure that the questionnaire was suitable for patients with low literacy. No analysis of internal consistency was performed because the questionnaire was intended to generate an inventory of opinions rather than to categorize the outcomes. Finally, the questionnaire was completed by a diverse group of women with and without recurrent UTI to assess its readability. Any resulting changes were made according to the feedback received.

Results

Saturation was reached after six interviews (four face-to-face and two by telephone) lasting 35–60 min each. The women were aged 32–86 years and all had suffered recurrent UTI for at least 1 year. The presenting symptoms consisted of dysuria, abdominal pain, frequency, urinary incontinence, and occasional fever. Analysis of the interviews yielded three main themes: medical route, knowledge of the condition, and social and psychological impact. The following sections describe each theme in turn.

Medical route

All respondents described that their general practitioner (GP) had tested their urine for a UTI when they had symptoms of a UTI and prescribed antibiotics when positive. They reported having received antibiotic treatment more than once for UTI, but also noted that some antibiotics worked better than others. Some respondents reported a delay in antibiotic treatment because they had to wait for the results of the urine culture before a GP was willing to start antibiotic therapy.

Well then, that is what you do at the GP. You bring

in your urine and after a day you're supposed to make a call. It always makes me feel like: oh, time to call again.

Some respondents had undergone physical examination, and only one reported completing a voiding diary.

Interviewer: What tests were done by the GP?
Respondent: Well actually, well yes, not internally. He has occasionally patted me on the back asking if I felt pain here or there.

None of the respondents had used antibiotics prophylactically, although one patient was aware that this was a therapeutic option.

Well, I thought that he maybe, that you maybe had–for example–a standard antibiotic treatment, because I've heard that you could preventively take something like two antibiotic pills.

All respondents were given advice about prophylaxis by their GPs, such as taking cranberry tablets, ensuring adequate fluid intake, and performing post-coital voiding.

And I've had it prescribed by the GP. But nowadays I just get them at my local pharmacy, those Cranberry tablets, because they are a lot cheaper there; but yes, I do make use of them.

Some respondents described repeatedly asking their GP for a urology referral, but having to wait up to 2 months for an appointment after the referral was made.

Yes, yes, I did visit there, but of course I insisted on it.

One respondent stated that her GP advised that a urology referral was needed and that she agreed because she felt like there had to be something wrong to get so many UTIs.

And then I told them my story and that I've had it all so and so. And then they said, "well it's about time that you visit a urologist." And then I responded, "yes, I happen to agree, now that I've had it so often in succession and it still isn't gone, there is probably something not completely in order indeed."

Full recovery was not always the main goal of patients. Some described that they would be satisfied with a reduction in the frequency of UTIs.

Interviewer: And when would you be satisfied?
Respondent: Well yeah, if I notice any results.
Interviewer: So, if you only had cystitis once a year, would you say the treatment was successful?
Respondent: Yes.

Another described that they would be satisfied with a clarification about their UTI.

Interviewer: And when would you be satisfied?
Respondent: Well at first instance I would say, with regard to tomorrow's examination, that I would be happy if I just had more clarity about my condition.

Patient knowledge of the condition

Respondents described a variety of measures they had adopted to prevent recurrence, including taking cranberry tablets and ensuring adequate fluid intake, post-coital voiding, and intimate hygiene. Some respondents were able to list all preventive measures, while others only named one or two. Most respondents had looked for information about recurrent UTI on the internet, but others did not want to because they feared what they would find.

No, no, no I totally can't. Yes, I have such a tablet but no, I don't look up anything. No, not at all. Oh, no I don't, I really don't want to know.

There were also differences in the information wanted by respondents. Some only wanted information about the causes, some only wanted information about the therapeutic options, and others wanted both. All respondents stated that they received information from the hospital about their appointment and were able to explain both the voiding diary they had to complete and the uroflowmetry to be performed. They felt like they had received enough information on these matters before the consultation.

Alright. And what exactly is this "pot" research? Well it goes, that's exactly it, it measures how fast or how slowly I pee, how much leaves my bladder and what its composition is, so to speak.

Most respondents did not know about other potential diagnostic tests. One respondent was aware of cystoscopy because she had been referred previously.

He'll probably have to look into the bladder anyway. Because that's what happened the last time. And then you can really see that a bladder isn't quite ... clean from the inside either.

Social and psychological impact

All respondents described that their daily lives were affected by the symptoms of recurrent UTI. They all had active social lives and some had needed to take measures in the event of urinary incontinence when they visited someone (such as taking sanitary napkins or clean underwear). The hospital visit was also a burden for some because they were unable to arrive with a full bladder because of symptoms. Others reported that they could not talk about their problems with relatives because they felt this was inappropriate.

> *And urology is of course still a subject that isn't that openly discussed at parties and the like.*

Another respondent felt guilty because she regularly handed her urine into the general practice and thought that she was complaining too much.

> *But sometimes I do get the feeling that you're a bit of a whiner. That's not how my GP responds, but I do feel like we, as patients, while we are confronted with the hindrance and pain and constant annoyance of having to pee so often, invoke a reaction of: "oh here comes another one with his pee." Yeah then they shouldn't have invented them in the first place, urologists.*

Respondents described a variety of worries. The most common was about taking regular antibiotics, which many felt was harmful to their bodies.

> *Because I don't want to take antibiotics every time since that isn't good for your body either.*

Another common worry was about the cause of the recurrent UTI. Respondents felt that there had to be something wrong with their bodies to be getting so many UTIs.

> *Why do you get a cystitis every time? There has to be something wrong somewhere.*

The questionnaire of patient expectations

We formulated a 32-item questionnaire based on the major themes identified in the participant interviews. The questions varied in style, including statements that required a yes or no answer, statements that required answers on 5-point Likert scales, open-end questions and questions that required multiple answers with room for free text responses. Next, we tested the questionnaire in interviews with five patients and five non-patients. This revealed that three questions needed to be withdrawn due to similarities with other questions and that ten questions needed to be rewritten to improve comprehensibility. The final questionnaire consisted of 32 questions and was entitled the ESC-rUTI questionnaire (Expectations of Treatment in Secondary Care–Recurrent UTI). A copy of the English translation is provided in Additional file 2.

Discussion

This is the first study to explore patient expectations of secondary care assessment and treatment for recurrent UTI. Thematic analysis of interview data uncovered three themes: medical route, patient knowledge of the condition, and social and psychological impact.

Medical route

The first theme concerned pathways taken by patients and broadly covered the trajectory from symptom onset to referral. The most notable finding was that none of the respondents received prophylactic antibiotics from their GP, despite this being a clear recommendation in the Dutch General Practitioner guideline [8]. We plan to investigate this further in a future questionnaire-based study among GPs.

Some respondents reported that they had frequently asked their GP for a urology referral, indicating that referral is not always deemed necessary by the GP. A prospective survey of all referrals over a 5-month period from generalists to four selected academic sub-specialisms in the United States concluded that one-fifth of referral decisions were influenced by patient requests [9]. Furthermore, we found indicators that not all patients expect to achieve complete cure.

Patient knowledge of the condition

Although all respondents were able to name some preventive measures for their recurrent UTI, only some were able to mention all of them, indicating room for improvement in patient education. Most respondents wanted more information on either what they could do to prevent UTI, what causes UTI or both. Both these findings are supported by a recent qualitative study in the primary care setting regarding UTI [10]. Most respondents took the initiative to search for the information they needed, but some were afraid to do so because of what they would find. All respondents were able to explain the diagnostic procedures that would initially be performed in the hospital based on the information they had been sent, though only one was able to explain cystoscopy. Overall, there was a lack of knowledge among respondents, which indicated a need for reliable information about the diagnostic and treatment options for recurrent UTI.

Social and psychological impact

All respondents in our study described that their social lives had been greatly affected by their UTIs. This finding is supported by a large web base study that showed that recurrent UTI have a significant impact on quality of life [11]. Some were concerned about the cause of their UTI because they felt that there had to be something wrong with them to have UTIs on such a regular basis. Others were worried that regularly taking antibiotics would harm their bodies. These worries have previously been described in a qualitative study regarding public beliefs about antibiotics, infection, and resistance [12].

Strengths and limitations

The strengths of this study include the use of qualitative semi-structured interviews until saturation. The responses highlighted the important issues and expectations among patients concerning the management of recurrent UTI. However, this study also had several limitations. It was notable, for example, that the findings were based on data from a single center, meaning that we cannot be certain if they can be extrapolated to the general population. Although one respondent had already been seen in this clinic for recurrent UTI, her expectations were similar to those expressed by the other respondents Patient inclusion in our study might have introduced a certain response bias, as nearly all patients will report some level of bother. However, the level of bother may well differ between patients, and impact their expectations. Future research will elucidate this. Although the results of open-end questions are more difficult to interpret we chose to use them in order to test knowledge and not recognition. It also helps to gain knowledge in misconceptions.

Though this questionnaire will not change patient expectations, we think that knowledge of such expectations, may be helpful to adjust assessment and treatments to individual needs. Gaining insight in the expectations of the group of patient helps us align general patient information with this.

The final questionnaire

Despite these limitations, we were able to create the 32-item ESC-rUTI questionnaire. We anticipated that this will prove useful in providing information about a given patient's trajectory from symptom onset to referral, knowledge of the disease, concerns about the social and psychologic impact of the disease, and expectations for the hospital visit. However, we opted not to perform test–retest analyses because we do not plan to use the questionnaire to measure treatment effects. Instead, the questionnaire will only be used to create an inventory of expectations before an outpatient visit; thus, we believe that additional validation is not necessary. The final questionnaire covers a variety of relevant subjects, including the impact of symptoms on daily life, satisfaction with the GP, peer support, and expectations regarding diagnostics, education, treatment, and recurrent UTI (Additional file 2).

As the questionnaire was developed to be used in the Netherlands, the English version was not tested for readability with native English speakers. This needs to be done before using the English version.

Conclusion

This study provides insights into the expectations of newly referred patients with recurrent UTI. Follow-up research using the developed questionnaire has already been started to quantify these expectations and to see how they affect the care we provide.

Abbreviations

UTI: Urinary tract infection; AUA: American Urology Association; CUA: Canadian Urology Association; SUFU: Society of Urodynamics, Female Pelvic Medicine and Urogenital Reconstruction; GP: General Practitioner; ESC-rUTI: Expectations of Treatment in Secondary Care–Recurrent UTI.

Acknowledgements

We thank Dr. Robert Sykes (www.doctored.org.uk) for providing editorial services in the preparation of the final drafts of this manuscript.

Authors' contributions

All authors made substantial contributions to the design of the work. TvdA conducted the interviews. TvdA and JJP performed the analysis. JJP drafted the work. MHB, MGS and LPW substantively revised it. All authors approved the submitted version. All authors agreed both to be personally accountable for the author's own contributions and to ensure that questions related to the accuracy or integrity of any part of the work, even ones in which the author was not personally involved, are appropriately investigated, resolved, and the resolution documented in the literature. All authors read and approved the final manuscript.

Competing interests

The authors declare that they have no competing interests.

Author details

[1] Department of Urology, ISALA Clinics, Dokter van Heesweg 2, 8025 AB Zwolle, The Netherlands. [2] Department of General Practice, University of Groningen, University Medical Centre, Groningen, Hanzeplein 1, 9713 GZ Groningen, The Netherlands.

References

1. Nederlandse vereniging voor urologie. Richtlijn bacteriële urineweginfecties bij adolescenten en volwassenen. 2009. https://www.nvu.nl/Portals/_default/Skins/NVU/DocumentHandlerPublic.ashx?id=817db8b4-e657-40d0-bc20-52ebc1d286ff&filename=bijlage%20C58%20urineweginfectie%202009.pdf. Accessed 23 May 2018.
2. Albert X, Huertas I, Pereiro II, Sanfelix J, Gosalbes V, Perrota C. Antibiotics for preventing recurrent urinary tract infection in non-pregnant women. Cochrane Database Syst Rev. 2004;(3):CD001209.
3. Ikaheimo R, Siitonen A, Heiskanen T, Karkkainen U, Kuosmanen P, Lipponen P, et al. Recurrence of urinary tract infection in a primary care setting: analysis of a 1-year follow-up of 179 women. Clin Infect Dis. 1996;22(1):91–9.
4. Bonkat G, Pickard R, Bartoletti R, Cai T, Bruyère F, Geerlings SE, et al. Guidelines on urological infections. 2018. https://uroweb.org/guideline/urological-infections/#3. Accessed 23 May 2018.
5. Dason S, Dason JT, Kapoor A. Guidelines for the diagnosis and management of recurrent urinary tract infection in women. Can Urol Assoc J. 2011;5(5):316–22.
6. Anger J, Lee U, Ackerman AL, Chou R, Chughtai B, Clemens JQ, et al. Recurrent uncomplicated urinary tract infections in women: AUA/CUA/SUFU guideline. J Urol. 2019;202(2):282–9.
7. McKinley RK, Middleton JF. What do patients want from doctors? Content analysis of written patient agendas for the consultation. Br J Gen Pract. 1999;49(447):796–800.

8. van Pinxteren B, Knottnerus BJ, Geerlings VE, Visser HS, van der Weele, G M, Verduijn MM, et al. NHG-Standaard Urineweginfecties. 2013. https://www.nhg.org/standaarden/volledig/nhg-standaard-urineweginfecties. Accessed 23 May 2018.
9. Donohoe MT, Kravitz RL, Wheeler DB, Chandra R, Chen A, Humphries N. Reasons for outpatient referrals from generalists to specialists. J Gen Intern Med. 1999;14(5):281–6.
10. Lecky DM, Howdle J, Butler CC, McNulty CA. Optimising management of UTIs in primary care: a qualitative study of patient and GP perspectives to inform the development of an evidence-based, shared decision-making resource. Br J Gen Pract. 2020;70(694):e330–8.
11. Wagenlehner F, Wullt B, Ballarini S, Zingg D, Naber KG. Social and economic burden of recurrent urinary tract infections and quality of life: a patient web-based study (GESPRIT). Expert Rev Pharmacoecon Outcomes Res. 2018;18(1):107–17.
12. Norris P, Chamberlain K, Dew K, Gabe J, Hodgetts D, Madden H. Public beliefs about antibiotics, infection and resistance: a qualitative study. Antibiotics (Basel). 2013;2(4):465–76.

Biofilm reduction potential of 0.02% polyhexanide irrigation solution in several types of urethral catheters

Florian H. H. Brill[1*], Julia Hambach[1,2], Christian Utpatel[3], Diana C. Mogrovejo[1], Henrik Gabriel[1], Jan-Hendrik Klock[1], Joerg Steinmann[4] and Andreas Arndt[5]

Abstract

Background: Long-term use of urethral catheters is associated with high risk of urinary tract infection (UTI) and blockage. Microbial biofilms are a common cause of catheter blockage, reducing their lifetime and significantly increasing morbidity of UTIs. A 0.02% polyhexanide irrigation solution developed for routine mechanical rinsing shows potential for bacterial decolonization of urethral catheters and has the potential to reduce or prevent biofilm formation.

Methods: Using an in vitro assay with standard market-leading types of catheters artificially contaminated with clinically relevant bacteria, assays were carried out to evaluate the biofilm reduction and prevention potential of a 0.02% polyhexanide solution versus no intervention (standard approach) and irrigation with saline solution (NaCl 0.9%). The efficiency of decolonization was measured through microbial plate count and membrane filtration.

Results: Irrigation using a 0.02% polyhexanide solution is suitable for the decolonization of a variety of transurethral catheters. The effect observed is significant compared to irrigation with 0.9% saline solution ($p = 0.002$) or no treatment ($p = 0.011$). No significant difference was found between irrigation with 0.9% saline solution and no treatment ($p = 0.74$).

Conclusions: A 0.02% polyhexanide solution is able to reduce bacterial biofilm from catheters artificially contaminated with clinically relevant bacteria in vitro. The data shows a reduction of the viability of thick bacterial biofilms in a variety of commercially available urinary catheters made from silicone, latex-free silicone, hydrogel-coated silicone and PVC. Further research is required to evaluate the long-term tolerability and efficacy of polyhexanide in clinical practice.

Keywords: Bacterial decolonization, Biofilm, Polyhexanide, Urinary catheter, Urinary tract infection, Transurethral catheter

Background

Urinary tract infections are among the most common nosocomial infections. In Germany, for instance, it was estimated that approximately 155,000 nosocomial urinary tract infections occur every year, and the majority of these cases are catheter-associated [1]. Catheters, as many inserted medical devices, are heavily prone to microbial biofilm formation [2]. A variety of pathogens

*Correspondence: florian.b@brillhygiene.com
[1] Dr. Brill + Partner GmbH Institute for Hygiene and Microbiology, Stiegstück 34, 22339 Hamburg, Germany
Full list of author information is available at the end of the article

are able to colonize catheters: commensal species of bacteria from the gastrointestinal tract or ascending from the urethra, or bacteria transferred from the insertion site [2, 3].

Pathogens such as *Escherichia coli, Enterobacter* spp., *Pseudomonas* spp., *Enterococcus* spp., *Staphylococcus aureus*, coagulase-negative staphylococci and yeasts are common causes of urinary tract infections and catheter blockage [3, 4] and the most commonly reported species forming biofilms on urethral catheters are *Candida* spp., *Pseudomonas aeruginosa, Proteus mirabilis, E. faecalis*, and *S. aureus* [2, 3]. Scanning electron microscopy performed on biofilms formed on indwelling catheters has shown depths ranging from 3 to 490 μm and up to 400 visible bacterial cells deep [5].

In a biofilm, microbes are attached to the catheter surfaces in a manner that prevents their removal with gentle rinsing and would require mechanical removal. In fact, biofilms formed in catheters often lead to catheter encrustation and obstruction [5]. Biofilms in catheters have important implications for health as antibiotics are rarely able to penetrate the superficial layers of the biofilm, complicating treatment [5]. Moreover, microbial biofilms are known to be up to 1500 times more resistant to antibiotic therapy compared to planktonic, free-living bacteria [3, 6]. Biofilms on catheters can lead to significant complications and unfavorable outcomes for the patients' health [3] and for this reason, the development of effective methods and compounds for the prevention of biofilm formation or their reduction is of great importance [2, 3, 7].

Polyhexanide (polyhexamethylene biguanide or PHMB) is a polymer frequently used as an antiseptic with broad antibacterial activity, good tissue tolerability and, to date, shows no development of bacterial resistance [8]. Polyhexanide has been used for mechanical rinsing and removal of biofilms across a range of applications [4, 7, 9]. In this study, we investigated the potential of a polyhexanide solution to reduce and prevent biofilm formation under in vitro conditions in a variety of artificially colonized catheters.

Methods

All experiments were performed using a mixed culture of the following bacterial strains: *Escherichia coli* (ATCC® 11229), *Proteus mirabilis* (ATCC® 14153, DSM 778) and *Staphylococcus aureus* (ATCC® 6538). An overnight culture plate in nutrient agar (OXOID, Germany) of each bacterium was washed away in 10 mL NaCl peptone and transferred to a sterile flask with glass beads. This suspension was homogenized for 2 min at 1500 rpm on a mechanical shaker and adjusted to 10^9 CFU per mL using standard plate count methods (data not shown).

Five different types of catheters were used, as shown in Table 1. These different catheters were selected to cover a broad range of commercially available products and observe the performance of the treatments in all of them. Due to its popularity as biomaterial [10–12], 4 catheters made of silicone out of the 5 were used in this study. Of these, Catheter A is the only one to have a hydrogel coating.

Thirty (30) catheters of each type were used for the decolonization test. The catheters were incubated with 5 ml of the mixed bacterial suspension for 4 h at 37 °C, after which the catheters were irrigated 2 × 400 ml of an organic load suspension (0.3% bovine albumin + 3.0% urea, reagents from Carl Roth Germany) per day to simulate the process of contamination with urine and organic materials. After 72 h, ten of the catheters were irrigated with 100 mL Uro-Tainer® 0.02% PHMB (B. Braun Medical, Switzerland) with 5 min exposure time, ten catheters were irrigated with 100 mL Uro-Tainer® 0.9% NaCl (B. Braun Medical, Switzerland) with an exposure time of 5 min and 10 catheters were not treated (controls).

After treatment, the microbial count was determined by irrigation of the catheters with 100 ml of a TLH-SDS neutralizer solution (0.1% polysorbat 80, 0.1% g/L lecithin, 0.1% histidine, 0.2% SDS, all reagents from Carl Roth Germany) and membrane filtration (0.45 μm pore size, MF-Millipore USA) of 50 mL via serial dilution method on trypticase soybean agar (TSA, OXOID Germany). No measurements of pH were made for the rinsed filtrates as the slightly acidic pH of the Uro-Tainer® 0.02% PHMB (pH at 20 °C of 5.5) was neutralized with the use

Table 1 Characteristics of the catheters used in this study

Reference for experiments	Specifications
Catheter A	2-way Foley catheter, latex-free silicone, Balloon 30 cc, 18Ch, hydrogel coating
Catheter B	Straight whistle tip catheter, silicone, 40 cm, 18Ch
Catheter C	Bladder catheter without balloon, PVC, 37 cm, 18Ch, latex-free
Catheter D	Transurethral Foley catheter, 2-way, latex-free silicone, 41 cm, 18Ch
Catheter E	Transurethral Foley Nelaton balloon catheter, latex-free silicone, 41 cm, 18Ch

of the TLH-SDS solution. We anticipated that the pH of the filtrates did not modify the pH of the culture media used in this study and therefore did not affect the growth of the surviving bacteria.

In addition, all catheters were cut and the material in the lumen was extracted with a sterile cotton swab. The swab was suspended in 0.9% NaCl solution (Carl Roth Germany) and the microbial count was determined via serial dilution method on TSA plates.

All nutrient media were incubated at 37 °C for 2 days. Mean values of microbial count ($\log_{10}$ CFU) after the different treatments were calculated as well as the reduction factors for the Uro-Tainer® 0.02% PHMB solution compared to Uro-Tainer® 0.9% NaCl and no treatment. Statistical analyses were done using the two-tailed Student's '*t*' test and *p* values of ($* \leq 0.05$) were considered as significant.

Results

We observed that treatment with the Uro-Tainer® 0.02% PHMB solution effectively reduced the biofilms artificially formed in the different catheter types as measured in after rinsing/membrane filtration (Fig. 1a) as well as in the swab samples (Fig. 1b). In general, the effect of irrigation with Uro-Tainer® 0.02% PHMB solution is superior compared to the untreated catheters ($p=0.011$) as well as compared to those treated with Uro-Tainer® 0.9% NaCl solution ($p=0.002$) while there was no significant effect of irrigation with 0.9% NaCl compared with no treatment at all ($p=0.74$) (Additional file 1: Table S1). Reductions factors (Table 2) ranged from 0.3 in the case of the type B catheter with no treatment to 4.6 for the type C catheter treated with Uro-Tainer® 0.9% NaCl.

Discussion

In natural, clinical, and industrial environments, the formation of biofilms is a basic microbial survival strategy. Medical devices such as suprapubic and indwelling catheters used in clinical settings are frequently colonized by biofilms of a variety of microbial species with detrimental consequences for the patients [13]. Research is focused on decolonization of urethral catheters via treatment with a range of systemic antibiotic regimens [14] even though antibiotic resistance and drug adsorption are heavily modified in biofilms [3, 4, 13]. In fact, antimicrobial compounds are usually not able to penetrate the full depth of the microbial biofilms, reducing the available options for effective therapy [15]. Treatment is further complicated by the fact that biofilms are frequently composed of a variety of species, as demonstrated from urine samples of colonized-catheters [16].

Besides antimicrobial therapy, the treatment of infections caused by bacterial biofilms in catheters requires the removal of the bacteria attached to the devices or at least, a noticeable reduction of the bacterial load [17]. Alternative methods and compounds for reduction and prevention of biofilms in catheters are necessary as altered catheter surfaces have proven ineffective at inhibiting microbial attachment [3, 15, 18].

In this regard, polyhexanide is considered one of the "most promising substances available" for clinical applications [19]. Mechanical rinsing with 0.9% NaCl solution and a 0.02% solution of polyhexanide has been observed to significantly and consistently reduce bacterial colonization, providing an effective, non-systemic approach to biofilm formation on urinary catheters [4]. Other studies have also confirmed the antiseptic efficacy and antibacterial effect of polyhexanide in the treatment of skin wounds, as an ingredient in mouthwash solutions or as a supplement of cleansing solutions [19]. Furthermore, observational studies in patients with indwelling catheters in which the Uro-Tainer® 0.02% PHMB solution was used for rinsing, showed no serious adverse events for the patients [20].

Here, the reduction of biofilms in artificially colonized commercially available catheters using Uro-Tainer® 0.02% PHMB solution was tested in an in vitro assay. The study confirms the efficacy of the solution on a range of catheters types. Our results showed that rinsing the catheters reduces colonization and the treatment with polyhexanide was more effective compared to rinsing with saline solution or no rinsing at all ($p=0.002$ and $p=0.011$, respectively), in all 5 types of catheters tested. These results go in accordance to previous reports of the usefulness of polyhexanide [19, 21–23] and confirms the efficacy of a 0.02% polyhexanide solution to reduce and prevent the formation of biofilms in catheter systems in vitro [4].

The formation of biofilms in urethral catheters is aided by the deposition of organic molecules from the urinary components, such as proteins and electrolytes [16]. The inert materials of catheters make them susceptible to microbial colonization [16], as they cannot produce the immunological response triggered in the mucosa of living tissue responsible for neutralizing colonizing microbes. While some bacteria have proven to adhere less to certain materials, as is the case of *E. coli* and *Klebsiella pneumoniae* in siliconized-rubber catheters [16, 24], with enough time the microflora inevitably finds a way to colonize the catheter. Thus, the characteristics of the catheter material is critical for both the biocompatibility of the device as well as for reducing and/or avoiding bacterial adhesion [17]. The interactions between bacteria and the polymers in the biomaterials are mediated by forces such as hydrophobic interactions between surfaces [25] or fimbrial interactions [10]. The initial adherence seems to

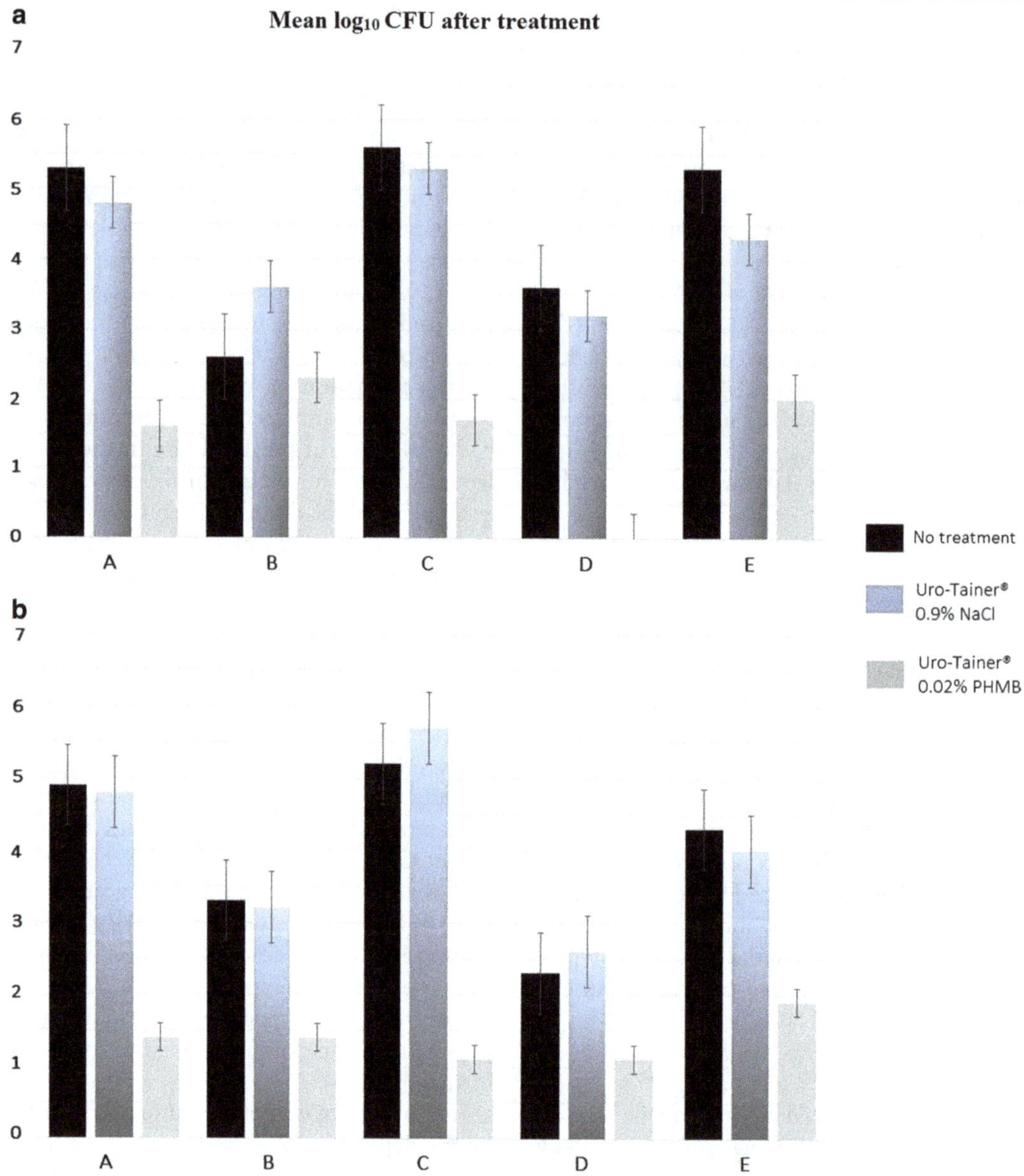

Fig. 1 Cell counts after filtration of **a** rinsing solutions and **b** after swab sampling of catheters treated with different irrigation solutions. The values of $\log_{10}$ CFU are shown as the mean of 10 parallel replications

depend mainly on the catheter biomaterial and it is later influenced in vivo by other factors such as the presence of proteins, fluids and host cells [25]. Moreover, the composition of already-formed microbial biofilms does not appear to be influenced by the biomaterial [26].

In our study, the result of the decolonization treatment with 0.02% PHMB was significantly different from the treatment with 0.9% NaCl in all the catheters tested, confirming the efficacy of polyhexanide in a variety of biomaterials, such as silicone, latex-free silicone, hydrogel-coated silicone and PVC besides its efficacy already proven in polyurethane catheters [4]. We observed a similar behavior between the hydrogel-coated silicon catheter A, the PVC catheter C and the silicone catheter E (Fig. 1).

Silicone is the most popular material in catheters [10–12] followed by other materials like PVC, polyurethane and latex. Hydrogel-coated catheters, while useful to decrease the mucosal trauma derived from catheter use, are comparable to other catheters in the formation of biofilm [27]. A review of the literature suggests that not one material is significantly better than another in preventing

Table 2 Biocidal activity of Uro-Tainer® 0.02% PHMB compared to Uro-Tainer® 0.9% NaCl and no treatment represented by Reduction factors of log_{10} CFU

Catheter	Reduction factors using Uro-Tainer® 0.02% PHMB compared to			
	Uro-Tainer® 0.9% NaCl	No treatment	Uro-Tainer® 0.9% NaCl	No treatment
	Cell counts after filtration		Cell counts after swab sampling	
Catheter A	3.2	3.7	3.4	3.5
Catheter B	1.3	0.3	1.8	1.9
Catheter C	3.6	3.9	4.6	4.1
Catheter D	1.2	1.6	1.5	1.2
Catheter E	2.3	3.3	2.1	2.4

the encrustation of long-term inserted medical devices [28], although smooth non-sticky materials such as silicone appear to behave more favorably while latex-based catheters seem to favor biofilm formation more often due to their uneven surfaces and irregularities [27]. On the other hand, there is insufficient scientific evidence for a decreased frequency of bacteriuria or catheter-associated UTI due to obstruction in silicone compared to latex catheters [27]. Hence the importance of methodologies that, besides improvements on catheter material, allow the reduction of the bacterial load in nascent biofilms.

Some materials contain additives meant to improve the properties of the device [17] but have been shown to bloom to the surface with natural aging where they are metabolized by organisms and facilitate their attachment, e.g. polyurethane and PVC [17, 29]. Combinations of materials, such as polyurethane and polycarbonate, seem to provide a solution for blooming [30]. Other materials, such as PVC and siliconized latex, appear to intrinsically favor the adherence of bacteria [25] even allowing growth in the absence of conventional nutrients [31]. In this study, the specifications of Catheter B did not indicate whether latex was used for its fabrication and perhaps the presence of this biomaterial could explain the lowest reduction factor observed (RF = 0.3) when the treatment with 0.02% PHMB was compared to no treatment at all (Table 2). However, we also observed higher reduction factors for catheter C, the only one made of PVC, along with the hydrophobic, hydrogel-coated catheter A, confirming that many other factors influence bacterial adherence to catheters besides biomaterial [25].

This study provides evidence of the efficacy of Uro-Tainer® 0.02% PHMB to reduce biofilms possibly through a combination of mechanical and antibacterial effects and independently of the catheter characteristics. Our results show significant reductions of the log_{10} CFU in all tested catheters. Such efficacy is of great importance as catheter material generally does not diminish the ability of microbes to form biofilms within them, except in the setting of short-term catheterization [16].

Additional research is recommended to investigate whether the presented results can be transferred into practice and lead to a reduction in urinary tract infections in clinical settings. Parameters such as the pH of patients' urine as well as retrograde bacterial growth into the bladder could be investigated further to determine their effect on the efficacy of polyhexanide.

Conclusion

Our experiments show that rinsing with Uro-Tainer® 0.02% PHMB on artificially colonized silicone catheters, latex-free silicone catheters, latex-free PVC catheters and latex-free hydrophobic (hydrogel-coated) silicone catheters, is significantly more effective compared to rinsing with saline solution or no rinsing at all.

The use of a polyhexanide solution constitutes a strategy for the reduction of the viability of thick bacterial biofilms in a variety of commercially available urinary catheters.

Abbreviations

UTI: Urinary tract infection; PHMB: Polyhexanide (polyhexamethylene biguanide); spp.: Species; mL: Milliliter; nm: Nanometer; µm: Micrometer; h: Hour(s); min: Minutes; g/L: Grams per liter; rpm: Revolutions per minute.

Acknowledgements

The authors would like to acknowledge the help and logistic support received by their teams at their host institutions.

Authors' contributions

FHHB, CU, HG, J-HK, JS were involved in the development of the methods and the planning of the laboratory tests. AA was involved in the study design. JH, CU carried out the experiments. HG and J-HK were responsible for data analysis. DCM drafted the original manuscript. All authors reviewed, edited, and approved the final version of the manuscript.

Competing interests

FHHB was an employee for B. Braun Medical Ltd. between 2006 and 2010. FHHB is Managing Director of Dr. Brill + Partner GmbH Institute for Hygiene and Microbiology. DCM, HG, JHK are currently employed at Dr. Brill + Partner GmbH. AA is an employee of B. Braun Medical Ltd. All authors declare no competing interests.

Author details

[1] Dr. Brill + Partner GmbH Institute for Hygiene and Microbiology, Stiegstück 34, 22339 Hamburg, Germany. [2] Institute of Immunology, University Medical Center Hamburg-Eppendorf, Hamburg, Germany. [3] Molecular and Experimental Mycobacteriology, Research Center Borstel – Leibniz Lung Center, Borstel, Germany. [4] Klinikum Nürnberg, Institute of Clinical Hygiene, Medical Microbiology and Infectiology, Paracelsus Medical University, Nuremberg, Germany. [5] Department of Research and Development, B. Braun Medical Ltd., Sempach, Switzerland.

References

1. Gastmeier P, Geffers C. Nosokomiale infektionen in Deutschland: Wie viele gibt es wirklich? Eine schätzung für das jahr 2006. Dtsch Medizinische Wochenschrift. 2008;133(21):1111–5.
2. Bonkat G, Widmer AF, Rieken M, van der Merwe A, Braissant O, Müller G, et al. Microbial biofilm formation and catheter-associated bacteriuria in patients with suprapubic catheterisation. World J Urol. 2013;31(3):565–71.
3. Tenke P, Köves B, Nagy K, Hultgren SJ, Mendling W, Wullt B, et al. Update on biofilm infections in the urinary tract. World J Urol. 2012;30(1):51–7.
4. Brill FHH, Gabriel H, Brill H, Klock JH, Steinmann J, Arndt A. Decolonization potential of 0.02% polyhexanide irrigation solution in urethral catheters under practice-like in vitro conditions. BMC Urol. 2018;18(1):1–6.
5. Saint S, Chenoweth CE. Biofilms and catheter-associated urinary tract infections. Infect Dis Clin N Am. 2003;17(2):411–32.
6. Vergidis P, Patel R. Novel approaches to the diagnosis, prevention and treatment of medical device-associated infections. Infect Dis Clin N Am. 2012;26(1):173–86.
7. Harbs N, Siebert J. In vitro efficacy of octenidine and polihexanide against biofilms composed of *Pseudomonas aeruginosa*. GMS Krankenhhyg Interdiszip. 2007;2(2):2–4.
8. Saleh K, Sonesson A, Persson K, Riesbeck K, Schmidtchen A. Can dressings soaked with polyhexanide reduce bacterial loads in full-thickness skin grafting? A randomized controlled trial. J Am Acad Dermatol. 2016;75(6):1221-1228.e4. https://doi.org/10.1016/j.jaad.2016.07.020.
9. Gray D, Barrett S, Battacharyya M, Butcher M, Enoch S, Fumerola S, et al. PHMB and its potential contribution to wound management. Wounds UK. 2010;6(2):40–6.
10. Siddiq DM, Darouiche RO. New strategies to prevent catheter-associated urinary tract infections. Nat Rev Urol. 2012;9(6):305–14. https://doi.org/10.1038/nrurol.2012.68.
11. Verma A, Bhani D, Tomar V, Bachhiwal R, Yadav S. Differences in bacterial colonization and biofilm formation property of uropathogens between the two most commonly used indwelling urinary catheters. J Clin Diagn Res. 2016;10:1–3.
12. Al-Qahtani M, Safan A, Jassim G, Abadla S. Efficacy of anti-microbial catheters in preventing catheter associated urinary tract infections in hospitalized patients: a review on recent updates. J Infect Public Health. 2019;12(6):760–6. https://doi.org/10.1016/j.jiph.2019.09.009.
13. Stickler DJ. Bacterial biofilms in patients with indwelling urinary catheters. Nat Clin Pract Urol. 2008;5(11):598–608.
14. Buehlmann M, Bruderer T, Frei R, Widmer AF. Effectiveness of a new decolonisation regimen for eradication of extended-spectrum β-lactamase-producing Enterobacteriaceae. J Hosp Infect. 2011;77(2):113–7. https://doi.org/10.1016/j.jhin.2010.09.022.
15. Tenke P, Kovacs B, Jäckel M, Nagy E. The role of biofilm infection in urology. World J Urol. 2006;24(1):13–20.
16. Trautner BW, Darouiche RO. Role of biofilm in catheter-associated urinary tract infection. Am J Infect Control. 2004;32(3):177–83.
17. Pascual A, de Arellano ER, Martínez LM, Perea EJ. Effect of polyurethane catheters and bacterial biofilms on the in-vitro activity of antimicrobials against *Staphylococcus epidermidis*. J Hosp Infect. 1993;24(3):211–8.
18. Morris NS, Stickler DJ, McLean RJC. The development of bacterial biofilms on indwelling urethral catheters. World J Urol. 1999;17(6):345–50.
19. Hübner NO, Kramer A. Review on the efficacy, safety and clinical applications of polihexanide, a modern wound antiseptic. Skin Pharmacol Physiol. 2010;23(suppl 1):17–27.
20. Pannek J, Everaert K, Möhr S, Vance W, Van Der Aa F, Kesselring J. Tolerability and safety of urotainer® polihexanide 0.02% in catheterized patients: a prospective cohort study. BMC Urol. 2020;20(92):1–7.
21. Müller G, Kramer A. Biocompatibility index of antiseptic agents by parallel assessment of antimicrobial activity and cellular cytotoxicity. J Antimicrob Chemother. 2008;61(6):1281–7.
22. Werthén M, Davoudi M, Sonesson A, Nitsche DP, Mörgelin M, Blom K, et al. *Pseudomonas aeruginosa*-induced infection and degradation of human wound fluid and skin proteins *ex vivo* are eradicated by a synthetic cationic polymer. J Antimicrob Chemother. 2004;54(4):772–9.
23. Rosin M, Welk A, Bernhardt O, Ruhnau M, Pitten FA, Kocher T, et al. Effect of a polyhexamethylene biguanide mouthrinse on bacterial counts and plaque. J Clin Periodontol. 2001;28(12):1121–6.
24. Sugarman B. Adherence of bacteria to urinary catheters. Urol Res. 1982;10:37–40.
25. Lopez-Lopez G, Pascual A, Perea EJ. Effect of plastic catheter material on bacterial adherence and viability. J Med Microbiol. 1991;34(6):349–53.
26. Higgins M, Zhang L, Ford R, Brownlie J, Kleidon T, Rickard CM, et al. The microbial biofilm composition on peripherally inserted central catheters: a comparison of polyurethane and hydrophobic catheters collected from paediatric patients. J Vasc Access. 2020. https://doi.org/10.1177/1129729820932423.
27. Jordan RPC, Nicolle LE. Preventing infection associated with urethral catheter biofilms. In: Percival SL, Williams DW, Randle J, Cooper T, editors. Biofilms in infection prevention and control: a healthcare handbook. Amsterdam: Elsevier; 2014. p. 287–309. https://doi.org/10.1016/B978-0-12-397043-5.00016-5.
28. Tunney MM, Keane PF, Jones DS, Gorman SP. Comparative assessment of ureteral stent biomaterial encrustation. Biomaterials. 1996;17(15):1541–6.
29. Nouman M, Jubeli E, Saunier J, Yagoubi N. Exudation of additives to the surface of medical devices: impact on biocompatibility in the case of polyurethane used in implantable catheters. J Biomed Mater Res Part A. 2016;104(12):2954–67.
30. Pathak R, Bierman SF, D'arnaud P. Inhibition of bacterial attachment and biofilm formation by a novel intravenous catheter material using an in vitro percutaneous catheter insertion model. Med Devices Evid Res. 2018;11:427–32.
31. Franson TR, Sheth NK, Menon L, Sohnle PG. Persistent in vitro survival of coagulase-negative staphylococci adherent to intravascular catheters in the absence of conventional nutrients. J Clin Microbiol. 1986;24(4):559–61.

30

Prostate artery embolization has long term efficacy for treatment of severe lower urinary tract symptoms from giant prostatic hyperplasia

Alexander S. Somwaru[1*], Stephen Metting[2], Laura M. Flisnik[3], Michael G. Nellamattathil[4], Arjun Sharma[5] and Venkat S. Katabathina[6]

Abstract

Background: Patients with severe lower urinary tract symptoms (LUTS) from giant prostatic hyperplasia (GPH): prostate volume greater than 200 mL that do not respond to medical therapy may not be eligible for surgical treatments due to morbidities, technical challenges, and patient preference. This retrospective investigation examined the long-term efficacy and safety of prostatic arterial embolization (PAE) as a treatment option for severe LUTS due to GPH in a large patient cohort.

Methods: Of 529 patients who underwent PAE between January 2016 and January 2020, 72 patients had severe LUTS from GPH and were retrospectively evaluated. PAE was performed with two embolic agents in sequence: 100–250 μm particles followed by 2 mm and 3 mm coils. Clinical assessment was performed with international prostate symptoms score (IPSS), quality of life (QoL), peak flow rate (Qmax), post-void residual volume (PVR), and prostate specific antigen (PSA) measurements before and 12 months and 24 months after PAE. Prostate volume (PV) was measured by multiparametric magnetic resonance (MR) imaging before and 12 months and 24 months after PAE.

Results: Patients with severe LUTS from GPH experienced significant clinical improvements in IPSS, QoL, Qmax, PVR, PSA, and PV at 12 months and 24 months after PAE. Mean IPSS decreased from 26.5 to 18.0 ($P < 0.01$) to 10.5 ($P < 0.01$). Mean QoL decreased from 6.0 to 4.0 ($P < 0.01$) to 2.0 ($P < 0.01$). Mean Qmax increased from 8.0 to 14 mL/s ($P < 0.01$) to 18 mL/s ($P < 0.01$). Mean PVR decreased from 198.0 to 152.0 mL ($P < 0.01$) to 90 mL ($P < 0.01$). Mean PV decreased from 303.0 mL to 258.0 mL ($P < 0.01$) to 209.0 mL ($P < 0.01$). Mean PSA decreased from 11.2 ng/mL to 9.5 ng/mL ($P < 0.05$) to 7.9 ng/mL ($P < 0.05$). No major complications occurred.

Conclusions: PAE is a safe treatment with long term efficacy for severe LUTS from GPH. PAE may be a viable therapeutic option for patients with severe LUTS from GPH whom fail medical therapy and are not candidates for surgical treatments.

Keywords: Giant prostatic hyperplasia (GPH), Prostatic artery embolization (PAE), Lower urinary tract symptoms (LUTS)

Background

Patients with severe urinary tract symptoms (LUTS) from prostatic hyperplasia that is refractory to medical therapy are offered surgical treatment options that range from minimally invasive procedures to transurethral resection of the prostate (TURP) to simple prostatectomy [1–4]. The surgical treatment selection process is governed by prostate volume, presence of LUTS, comorbidities, risk–benefit profile, patient preference treatment

*Correspondence: alex.somwaru@gmail.com
[1] Department of Diagnostic, Molecular, and Interventional Radiology, Icahn School of Medicine At Mount Sinai, 1000 10th Avenue, New York, NY 10019, USA
Full list of author information is available at the end of the article

availability and physician expertise [1–4]. Prostate volume is a significant factor in surgical treatment selection [1–4]. TURP and minimally invasive procedures, such as photoselective vaporization, laser enucleation, transurethral vapor and microwave ablation, transurethral incision, and prostate urethral lift, are best suited for patients with prostate volumes less than 80 mL [1–4]. Large prostatic hyperplasia is defined as prostate volume greater than 100 mL and giant prostatic hyperplasia (GPH) is defined as prostate volume greater than 200 mL [1–9]. Patients with large and giant prostatic hyperplasia with severe LUTS may require simple prostatectomy however may have a higher risk of morbidity from blood loss that requires blood transfusion (8–15%), urinary incontinence (10%), and urinary bladder neck stenosis and urethral strictures (5%) [1–9)].

Prostate artery embolization (PAE) has emerged as a safe and efficacious treatment of patients with severe LUTS from prostatic hyperplasia with prostate volumes up to 100 mL, or large prostatic hyperplasia [5–13]. Numerous retrospective and prospective studies of large cohorts of patients have shown that PAE safely provides long term reduction in symptoms and prostate volume by inducing ischemic necrosis, diminished hormonal response, and reduced prostate innervation with consequent reduced smooth muscle tone [10–13].

GPH is defined as prostate volume greater than 200 mL [1–9, 14–19]. GPH has been described in several individual patients as case reports in a review of international scientific literature [1–9, 14–19]. Individual cases of patients with severe LUTS from GPH whom underwent treatment with surgery or minimally invasive ablative urological treatment have also been reported [20–26]. However the safety and long-term efficacy of PAE for treatment of large cohorts of patients with severe LUTS from GPH has not been examined. One study retrospectively reviewed eight patients and one case report reviewed one patient whom underwent PAE for severe LUTS from GPH [27, 28]. While these two studies reported short term efficacy: eight months and three months, respectively, for significant symptom relief, long term efficacy remains unknown [27, 28]. A prostate volume limit that may render PAE ineffective, due to unsuccessful symptom and prostate volume reduction, has also not been established [1–4, 27, 28]. This study evaluated the safety and long-term efficacy of PAE in the largest cohort of patients, to date, with severe LUTS due to GPH.

PAE has a steep learning curve because it requires both refined microvascular skills and detailed knowledge of highly variable anatomic anatomy to identify, catheterize, and embolize target prostatic arteries to attain successful outcomes and avoid adverse complications [5–8]. The variant origins and anatomies of the prostate artery have been, in turn, reported in a variable fashion across anatomic and angiographic literature. The most commonly reported origins are the internal pudendal artery, the superior vesical artery (with a common trunk), inferior vesical artery, the gluteal-pudendal arterial trunk, and the obturator artery [5–11]. Prostate artery anatomy origins, number, accessory branches, and extra-prostatic anastomoses of the prostate artery may vary from left to right pelvic side. The prostatic artery bifurcates into the central and capsular divisions. The superior and anterolateral pedicle, which is the primary arterial target of PAE, provides the dominant supply to the central gland and the inferior and posterolateral pedicle provides supply to the peripheral gland and prostate apex [5–12]. In hyperplastic prostate glands, the prostate artery is tortuous with intraglandular twists and spiral arterial branches, which are used as landmarks for angiographic identification and confirmation of catheter position during PAE [5–13]. Extra-arterial anastomoses commonly communicate with the internal pudendal artery, contralateral prostate artery, and superior and inferior vesical arteries [5–10, 12].

Clinical volume and experience allow the operator to develop a level of expertise in PAE, which is a technically challenging although safe and efficacious procedure, however complications may occur. PAE is performed under direct fluoroscopic guidance with cone-beam CT. Cone-beam CT is particularly useful to assist in the identification of the prostatic arteries, reduce ionizing radiation dose and procedural time, and minimize complications of nontarget embolization. Non-target embolization of pelvic organs, like the urinary bladder, urethra, rectum, and penis, is a source of complications such a hematuria, rectal bleeding, erectile dysfunction, penile skin changes and pain that usually resolve without intervention or surgery [1–5]. Acute urinary retention and dysuria may be caused increased pressure and compression of the intraprostatic urethra from swelling, edema, ischemia, and necrosis of the prostate gland that occur after embolization that may require temporary post-procedural catheterization of the urinary bladder until spontaneous urination resumes [1–5]. Urinary tract infections, also thought to be caused by increased pressure and compression of the intraprostatic urethra from swelling, edema, ischemia, and necrosis of the prostate gland, require outpatient antibiotic therapy [1–5]. Other self-limited complications include hematospermia, urethral pain, and soft tissue hematomas at the arterial access site [1–5].

Methods

Institutional review board (IRB) approval was received for this retrospective study. Written informed consent was obtained from the patients and any accompanying images. Patients gave consent for their personal or clinical details along with any identifying images to be published in this study. A review of the electronic medical records (EMR) from a single medical center was conducted on all patients (529) whom underwent PAE for severe LUTS between January 2016 and January 2020. Severe LUTS was classified as International Prostate Symptom Score (IPSS) greater than 18 points, urinary quality of life (QoL) greater than 3 points, and peak flow rate (Qmax) less than 12 mL/s. Patients were evaluated in this investigation if they underwent PAE for severe LUTS from GPH. GPH is defined as prostate volume greater than 200 mL. Patients that did not have GPH (prostate volumes less than 200 mL) were not evaluated in this investigation. Of the 529 patients that underwent PAE for severe LUTS, 72 patients had GPH and were evaluated in this investigation. At our institution, multiparametric MR imaging is performed on all patients before PAE for prostate volume (PV) measurements and to ensure the absence of any lesions suspicious for clinically significant cancers according to version 2.1 of Prostate Imaging-Reporting and Data System (PI-RADS) [29]. No patients underwent PAE if MR imaging revealed lesions suspicious for clinically significant cancer. MR imaging was also used to measure prostate volumes at 12 months and 24 months after PAE. Patients underwent PAE if they did not respond to 5-alpha-reductase inhibitor and/or alpha-1-adrenergic receptor antagonist medical therapy for at least 6 months or longer and were not eligible for surgery or refused surgery. Patients were not eligible for surgical treatment due to comorbidities and/or contraindications to surgery and/or general anesthesia 49 (68%) patients with cardiovascular disease on anticoagulation/antiplatelet therapy and 23 (32%) patients with chronic lung disease. IPSS, QoL, Qmax, PV, postvoid residual volume (PVR), and PSA were measured and collected before PAE and 12 months and 24 months after PAE. Because MR imaging is performed on all patients before PAE to ensure the absence of any lesions suspicious for clinically significant cancers in our institution, patients with PSA levels above 4 ng/mL were examined in this investigation. Before PAE, 5-alpha-reductase inhibitor therapy was stopped and alpha-1-adrenergic receptor antagonist therapy was tapered and stopped after one month after PAE. No patients underwent additional interventions after PAE.

Clinical metrics

Clinical assessment was performed in all patients before PAE and 12 months and 24 months after PAE with history and physical examination, IPSS and QoL questionnaires, uroflowmetry Qmax, PVR, and PSA levels measurements. These clinical metrics are routinely recorded for patient care, to optimize patient outcomes, and for quality improvement and performance.

Prostate MR imaging and volume measurement

The protocol at our institution is to perform multiparametric MR imaging for all patients before PAE for prostate gland volume measurements and to ensure the absence of clinically significant cancers before PAE. Prostate volumes were calculated using MR imaging obtained before PAE and 12 months and 24 months after PAE. At our institution, multiparametric prostate MR imaging is performed using 3.0 T magnet systems (Siemens Healthcare, Erlangen, Germany). Exams are performed with phased array torso coils using the following protocol (Table 1): axial, sagittal, and coronal T2-weighted turbo spin echo images; axial b50, b500, and b800 s/mm^2 diffusion-weighted images; synthetic extrapolated b1200,

Table 1 MRI acquisition protocol

Sequence	Plane	Slice/gap (mm)	TR/TE (ms)	FOV (mm)	Matrix	Flip angle
T2W TSE	Sagittal	5/1	4000/100	200 × 200	384 × 224	150
T2W TSE	Axial	3/0	4000/100	200 × 200	384 × 224	150
T2W TSE	Coronal	3/0	4000/100	200 × 200	384 × 224	150
DWI (b0, 50, 500, 800, 1200, 1500, 2000, 2500 s/mm^2)/ADC	Axial	3/1	3300/60	260 × 260	128 × 96	
T1W FS VIBE MRA	Coronal	5/1	3.85/1.42	260 × 260	256 × 180	70
T1W FS VIBE pre	Axial	5/1	3.85/1.42	260 × 260	256 × 180	100
T1W FS VIBE post dynamic × 3	Axial	5/1	3.85/1.42	260 × 260	256 × 180	2.5/10/20
T1W FS VIBE post whole pelvis	Axial	5/1	3.85/1.42	260 × 260	256 × 180	70

ADC apparent diffusion coefficient, *DWI* diffusion weighted imaging, *FOV* field of view, *FS* fat saturated, *MRA* magnetic resonance angiography, *TE* echo time, *TR* repetition time, *TSE* turbo spin echo, *VIBE* volumetric interpolated breath-hold examination b1500, b2000, and b2500 diffusion-weighted images; apparent diffusion coefficient (ADC) map; axial T1 pre-contrast fat saturated volumetric interpolated breath-hold examination (VIBE) images; coronal T1-precontrast fat-saturated MR angiographic VIBE images of the pelvis; serial dynamic axial T1 pre-contrast fat saturated VIBE images obtained after intravenous gadolinium contrast injection (Gadavist 0.1 mmol/kg; Bayer Healthcare Pharmaceuticals, Wayne, NJ, USA); axial fat-saturated T1-weighted delayed postcontrast VIBE images.

Two diagnostic radiologists with 12 and 6 years of experience in interpreting multiparametric prostate MR imaging, respectively, independently reviewed the MR imaging exams before and after PAE. The radiologists used DynaCAD software (InVivo, Philips Healthcare, Amsterdam, Netherlands) on two separate workstations to perform semiautomated prostatic volumetric measurements of the prostate using the MR T2-weighted images. Prostatic volumes were manually confirmed by calculation of the ellipsoid volume formula ($L \times W \times H \times \pi/6$). Discordant measurements were resolved by consensus agreement. The diagnostic radiologists also reviewed MR imaging before and after PAE for any prostate gland lesions suspicious for clinically significant cancer according to version 2.1 of Prostate Imaging-Reporting and Data System (PI-RADS) [29].

Prostate artery embolization

All PAE procedures were performed by a single operator with thirteen years of angiographic and embolization experience and four years of experience performing PAE. All patients received one dose of ciprofloxacin 400 mg administered intravenously for infection prophylaxis. All procedures were performed under moderate (conscious) sedation with local anesthesia in a therapeutic angiography unit. A unilateral left trans-radial arterial approach was utilized in all patients. Real time ultrasound was used to visualize patency and access of the left radial artery, which entered with a micropuncture set, 21-gauge needle, and a 5-French (-F) sheath. Patients underwent digital subtraction angiography (DSA) and PAE with a digital flat-panel detector fluoroscopy system (Innova 4100 IQ; General Electric Healthcare, Chicago, IL, USA) with nonionic intravenous contrast (Omnipaque 350 mg/mL; General Electric Healthcare, Chicago, IL, USA). Internal iliac arterial angiography in the ipsilateral oblique projection was performed to identify the right and left prostatic arteries, accessory prostatic arteries, and variant anatomy. Pelvic and prostatic arteries were catheterized using a combination of wires and catheters: 5-F Cobra 2 catheter (Cook Medical, Bloomington, IN, USA), 4-F Berenstein catheter (Merit Medical Systems, Incorporated, South Jordan, UT, USA), 2.4-F Progreat microcatheter (Terumo Interventional Systems, Tokyo, Japan) and 0.014-inch Transend microguide wire (Stryker Neurovascular, Fremont, CA, USA). The prostatic arteries were identified with DSA. Advanced imaging was performed with localized intraoperative cone-beam computed tomography (CT) with intravenous contrast (100 mL Isovue 370, Bracco Diagnostics, Milan, Italy) prior to embolization. Cone-beam CT images were transmitted, reconstructed in three dimensions, and reviewed to confirm prostatic arterial vascular anatomy, prostate gland vascular supply, and ensure the absence of vascular supply to adjacent anatomical structures, such as the urinary bladder, penis, and rectum. Bilateral PAE was then performed to stasis with a primary embolic agent: 100–250 µm Embospheres (Merit Medical Systems, Incorporated, South Jordan, UT, USA) and a secondary embolic agent: 2 mm and 3 mm CX coils (Boston Scientific, Marlborough, MA, USA). A band compression device was utilized to achieve radial arterial vascular access closure in all patients.

DSA, which was performed with a flat panel detector fluoroscopy system, and cone-beam CT both utilize photoelectric x-rays with ionizing radiation to visualize, identify, and catheterize the prostatic arteries during PAE. In accordance with the American College of Radiology, European Union of Radiology, and Society of Interventional Radiology, ionizing radiation was used in a fashion as low as reasonably achievable (ALARA) to minimize exposure of patients to radiation [30]. Low radiation doses to patients were maintained and further reduced with intraprocedural cone-beam CT in combination with three dimensional reconstruction that in turn abbreviated procedure times [30].

The Quality Improvement Guidelines for Percutaneous Transcatheter Embolization were used to classify complications after PAE; major complications are complications that require inpatient treatment and/or surgery and minor complications are complications that can be treated with conservative and/or outpatient treatment [31].

Statistical analysis

The clinical metrics of IPSS, QoL, Qmax, PVR, PV, and PSA were expressed as quantitative values with means and standard deviations (SD). These quantitative values were analyzed with a Wilcoxon signed rank test using SAS software, version 9.4 (SAS Institute Incorporated, Cary, NC, USA). A probability value of $P < 0.05$ or lower was considered statistically significant. We had no missing information for the patients and data that were presented in this study.

Results

72 patients with GPH were included with a mean baseline prostate volume of 303 mL (range 201–644 mL). Mean patient age was 71 years old (range 53–89 years); 72 males; 34 patients identified as European descent, 21 patients identified as African descent, 12 patients identified as Asian descent, and 5 patients identified with various descents.

Bilateral PAE was technically successful in all patients (Fig. 1: representative patient). Clinical metrics before PAE and 12 months and 24 months after PAE were collected (Table 2). Clinical metrics for each patient were retrieved from the EMR. Mean IPSS decreased from

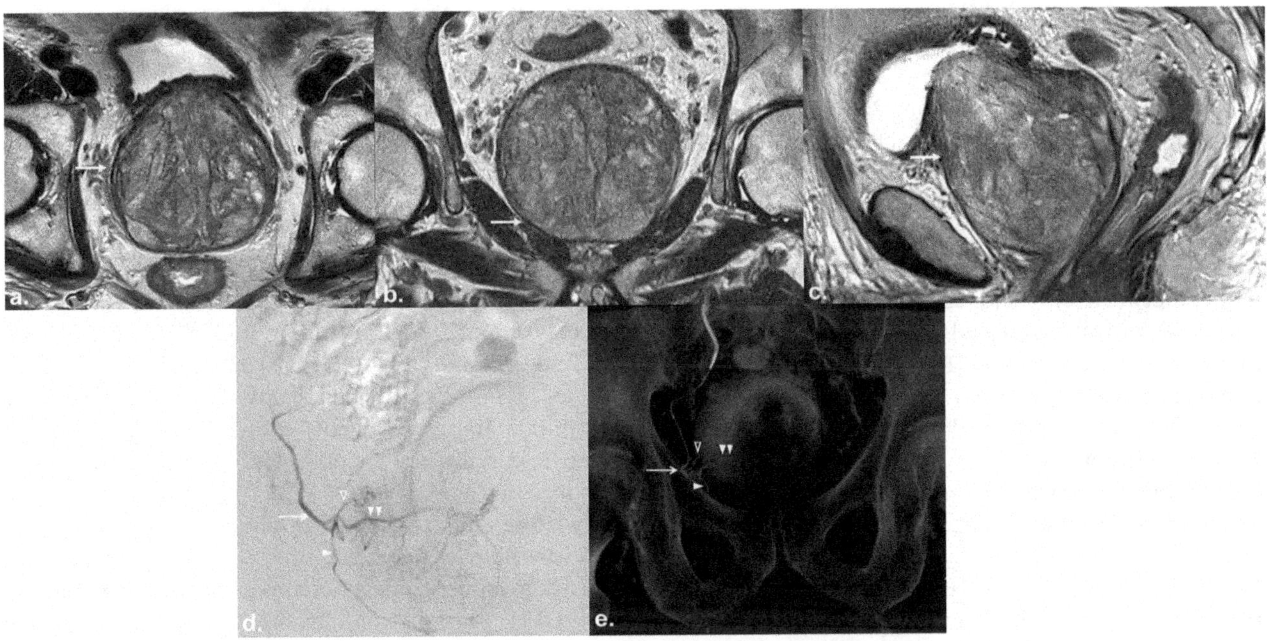

Fig. 1 A 71 year-old patient with severe lower urinary tract symptoms (LUTS) from giant prostatic hyperplasia (GPH) underwent prostate artery embolization (PAE). **a** Axial T2-weighted turbo spin echo (TSE) image, **b** coronal T2-weighted TSE image, and **c** sagittal T2-weighted image from multiparametric magnetic resonance (MR) imaging show giant hyperplasia of the prostate gland (arrow) that measures 312 mL in volume. **d** Digital subtraction angiography (DSA) of selective catheterization of the right internal iliac artery anterior division shows a common origin of the right prostatic artery (straight arrow), which is hypertrophied, and the right superior vesical artery (open arrowhead). The anterior/lateral prostatic artery (single arrowhead) and the posterior/lateral prostatic artery (double arrowheads) are hypertrophied with a corkscrew pattern of the intraprostatic arterioles. **e** Cone-beam computed tomography (CT) with intravenous contrast in the coronal plane after selective catheterization of the internal iliac artery anterior division shows the anatomy of the right prostatic artery: a common origin of the right prostatic artery (straight arrow) and the right superior vesical artery (open arrowhead), hypertrophy of the anterior/lateral prostatic artery (single arrowhead) and the posterior/lateral prostatic artery (double arrowheads), and no vascular supply to the adjacent anatomical structures, to include the urinary bladder, penis, and rectum

Table 2 Clinical metrics summary

Clinical metric	Before PAE Mean ± SD	12 months after PAE Mean ± SD	24 months after PAE Mean ± SD	*P* values
IPSS (points)	26.5 ± 5.0	18.0 ± 4.5	10.0 ± 4.0	< 0.01
QoL (points)	6.0 ± 1.0	4.0 ± 1.0	2.0 ± 1.0	< 0.01
Qmax (mL/sec)	8.0 ± 2.0	14.0 ± 5.0	18.0 ± 4.0	< 0.01
PVR (mL)	198 ± 20.0	152 ± 25.0	90 ± 15.0	< 0.01
PV (mL)	303 ± 20.0	258 ± 15.0	209 ± 15.0	< 0.01
PSA (ng/mL)	11.2 ± 2.5	9.5 ± 1.5	7.9 ± 1.5	< 0.05

IPSS International Prostate Symptom Score, *mL* milliliter, *PAE* prostate artery embolization, *PSA* prostate specific antigen, *PV* prostate volume, *PVR* postvoid residual volume, *Qmax* peak flow rate, *QoL* urinary quality of life, *SD* standard deviation

26.5 ± 5.0 (SD) to 18.0 ± 4.5 (P < 0.0.01) 12 months after PAE and decreased from 18.0 ± 4.5 to 10.5 ± 4.0 (P < 0.01) 24 months after PAE. Mean QoL decreased from 6.0 ± 1.0 to 4.0 ± 1.0 (P < 0.01) 12 months after PAE and decreased from 4.0 ± 1.0 to 2.0 ± 1.0 (P < 0.01) 24 months after PAE. Mean Qmax increased from 8.0 mL/s ± 2.0 mL/s to 14 mL/s ± 5.0 mL/s (P < 0.01) at 12 months to 18 mL/s ± 4.0 mL/s (P < 0.01) at 24 months. Mean PVR decreased from 198.0 mL ± 20.0 mL to 152.0 mL ± 25.0 mL (P < 0.01) at 12 months and decreased from 152.0 mL ± 25.0 mL to 90 mL ± 15.0 mL (P < 0.01) at 24 months. Mean PV decreased from 303.0 mL ± 20.0 mL to 258.0 mL ± 15.0 mL (P < 0.01) at 12 months and decreased from 258.0 mL ± 15.0 mL to 209.0 mL ± 15.0 mL (P < 0.01) at 24 months. Mean PSA decreased from 11.2 ng/mL ± 2.5 ng/mL to 9.5 ng/mL ± 1.5 ng/mL (P < 0.05) at 12 months to 7.9 ng/mL ± 1.5 ng/mL (P < 0.05) at 24 months.

Minor complications occurred in 55 (76%) patients, resolved between two and seven days after PAE, and were conservatively managed. 20 (28%) patients experienced acute urinary retention that required temporary urinary bladder catheterization, 14 (19%) patients experienced urethral pain and dysuria, 11 (15%) patients experienced hematuria, eight (11%) patients experienced hemospermia, and two (3%) patients experienced small hematomas at the radial arterial access site. No major complications occurred.

No lesion suspicious for clinically significant cancer was detected on multiparametric MR imaging obtained in patients before or after PAE. All patients had PI-RADS v2.1 scores of PI-RADS 1: very low (clinically significant cancer is highly unlikely to be present) and PI-RADS 2: low (clinically significant cancer is unlikely to be present); no patient had scores of PI-RADS 3: intermediate (the presence of clinically significant cancer is equivocal), PI-RADS 4: high (clinically significant cancer is likely to be present), or PI-RADS 5: very high (clinically significant cancer is highly likely to be present).

Discussion

Patients with LUTS due to prostatic hyperplasia that do not respond to medical therapy may be candidates for surgical and minimally invasive treatments. However patients with GPH have limited treatment options due to risks associated with these therapies. Simple prostatectomy, which is the gold standard, and minimally invasive urological procedures may have complications such as blood loss that requires transfusion, urinary incontinence, urinary bladder neck stenosis, and urethral strictures [5–8]. Moreover these surgical and minimally invasive treatments require general anesthesia, which has its own associated risks.

The current set of studies on the efficacy of PAE for treatment of LUTS from prostatic hyperplasia continues to grow. Our study can be added to the contemporary data. This investigation demonstrated the long term efficacy of PAE for treatment of severe LUTS from GPH: prostate volumes greater than 200 mL, in a large patient cohort at 12 months and 24 months after PAE. Mean value for IPSS, QoL, PVR, PV, and PSA significantly decreased and mean Qmax significantly increased at 12 months and at 24 months after PAE. The patients in our investigation continued to experience significant reductions in QoL, Qmax, PVR, and PSA after 12 months and at 24 months after PAE that may be potentially attributed to sustained long term hormonal downregulation and diminished neuromuscular feedback as well as greater initial prostate volumes (greater than 200 mL). These long term results are similar to prior investigations that illustrated the long term efficacy of PAE for treatment of LUTS due to prostate hyperplasia with prostate volumes 80–100 mL, in contrast to this investigation, which examined PAE treatment of LUTS from GPH with prostate volumes greater than 200 mL [5–13]. These studies demonstrated significant decreased severity of symptoms, improved quality of life, increased peak flow rates, and reduction in post void residual and prostate volumes and PSA levels [5–13]. Prior investigators have shown the efficacy of PAE in patients with LUTS from large prostatic hyperplasia: prostate volume greater than 100 mL however clinical outcomes specifically in patients with GPH, prostate volumes greater than 200 mL, have not been reported [5–13]. Bhatia et al. reported a single patient whom underwent PAE for treatment of severe LUTS from GPH had significant symptomatic relief at three months: IPSS decreased from 26.0 to 4.0, QoL decreased from 6.0 to 1.0, and PV decreased from 571 to 270 mL; PVR was not measured before PAE due to inability to void and was 50 mL after PAE.[27]. Mathevosian et al. showed similar success and short term efficacy in eight patients whom underwent PAE for severe LUTS from GPH and had sustained symptomatic relief at eight months: IPSS decreased from 20.5 to 3.8, QoL decreased from 4.4 to 1.4, and PV decreased from 318 to 212 mL [28]. However the limitations of these studies are small patient cohorts, one and eight, and short follow-up times, 3 months and 8 months [27, 28]. Larger cohorts of patients and long term efficacy have not been examined. Moreover an upper limit prostate volume for the efficacy of PAE has not been established. This upper limit volume number can be used to match patients to the appropriate therapy.

We confirmed that PAE is not only an effective treatment but also a safe therapy for severe LUTS in patients with GPH (prostate volumes greater than

200 mL) because no major complications occurred in 72 patients. No patient experienced a major complication, which required inpatient treatment and/or surgery. 76% of patients experienced at least one minor complication, which was either conservatively managed, treated in an outpatient or ambulatory fashion, or was self-limited and resolved. 20 (28%) patients experienced acute urinary retention that required temporary urinary bladder catheterization that was likely due to anticipated increased pressure and compression of the intraprostatic urethra from swelling, edema, and ischemic necrosis of the prostate gland after PAE. The urethral pain and dysuria in 14 (19%) patients, the hematuria in 11 (15%) patients, and the hematospermia in eight (11%) patients may have been caused by non-target embolization of the urethra and/or penis or passage of blood from ischemic necrosis of the prostate gland.

Our study has objective strengths with limitations. While we examined the largest number of patients whom underwent treatment of LUTS from GPH with PAE to date, results may be improved with larger cohorts. The length of follow-up time was longer than any other prior study: 24 months, which establishes sustainability, nevertheless longer-term follow-up studies may verify sustained patient outcomes. Our patients were referred from urologists and therefore subject to intrinsic referral bias. This bias was abated by blinding the interpreting radiologists to the indication for the multiparametric MR imaging exams. There were additional limitations to this investigation. This study was a single-institution, retrospective experience at a tertiary care academic medical center with urology, PAE, and MR availability and experience. Therefore our results may not be transferrable to all patient populations due to accessibility and contraindications. While no major complications occurred in 72 patients, this investigation was retrospective and therefore prospective safety may not be transitively established. PAE is a procedure that may not be widely available to all patients. Certain patients with LUTS from GPH may not be candidates for PAE. If a patient has a contraindication to receiving procedural anesthetic moderate sedation, then a patient cannot undergo PAE. Certain patients may have contraindications to undergo MR imaging, such as medical devices, hardware, or claustrophobia, for prostate volume measurement. In these patients, CT may be used for follow-up imaging for prostate volume measurement. Future research may be directed to prospective, multivariate comparisons of the efficacy of minimally invasive urological procedures and PAE in large patient cohorts for long follow-up times.

Conclusions

PAE is an efficacious and safe treatment that provides significant and sustained relief of severe LUTS in patients with GPH. PAE may play an important role in the treatment patients with severe LUTS from GPH in whom medical therapy has failed, are not candidates for surgical and minimally invasive treatments, or refuse surgical treatment. We hope that these results, along with future investigations directed to prospective, multivariate, comparative and randomized studies, may provide patients with the best treatment to optimize symptom relief, minimize morbidity, and achieve safe and successful outcomes.

Abbreviations

GPH: Giant prostatic hyperplasia; BPH: Benign prostatic hyperplasia; PAE: Prostatic artery embolization; LUTS: Lower urinary tract symptoms; IPSS: International Prostate Symptom Score; mL: Milliliter; PV: Prostate volume; PVR: Postvoid residual volume; QoL: QoL urinary quality of life; Qmax: Peak flow rate; PSA: Prostate specific antigen; MRI: Magnetic resonance imaging; ADC: Apparent diffusion coefficient; DWI: Diffusion weighted imaging; FOV: Field of view; FS: Fat saturated; MRA: Magnetic resonance angiography; TE: Echo time; TR: Repetition time; TSE: Turbo spin echo; VIBE: Volumetric interpolated breath-hold examination; F: French; DSA: Digital subtraction angiography; IRB: Institutional review board; EMR: Electronic medical records; HIPAA: Health Information Portability and Accountability Act.

Authors' contributions

ASS developed the concept and design, performed critical revision of the manuscript for intellectual content, performed imaging interpretations, acquired data, which was analyzed and interpreted, completed statistical analysis, supervised the investigation, and performed final approval. SM performed critical revision of the manuscript, performed imaging interpretations, and acquired data, which was analyzed and interpreted. LMF performed critical revision of the manuscript, performed imaging interpretations, and acquired data, which was analyzed and interpreted. MGN performed critical revision of the manuscript, performed imaging interpretations, and acquired data, which was analyzed and interpreted. AS performed critical revision of the manuscript, performed imaging interpretations, and acquired data, which was analyzed and interpreted. VSK performed critical revision of the manuscript, performed imaging interpretations, and acquired data, which was analyzed and interpreted. All authors read and approved the final manuscript.

Authors' information

A.S.S. is a board-certified, fellowship-trained radiologist. He is an Assistant Professor of Radiology in the Department of Diagnostic, Molecular, and Interventional Radiology at the Icahn School of Medicine at Mount Sinai in New York City, New York. His areas of clinical expertise are multiparametric MR imaging of the prostate and multivisceral transplants. His research has resulted in numerous exhibits at national and international conferences as well as several peer-reviewed publications and a textbook chapter. S.M. is a board-certified, fellowship-trained radiologist. He is the Director of MR imaging and CT at Valley Radiology Associates in San Jose, California. His research has resulted in multiple educational and scientific exhibits, peer-reviewed publication, and textbook chapters. L.M.F. is a board-certified, fellowship-trained radiologist. She is an Assistant Professor of Radiology in the Department of Radiology at New York Presbyterian/Weill Cornell Medicine. Dr. Flisnik's clinical expertise is in multi-parametric MR imaging of the prostate and PET-CT oncological staging and treatment response. Her research has resulted in exhibits at national and international conferences. She is a reviewer for a peer-reviewed journal. M. G. N. is a board-eligible physician in diagnostic radiology. Dr. Nellamattathil completes his residency in Diagnostic Radiology at MedStar Georgetown

University Hospital in 2021, where he was elected Chief Resident. He will complete his fellowship in Body Imaging at Northwestern Memorial Hospital in 2021. A.S. is a board-certified, fellowship-trained interventional radiologist at Beverly Radiology Medical Group in Los Angeles, California. Dr. Sharma's clinical expertise is in minimally invasive vascular interventions and interventional oncology. Dr. Sharma completed his fellowship in Interventional Radiology at Brigham and Women's Hospital in 2020. His research has resulted in numerous educational and scientific exhibits and peer-reviewed publications. V.S.K. is a board-certified, fellowship-trained radiologist. He currently works as an Associate Professor of Clinical Radiology in the Department of Radiology at the University of Texas Health Science Center San Antonio where he is the Director of Abdominal Imaging. He is academically very successful and presents scientific papers, posters, and educational exhibits at national radiology meetings. He is actively involved in teaching medical students, radiology residents, and abdominal radiology fellows and conducts clinical research.

Competing interests

The authors declare that they have no competing interests.

Author details

[1] Department of Diagnostic, Molecular, and Interventional Radiology, Icahn School of Medicine At Mount Sinai, 1000 10th Avenue, New York, NY 10019, USA. [2] Valley Radiology Medical Associates, San Jose, CA, USA. [3] Department of Radiology, New York Presbyterian/Weill Cornell Medical Center, New York, NY, USA. [4] Department of Radiology, MedStar Georgetown University Hospital, Washington, DC, USA. [5] Department of Interventional Radiology, Brigham and Women's Hospital, Boston, MA, USA. [6] Department of Radiology, University of Texas Health Science Center San Antonio, San Antonio, TX, USA.

References

1. American Urological Association Clinical Guidelines. Surgical management of lower urinary tract symptoms attributed to benign prostatic hyperplasia. 2018. https://www.auanet.org/guidelines/benign-prostatic-hyperplasia/lower-urinary-tract-symptoms (2018).
2. Oelke M, Bachmann A, Descazeaud A, Emberton M, Gravas S, Michel MC, et al. European association of urology: EAU guidelines on the treatment and follow-up of non-neurogenic male lower urinary tract symptoms including benign prostatic obstruction. Eur Urol. 2013;64:118–40.
3. Lourenco T, Pickard R, Vale L, Grant A, Fraser C, MacLennan G, et al. Benign prostatic enlargement team: minimally invasive treatments for benign prostatic enlargement: systematic review of randomised controlled trials. BMJ. 2008;337:a1662.
4. McWilliams JP, Bilhim TA, Carnevale FC, et al. Society of Interventional Radiology Multisociety Consensus Position Statement on Prostatic Artery Embolization for Treatment of Lower Urinary Tract Symptoms Attributed to Benign Prostatic Hyperplasia: From the Society of Interventional Radiology, the Cardiovascular and Interventional Radiological Society of Europe, Société Française de Radiologie, and the British Society of Interventional Radiology: Endorsed by the Asia Pacific Society of Cardiovascular and Interventional Radiology, Canadian Association for Interventional Radiology, Chinese College of Interventionalists, Interventional Radiology Society of Australasia, Japanese Society of Interventional Radiology, and Korean Society of Interventional Radiology. J Vasc Interv Radiol. 2019;30(5):627–37.
5. Pisco J, Bilhim T, Pinheiro LC, et al. Prostate embolization as an alternative to open surgery in patients with large prostate and moderate to severe lower urinary tract symptoms. J Vasc Interv Radiol. 2016;27:700–8.
6. de Assis AM, Moreira AM, de Paula Rodriguez VC, et al. Prostatic artery embolization for treatment of benign prostatic hyperplasia in patients with prostates greater than 90 grams: a prospective single center study. J Vasc Interv Radiol. 2015;26:87–93.
7. Kurbatov D, Giorgio IR, Lepetukhin A, et al. Prostatic artery embolization for prostate volume greater than 80 cm^3: results from a single center prospective study. Urology. 2014;84:400–4.
8. Pisco JM, Bilhim T, Pinheiro LC, et al. Medium and long term outcome on prostate artery embolization for patients with benign prostatic hyperplasia: results in 630 patients. J Vasc Interv Radiol. 2016;27:1115–22.
9. Bagla S, Smirniotopoulos JB, Orlando JC, et al. Comparative analysis of prostate volume as a predictor of outcome in prostate artery embolization. J Vasc Interv Radiol. 2015;26:1832–8.
10. Uflacker A, Haskal ZJ, Bilhim T, et al. Meta-analysis of prostatic artery embolization for benign prostatic hyperplasia. J Vasc Interv Radiol. 2016;27:1686–97.
11. Wang MQ, Guo LP, Zhang GD, et al. Prostatic arterial embolization for the treatment of lower urinary tract symptoms due to large (> 80 ml) benign prostatic hyperplasia: results of midterm follow-up from Chinese population. BMC Urol. 2015;15:33.
12. Bhatia S, Sinha VK, Harward S, et al. Prostate artery embolization in patients with prostate volumes of 80 mL or more: a single institution retrospective experience of 93 patients. J Vasc Interv Radiol. 2018;29:1392–8.
13. Bhatia S, Sinha VK, Kava B, et al. Efficacy of prostatic artery embolization for catheter-dependent patients with large prostate sizes and high comorbidity scores. J Vasc Interv Radiol. 2018;29:78–84.
14. Ashamalla GR, Ahmed AM. Giant prostatic hypertrophy. Arch Surg. 1972;105:769–70.
15. Fishman JR, Merrill DC. A case of giant prostatic hyperplasia. Urology. 1993;42:336–7.
16. De Silva-Gutiérrez A, Pérez-Evia CA, Alcocer-Gaxiola B, Martínez-Méndez ME. Giant prostatic hyperplasia. A case report and literature review. Rev Mex Urol. 2010;70:183–6.
17. Wang L, Davis P, McMillan K. A case of giant prostatic hyperplasia. Asian J Urol. 2016;3(1):53–5.
18. Domínguez A, Gual J, Muñoz-Rodríguez J, et al. Giant prostatic hyperplasia: case report of 3987 mL. Urology. 2016;88:e3–4.
19. Aghamir SMK, Khatami F, Rahimi MR, Guitynavard F. Giant benign prostatic hyperplasia: a case report. Urol Case Rep. 2019;28:101051.
20. Lacy JM, Bole R, Hendrix L, Strup S. Retropubic prostatectomy for giant benign prostatic hyperplasia. Can J Urol. 2015;22(5):8000–2.
21. Ogawa S, Manome M, Yabe M, et al. A giant prostatic hyperplasia treated by open surgery. Int J Gen Med. 2012;5:1009–12.
22. Zeng QS, Zhao YB, Wang BQ, et al. Minimally invasive simple prostatectomy for a case of giant benign prostatic hyperplasia. Asian J Androl. 2017;19(6):717–8.
23. Learney RM, Malde S, Downes M, Shrotri N. Successful minimally invasive management of a case of giant prostatic hypertrophy associated with recurrent nephrogenic adenoma of the prostate. BMC Urol. 2013;13:18.
24. Sevryukov FA, Nakagawa K, Kochkin AD, et al. A case of successful plasma transurethral enucleation of benign prostatic hyperplasia the size of 530 cm^3. Urologiia. 2019;2:59–63.
25. Glybochko PV, Rapoport LM, Enikeev ME, Enikeev DV. Holmium laser enucleation of the prostate (HoLEP) for small, large and giant prostatic hyperplasia: tips and tricks. Urologia. 2017;84(3):169–73.
26. Enikeev DV, Glybochko PV, Alyaev YG, et al. Holmium laser enucleation of the prostate (HOLEP) for small, large and giant prostatic hyperplasia. Practice guidelines. Experience of more than 450 surgeries. Urologiia. 2016;4:63–9.
27. Bhatia S, Kava B, Pereira K, et al. Prostate artery embolization for giant prostatic hyperplasia. J Vasc Interv Radiol. 2015;26(10):1583–5.
28. Mathevosian S, Plotnik AN, McWilliams JP. Prostate artery embolization for giant prostatic enlargement: short-term efficacy and safety. J Vasc Interv Radiol. 2019;30(11):1820–3.
29. Weinreb JC, Barentsz JO, Choyke PL, et al. PI-RADS Prostate imaging—reporting and data system: 2015, Version 2. Eur Urol. 2016;69:16–40.
30. Schott P, Katoh M, Fischer N, Freyhardt P. Radiation dose in prostatic artery embolization using cone-beam CT and 3D roadmap software. J Vasc Interv Radiol. 2019;30(9):1452–8.
31. Angle JF, Siddiqi NH, Wallace MJ, Kundu S, Stokes L, Wojak JC, et al. Quality improvement guidelines for percutaneous transcatheter embolization: Society of Interventional Radiology Standards of Practice Committee. J Vasc Interv Radiol. 2010;21:1479–86.

31

The incidence and prevalence of upper tract urothelial carcinoma

Ahmed Soualhi[1*], Elke Rammant[2,3], Gincy George[2], Beth Russell[2], Deborah Enting[4], Rajesh Nair[5], Mieke Van Hemelrijck[2] and Cecilia Bosco[2]

Abstract

Background: Upper tract urothelial carcinoma (UTUC) is a rare urological cancer that is still an important public health concern in many areas around the world. Although UTUC has been linked to a number of risk factors, to our knowledge no systematic review has been published on the overall incidence and prevalence of de-novo UTUC. This review aimed to examine the global epidemiology of UTUC to provide clinicians and public health specialists a better understanding of UTUC.

Methods: A systematic search was conducted on MEDLINE, Embase, and the Web of Science using a detailed search strategy. Observational epidemiological studies describing the incidence and prevalence of de-novo UTUC in adults were included, and the Joanna Briggs Institute checklist was used for critical appraisal and data extraction of the studies selected.

Results: The systematic search identified 3506 papers, of which 59 papers were included for qualitative synthesis. The studies selected included data ranging from the years 1943 to 2018. A comprehensive qualitative synthesis of the data was performed. UTUC incidence generally varied according to age (higher with increasing age), sex (unclear), race (unclear), calendar time (increased, stable, or decreased according to region), geographical region (higher in Asian countries), occupation (higher in seamen and printers), and other population characteristics. Prevalence was only reported by one study, which showed UTUC to have the highest incidence of the rare urogenital cancers in Europe.

Conclusion: This systematic review highlights an increased incidence of UTUC in certain groups, including increasing age and certain occupations such as seamen. The incidence of UTUC also varies between certain geographical regions. The trend of UTUC incidence for sex, race, and calendar time is less clear due to a wide variety of metrics used by the studies identified. More studies are also required on the prevalence of UTUC to understand its disease burden.

Keywords: Epidemiology, Incidence, Upper tract urothelial carcinoma, Urological oncology

Background

Upper tract urothelial carcinoma (UTUC) is a relatively rare cancer of the urinary tract. UTUC describes a cancer originating in the renal pelvis, renal calices, and the ureter. Smoking and aristolochic acid are the two most common risk factors for UTUC [1, 2]. UTUC has been genetically linked to hereditary non-polyposis colorectal cancer (HNPCC), also known as Lynch syndrome, through mutations in DNA mismatch repair genes [3]. The link between UTUC and bladder cancer has also been studied, with both cancers being called 'disparate twins' for their similarities in histology and origins yet differences in diagnosis and treatment [4].

*Correspondence: asoualhi@doctors.org.uk
[1] University Hospital Hairmyres, Glasgow, UK
Full list of author information is available at the end of the article

Understanding the epidemiology of UTUC can help aid clinical diagnosis and can be used to highlight high-risk groups that can be targeted with strategies to prevent such groups from developing UTUC [5]. However, whilst systematic reviews on the epidemiology of other urological cancers have been performed [6, 7], to our knowledge a systematic review of the incidence and prevalence of de-novo UTUC has never been published. The incidence of UTUC has been estimated at 1–2 cases per 100,000 [8], although this varies between age, geographical region, occupation, and other factors. This paper aims to provide a more comprehensive assessment of the global incidence and prevalence of UTUC in order to support guidance for future studies on its epidemiology.

Methods

A detailed search strategy (Additional file 1) was developed using the Peer Review of Electronic Search Strategies (PRESS) checklist. Three databases were searched for this systematic review: MEDLINE, Embase, and the Web of Science Core Collection. No limitations on dates were applied, and the final search was done on 4th February 2021. This review was registered on PROSPERO (Registration Number CRD42019134255).

Observational studies (cross-sectional and cohort) describing the incidence and prevalence of de-novo UTUC in adults ($\geq$ 18 years of age) were included. Studies that reported both lower and upper urinary tract carcinomas were only included if data for UTUC was separately reported. No further exclusion criteria were set for study setting and demographic factors. Studies were excluded if no full text was available, or if the abstracts were in any other language than English. There was no language restriction for full texts; translations were carried out if necessary. The reference lists of the papers selected were manually searched for further relevant studies to include in the data extraction.

Results from the database searches were managed in Mendeley and imported into Rayyan QCRI [9], where two independent authors (AS and ER) screened the titles and abstracts. Any remaining conflicts were resolved by a third author (CB). Both authors (AS and ER) then screened the full texts of the selected papers for relevance and bias using the Joanna Briggs Institute (JBI) Checklist for Prevalence Studies [10]. Any further conflicts were resolved by a third author (CB).

Data extraction from the selected papers was performed using the JBI Checklist and managed using Microsoft Excel. The following data were extracted: study title, study author(s), year of publication, journal, country, aim of study, population, setting, study design, study duration, outcomes measured, diagnostic criteria used, ethical approval, methods of data analysis, incidence (and 95% confidence interval), and prevalence (and 95% confidence interval).

Some papers did not report incidence data in numbers, instead showing only a graph. The authors of these studies were contacted for raw data, which are included in this review. Where raw data was unavailable, data from graphs in the selected articles were extracted using WebPlotDigitizer, a software tool that allows reverse data extraction from both linear and logarithmic graphs [11].

The data from the selected studies was found to be heterogeneous and hence a meta-analysis could not be conducted. Therefore, a narrative synthesis of the data was done according to the following subgroups: age, sex, race, geographic region, calendar time, occupation, Lynch syndrome, and other population characteristics.

Results

The results of the database searches, title and abstract screening, and full-text screening are outlined in Fig. 1. The search strategy identified 3506 papers after duplicates were removed. After title, abstract, and full-text screening, 117 titles were excluded for a number of reasons, and 59 papers were included for this review (Table 1).

The studies selected included data ranging from the years 1943 to 2018. Europe had the greatest number of studies (n = 26, 44%), followed by Asia (n = 15, 25%), North America (n = 14, 24%), Australia (three studies), and one worldwide study. Of the studies from Europe, 14 (54%) were conducted in the Nordic countries of Denmark, Finland, Iceland, Norway, or Sweden. Of the studies from Asia, seven (47%) were conducted in Taiwan. Nearly all studies employed a retrospective cohort study design except for two studies: Mok et al. and Aparicio et al., which were prospective cohort studies [12, 13]. Similarly, nearly all studies focused on the incidence of UTUC, with only one study by Visser and colleagues [14] reporting incidence together with prevalence.

The studies selected for this review included a wide variety of cancer registries and patient populations. Eleven studies (19%) used data from the SEER (Surveillance, Epidemiology, and End Results) registry in the USA. In total, 38 studies (64%) used International Classification of Diseases (ICD) codes to identify patients with a diagnosis of UTUC.

Seven corresponding authors were contacted for the raw data of graphs in their respective articles, to which four authors [15–18] replied with this data. In total, eight papers required data extraction using WebPlotDigitizer (Additional file 2).

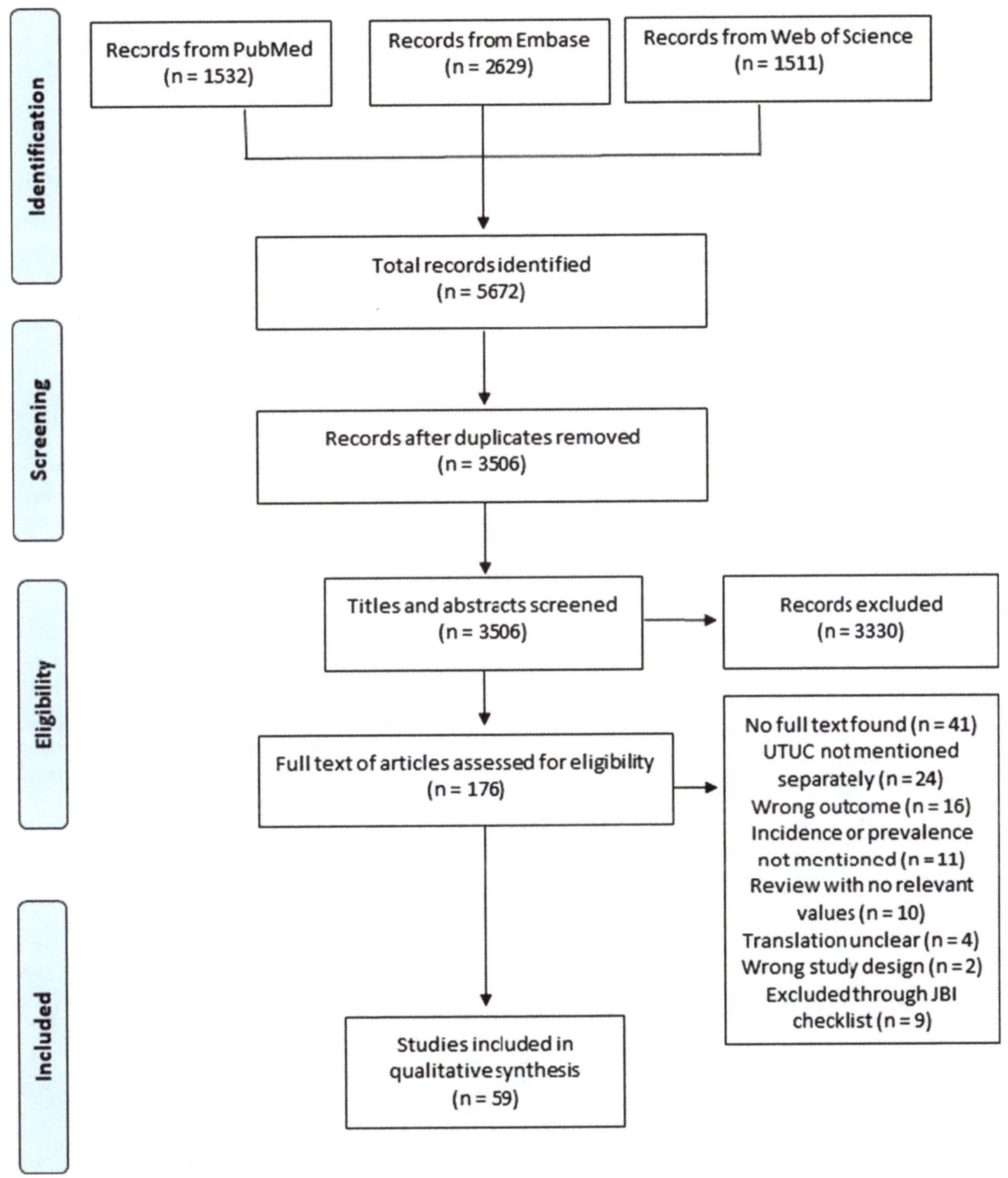

Fig. 1 PRISMA flow diagram

Incidence by age

In total, 12 studies reported incidence of UTUC according to age [14, 17–28]. The measures used to report incidence varied widely between different studies. For example, the study by Visser et al. used rate per million persons, whereas Cheon and colleagues used rate per 100,000 persons [14, 22]. Other measures used in other studies include incidence density per 10,000 person-years and standardised incidence ratios.

Overall, there appeared to be a higher incidence of UTUC with increasing age. This was seen in both males and females. Stoyanov and colleagues [19] reported an incidence of 11.22 per 100,000 persons in male 30–39 year olds, which increased to 17.30 per 100,000

Table 1 Study descriptives of all studies selected

Study	Country	Setting	Duration	Factors reported
Noone et al. [35]	USA	SEER Registry	1992–2013	Race
Yu et al. [64]	South Korea	Samsung Medical Center	1995–2016	Overall incidence
Chernozemsky et al. [47]	Bulgaria	27 villages in the Vratza district	1965–1974	Calendar time
Kockelbergh et al. [15]	England	National Cancer Registration and Analysis Service	2001–2013	Calendar time
Chen et al. [65]	Taiwan	Longitudinal Health Insurance Database	1997–2011	Overall, other population characteristics
Stoyanov et al. [19]	Bulgaria	15 villages in the Vratza district	1965–1974	Sex, age
Visser et al. [14]	Europe	RARECARE database	1995–2002	Sex, age, geographical region
Wang et al. [20]	Taiwan	NHIR database	1997–2002	Overall, sex, age
Joung et al. [21]	South Korea	Korea National Cancer Incidence Database	1999–2012	Overall, sex, age
Janbabaei et al. [32]	Iran	Population-based cancer registry system of Mazandaran University of Medical Sciences	2014	Overall, sex
Sun et al. [54]	Taiwan	NHIR database	1997–2010	Overall, other
Cheon et al. [22]	South Korea	Pathologic records of 46 hospital and clinics	1985–1999	Overall, sex, age, calendar time
Chow et al. [23]	Sweden	Swedish Cancer Registry	1965–1983	Overall, sex, age, other
Balaji et al. [66]	USA	Memorial Sloan-Kettering Cancer Center	1989–1997	Overall
Kang et al. [67]	Taiwan	Tumour registry of Chang Gung Memorial Hospital	1992–2001	Overall
Holmäng et al. [39]	Sweden	Swedish Cancer Registry	1971–1998	Calendar time
Bermejo et al. [33]	Sweden	Swedish Cancer Registry	1961–2006	Sex
Hsiao et al. [24]	Taiwan	NHIR database	2000–2012	Overall, sex, age, geographical region, occupation, other
Raman et al. [40]	USA	SEER Registry	1973–2005	Overall, calendar time
Nakata et al. [25]	Japan	62 hospitals and clinics	1985–1994	Age, calendar time
Wihlborg and Johansen [41]	Denmark	Danish Cancer Registry	1944–2003	Calendar time
Wang et al. [42]	Taiwan	NHIR database	1997–2008	Calendar time
Shinka et al. [68]	Japan	Wakayama Medical College	1969–1984	Overall
Wright et al. [69]	USA	SEER Registry	1988–2003	Overall
Eylert et al. [16]	England	National Cancer Data Repository	1985–2009	Overall, calendar time
Antoni et al. [34]	Australia	Population-based cancer registries in five Australian states	1983–2007	Sex, calendar time, geographical region
Cauberg et al. [43]	Netherlands	Association of Comprehensive Cancer Centres population-based cancer registry	1995–2003	Calendar time
Woodford et al. [18]	Australia	Victorian Cancer Registry	2001–2011	Overall, age, calendar time
Mellemgaard et al. [28]	Denmark	Danish Cancer Registry	1943–1988	Age, calendar time
Yang et al. [70]	Taiwan	Taipei Veterans General Hospital	1983–1998	Overall
Huguet-Pérez et al. [71]	Spain	Fundació Puigvert	1980–1994	Overall
Munoz et al. [44]	USA	SEER Registry	1973–1976	Calendar time
Furukawa et al. [72]	Japan	Kobe University Graduate School of Medicine hospitals	1995–2003	Overall
Amar and Das [73]	USA	Kaiser Permanente Medical Center	-	Overall, other
Millán-Rodríguez et al. [74]	Spain	Fundació Puigvert	1968–1996	Overall, other
Hurle et al. [75]	Italy	United Hospitals of Bergamo	1986–1992	Overall, other
Schwartz et al. [76]	USA	Montefiore Medical Center	1972–1982	Overall, other
Pukkala et al. [48]	Denmark, Finland, Iceland, Norway, Sweden	Computerised population census in the countries listed	1943–1990	Occupation

Table 1 (continued)

Study	Country	Setting	Duration	Factors reported
Friis et al. [77]	Denmark	Prescription Database of North Jutland County; Danish Cancer Registry	1989–1995	Overall, other
McLaughlin et al. [50]	USA	Valley Forge satellite manufacturing complex in Pennsylvania	1962–2008	Occupation
Mok et al. [12]	South Korea	Korean Heart Study	1996–2012	Other
Christensen et al. [30]	Denmark	Danish Cancer Registry	1968–2012	Sex, other
Yang et al. [36]	USA	SEER Registry	1973–2010	Overall, race, other
Mathew et al. [37]	Worldwide	SEER Registry, Cancer Incidence in Five Continents	1973–1992	Race, geographical region
Lynch and Cohen [26]	USA	SEER Registry	1973–1987	Age, calendar time
McLaughlin et al. [50]	Sweden	Swedish Cancer-Environment Registry	1960–1979	Occupation
Devesa et al. [78]	USA	SEER Registry	1975–1985	Race
Lynge et al. [51]	Denmark	Danish Cancer Registry	1970–1987	Occupation
Chow et al. [38]	USA	SEER Registry	1975–1995	Race
Ericson et al. [53]	Sweden	Swedish Cancer Registry	1961–1999	Lynch syndrome
Premuzic et al. [29]	Croatia	University Hospital Centre Zagreb	2011–2016	Sex
Michalek et al. [27]	Denmark, Iceland, Finland, Norway and Sweden	Respective national cancer registries	1961–2005	Age, occupation, calendar time
Medunjanin et al. [31]	Croatia	Croatian National Cancer Registry	2001–2011	Sex, geographical region
Aragon-Ching et al. [79]	USA	SEER Registry	2000–2014	Overall
Wu et al. [42]	USA	SEER Registry	1988–2015	Calendar time
Fernandez Aparicio et al. [80]	Spain	31 hospitals in Spain	2017–2018	Overall
Tempo et al. [46]	Australia	South Australia Cancer Registry	1977–2013	Calendar time
Almås et al. [17]	Norway	Cancer Registry of Norway	1999–2018	Overall, age, calendar time
Michalek et al. [27]	Denmark, Iceland, Finland, Norway and Sweden	Respective national cancer registries	1961–2005	Occupation

persons in males aged 70+. In females, the increase seen in age was higher, from 21.28 to 277.78 per 100,000 persons between 30 and 39 year olds and 70+, respectively. A similar increasing trend with age was reported by Visser et al. [14], with an incidence of 1.8 (standard error [SE] 0.1) per million persons in patients <55 years old compared to 73.6 (SE 1.1) per million persons in 75+year olds.

Incidence by sex

The calculation of age-standardised rates (ASRs) varied according to what population was used in standardisation. In the 13 studies that reported on incidence of UTUC according to sex [14, 19–24, 29–34], the ASR values were adjusted based on different populations, including a European population [14], a standard world population [21], the World Health Organisation (WHO) standard population [32], the 1995 South Korean population [22], and population data from the Australian Bureau of Statistics [34].

The comparative incidence between males and females was not clear from the studies. Some studies reported a higher incidence in males than females. For example, Joung and colleagues [21] reported an ASR of 1.39 (males) vs. 0.49 (females) per 100,000 persons. Others such as Wang and colleagues [20] reported a higher incidence in females than males, with a standardised incidence ratio (SIR) of 15.2 (95% CI 12.7–17.9) for females vs. 8.1 (95% CI 6.5–10.2) for males.

Incidence by race

Four studies compared incidence between different races [35–38]. The most comprehensive study was by Mathew and colleagues [37], who reported worldwide incidence of UTUC between 1973 and 1992. The study reported SIR values for, among others, Black Americans, White Americans, Jewish Israelis, and Chinese Singaporeans. The highest SIR for renal pelvis cancers in this study was seen in White Americans (0.79 per 100,000 person-years for males). Another study by Chow and colleagues [38] reported a lower ASR in Black American males (0.8 per 100,000 person-years) compared to White American males (1.5 per 100,000 person-years). This was similarly seen in Black American females (0.5 per 100,000 person-years) vs. White American females (0.7 per 100,000 person-years).

Another study by Li and colleagues, [36] which covered an even wider period (1973–2010) but focused on colorectal cancer survivors, reported a higher SIR of renal pelvis cancers in Black compared to White Americans (1.73 [95% CI 0.56–4.04] vs. 1.29 [0.97–1.69], respectively). The opposite was seen in ureter cancers, with White Americans having a higher SIR than Black Americans (1.49 [1.18–1.86] vs. 1.32 [0.16–4.78], respectively).

Incidence by geographical region

Five studies reported on incidence of UTUC according to specific geographical regions [14, 24, 31, 34, 37]. The study by Mathew et al. [37] covered 10 regions for both males and females, and a further five regions for males. This study used data from the Cancer Incidence in Five Continents resource and found that the region with the highest SIR of renal pelvis cancers between 1973 and 1992 was the Bas-Rhin region in eastern France, with an SIR of 15.5 per 100,000 person-years in males.

Visser et al. [14] further reported incidence in different regions of Europe between 1995 and 2002 and found northern Europe to have the highest ASR of 12.8 (SE 0.3) per million persons. The high incidence of UTUC in regions with a high prevalence of Balkan endemic nephropathy (BEN) was studied by Medunjanin and colleagues [31], who reported a high incidence in Croatia geographically associated with a high prevalence of BEN, specifically in the Brod-Posavina county.

Differences between regions within countries were also studied. Hsiao et al. [24] studied UTUC incidence in Taiwan in patients who had undergone haemodialysis, finding the highest incidence in southern Taiwan for both patients who had haemodialysis and those who did not (38.6 and 1.35 per 10,000 person-years, respectively). Other regions in Taiwan followed a similar pattern, with northern Taiwan having the lowest incidence of UTUC in both groups of patients (11.3 and 0.33 per 10,000 person-years, respectively). In Australia, Antoni et al. [34] studied the incidence of renal pelvis cancer in five Australian states and reported the highest ASRs in New South Wales and Queensland.

Incidence by calendar time

Nineteen studies compared UTUC incidence based on calendar time [15–18, 22, 25–28, 34, 39–47]. For three of these studies, more accurate numbers were obtained by contacting the study authors. The first of these studies was by Eylert and colleagues [16], who used data from the National Cancer Data Repository (NCDR) of England between 1985 and 2009 and found an overall increase throughout time in UTUC incidence for males, females, and both sexes combined. Similarly, Kockelbergh and colleagues [15] studied the National Cancer Registration and Analysis Service (NCRAS)—which contains data from the NCDR—from 2001 to 2013 and reported a similar overall increase in incidence throughout time. The third study with accurate numbers obtained from the study authors was by Woodford and colleagues [18], who studied the Victorian Cancer Registry of Australia from 2001 to 2011 and found the incidence of UTUC to be stable throughout time.

Other studies that showed a decreased incidence over time include the study by Antoni et al. [34], which reported a reduction in incidence in all five cancer registries in Australia that were studied from 1983–1987 to 2003–2007. The study by Wang et al. [42], which used data from the National Health Insurance Research Database in Taiwan and focused on patients with end-stage renal disease under maintenance dialysis, reported a reduced $SIR_{40\text{-}84}$ of UTUC in males from 1998 (13.0 [95% CI 6.2–27.3]) to 2008 (9.5 [7.3–12.3]), but an increased $SIR_{40\text{-}84}$ in females from 1998 (9.5 [7.3–12.3]) to 2008 (13.6 [11.4–16.4]).

Incidence by occupation

Seven studies reported on UTUC incidence according to occupation [24, 27, 48–52]. Five of these studies were based on the national cancer registries and censuses of Nordic countries [27, 48, 50–52]. A total of 54 occupational categories are included in the comprehensive study by Michalek and colleagues [27] on five Nordic countries (Denmark, Iceland, Finland, Norway and Sweden) between 1961 and 2005. The occupation categories with the highest SIR were seamen (1.51 [95% CI 1.23–1.82]), printers (1.39 [1.11–1.71]), and welders (1.37 [1.03–1.78]). The study further classified occupations according to age at diagnosis, and the highest SIR was observed in seamen aged 30–49 years old (1.75 [0.96–2.94]). Michalek et al. published another study [52] using smoking prevalence data to adjust for smoking in males when reporting UTUC incidence. This study found the highest statistically significant smoking-adjusted SIR to be in physicians (1.63 [1.16–2.23]).

The study by Pukkala and colleagues [48] on the same five Nordic countries between 1943–1990 reported a similarly high SIR in seamen of 1.52 (1.26–1.85), while the highest SIR in women was seen in clerical workers (1.19 [1.08–1.31]). Moreover, McLaughlin et al. [50] reported SIR of renal pelvis cancers in 34 different occupations between 1960 and 1979 in Sweden, with the highest incidence found to be in judges (9.16), engineers and technicians in mining and metallurgy (3.29), and plumbers (2.17).

Incidence by Lynch syndrome

Our search of the literature found only one epidemiological study on the incidence of UTUC in patients with Lynch syndrome. Many studies were excluded that focused instead on the incidence of Lynch syndrome in patients with UTUC, with other studies investigating the risks and survival rates of these patients.

The study by Ericson and colleagues [53] set out to assess cancer risk in patients whose parents developed any tumour associated with Lynch syndrome. The study used data from the Swedish Cancer Registry between 1961 and 1999. Patients were categorised according to familial risk groups, as well as the type of malignancy present in the parent. The overall SIR of UTUC in all patients was 1.2 (95% CI 0.9–1.5). The highest incidence of UTUC was seen in patients whose parent and sibling had an HNPCC-associated cancer, one of whom was under 50 years old when diagnosed—the SIR in this group was 29.6 (8.1–75.9).

Incidence by other population characteristics

A number of studies included in this review reported an increased UTUC incidence in different populations and patient groups. For example, Sun et al. [54] studied patients with a recent urinary tract infection (UTI) diagnosis and found a higher incidence of UTUC in patients who had an upper UTI (1.38 per 10,000 person-years) compared to those who had a lower UTI (1.12) and no UTI (0.27). Another study by Chow et al. [23] to assess whether UTUC is linked to kidney and ureter stones reported a higher SIR of UTUC in patients who had a UTI at their index visit (6.7 [95% CI 2.4–14.5]) compared to those who did not (2.2 [1.6–3.0]).

Prospective cohort studies

There were only two prospective cohort studies included in this review. Mok et al. [12] reported a higher incidence of ureter cancer in patients with a low estimated glomerular filtration rate (eGFR) of <45 (13.7 per 10,000 person-years) compared to patients with a higher eGFR of ≥ 90 (0.3). The second study by Aparicio et al. [13] was a multicentre study of 31 institutions in Spain utilising a centralised database to report cases of UTUC prospectively. This study reported a relatively high incidence rate of 3.27 (95% CI 2.93–3.61) per 100,000 person-years, which the authors conclude is due to the prospective nature of their study.

Prevalence

The only study to report on prevalence values for UTUC included in this review was by Visser et al. [14], which used the RARECARE database of rare cancers in Europe. However, estimated complete prevalence was only available for the index year 2003, and data was only used from 22 registries in 12 countries as representative of the EU27 countries. In total, the estimated complete prevalence for epithelial tumours of the renal pelvis and ureter was 101.0 (SE 1.5) per million persons. This was nearly double that of epithelial tumours of the penis, which was the next most prevalent cancer at 55.4 (SE 1.1) per million persons. The most common subtype of UTUC was transitional cell carcinoma at 93.2 (SE 1.4) per million persons, followed by adenocarcinoma at 1.4 (SE 0.2) per million persons, then squamous cell carcinoma (prevalence not reported).

Discussion

Data from the 59 papers included in this review highlight a number of trends in the epidemiology of UTUC. Overall, there is an increase in incidence with age and specific occupations such as seamen and printers. The trend in incidence seen in other factors—sex, race, geographical region, and calendar time—was less clear. Single studies reported a high incidence of UTUC in patients with a history of an upper UTI, and patients with a low eGFR. Prevalence of UTUC was only reported by one study, which showed UTUC to be the most common of the rare urogenital cancers. Similarly, only one study reported the incidence of UTUC in patients with Lynch syndrome, and although this was limited to data obtained only from the Swedish Cancer Registry, it included data from a period of 40 years.

The general increase in UTUC incidence across time reported by some studies can be attributed to the introduction of computed tomography (CT) urography in the detection of UTUC [15]. CT urography is a recent introduction in the diagnosis of UTUC, which for many decades was dominated by intravenous urography. Several guidelines have only recently changed to reflect the higher diagnostic accuracy provided by CT urography, which is now the first-line imaging modality for investigating UTUC [55].

The relatively high incidence of UTUC reported in seamen has been proposed to be due to increased exposure to asbestos fibres in ships [27]. The association between occupational exposure and other urological cancers has been studied, with a high incidence of bladder cancer in seamen reported in a study on the Nordic Occupational Cancer cohort [56]. Exposure to other chemicals, such as the azo dyes used in the printing and dyeing industry, have also been linked to increased bladder cancer incidence [57]. This could explain the increased UTUC incidence observed in printers in the study reported by Michalek et al. [27]. A further aspect of occupational exposure was proposed by Michalek et al. [52] in their study of smoking-adjusted incidence, with the suggestion that exposure to phenacetin and X-rays/gamma rays could be the cause of a statistically significant high smoking-adjusted SIR in physicians, although this was also suggested to be due to surveillance bias and increased awareness of urothelial cancer symptoms by physicians.

The studies that reported values on race generally found a mixed picture in the incidence of UTUC between Black and White Americans. Mathew et al. and Chow et al. reported a higher SIR for renal pelvis cancers in White Americans compared to Black Americans [37, 38]. Racial disparities between Black and White Americans have been studied and have been found to exist in other urological cancers [58, 59]. The reason for this disparity is difficult to quantify, as it could be attributed to genetics, lifestyle factors such as smoking, or poorer access to healthcare.

Studies based in Taiwan report a relatively high incidence of UTUC due to the widespread consumption of aristolochic acid, an established risk factor for UTUC. This carcinogenic and nephrotoxic agent, which was banned in Taiwan in 2003, is present in herbal medicines and has been linked to an increased risk of urinary tract cancers [60]. Exploring the effect of the ban of aristolochic acid on UTUC incidence, Wang et al. [42] reported a decrease in the $SIR_{40\text{-}84}$ in both males and females after the introduction of the ban, although the authors note that there remains another carcinogenic and nephrotoxic agent (Xi-Xin) similar to aristolochic acid in circulation in Taiwan that requires further study.

The SEER (Surveillance, Epidemiology, and End Results) Program is a database that collects data on cancer incidence in the USA and is a common tool used in epidemiological studies of cancer [61]. However, many excluded studies from this review considered the SEER category of 'kidney and renal pelvis' cancers as cancers of the renal pelvis. Kidney and renal pelvis cancers are not alike as they originate from different tissues and are histologically different, namely, renal cell carcinoma and urothelial carcinoma. This is reflected in the different ICD-10 codes assigned to each cancer: C64 (Malignant neoplasm of kidney, except renal pelvis), C65 (Malignant neoplasm of renal pelvis), and C66 (Malignant neoplasm of ureter) [62].

Similarly, many of the studies excluded from this review cite the comprehensive study by Siegel and colleagues [63], but this paper has the same limitation as above in that renal pelvis cancers are grouped together with kidney cancers. Moreover, studies that mention a high incidence of UTUC in endemic areas of blackfoot disease do not report UTUC separately, instead grouping UTUC with other urinary cancers. Future studies reporting on renal pelvis cancers should ensure that there is a clear delineation between these two types of cancers with a different aetiology and histology.

Full-text screening identified only one study [14] reporting on the prevalence of UTUC that met our inclusion criteria. While data on the incidence of UTUC is useful in identifying trends, the lack of prevalence studies on UTUC needs to be addressed in order to provide a better picture of the burden of UTUC in different populations.

A notable limitation that was identified through the use of the JBI checklist was that many studies did not report the 95% confidence intervals of their incidence values. Furthermore, the JBI checklist also highlighted that many papers in our review did not mention ethical approval, which should be required even if the study design is observational, as databases with personally identifiable information may be used during the study. Future epidemiological studies should ensure that appropriate ethical approval is obtained before commencing the study.

A limitation of this review is that the data from the studies selected was found to be heterogeneous, and hence a qualitative synthesis of the data was done in place of a meta-analysis to reflect the nature of the data. Future studies on the epidemiology of UTUC should consider reporting incidence data using similar metrics (such as those for age standardisation) in order to allow for a more accurate quantitative comparison.

Conclusion

Although UTUC is a relatively rare urological cancer, it is still an important public health concern in many areas and patient populations around the world. The present review highlights an increased incidence of UTUC seen in certain groups, including increasing age and certain occupations such as seamen. UTUC is more endemic in certain geographical regions of the world where there are associated risk factors. The trend of UTUC incidence for sex, race, and calendar time is less clear due to a wide variety of measures used to report incidence. There is also sparse literature on the prevalence of UTUC, and further studies using this important epidemiological metric are needed to know the true disease burden of UTUC. The results of this review provide epidemiologists, public health specialists, and clinicians a better understanding of the epidemiology of UTUC in order to guide diagnosis and prevention.

Abbreviations

UTUC: Upper urinary tract urothelial carcinoma; JBI: Joanna Briggs Institute; SEER: Surveillance, Epidemiology, and End Results; CI: Confidence interval; ASR: Age-standardised rate; SIR: Standardised incidence ratio; SE: Standard error; UTI: Urinary tract infection.

Authors' contributions

Conception and design: AS, ER, CB, MVH. Acquisition of data: AS, ER, CB. Analysis and interpretation of data: AS, ER, CB. Drafting of manuscript: AS. Critical revision of the manuscript for important intellectual content: ER, CB, GG, BR, DE, RN, MVH. All authors read and approved the final manuscript.

Competing interests

The authors declare that they have no competing interests.

Author details

[1]University Hospital Hairmyres, Glasgow, UK. [2]Translational Oncology and Urology Research, School of Cancer and Pharmaceutical Sciences, King's College London, London, UK. [3]Department of Human Structure and Repair, Ghent University, Ghent, Belgium. [4]Department of Oncology, Guy's Hospital, Guy's and St Thomas' NHS Foundation Trust, London, UK. [5]Department of Urology, Guy's Hospital, Guy's and St Thomas' NHS Foundation Trust, London, UK.

References

1. Crivelli JJ, Xylinas E, Kluth LA, Rieken M, Rink M, Shariat SF. Effect of smoking on outcomes of urothelial carcinoma: a systematic review of the literature. Eur Urol. 2014;65:742–54.
2. Cosyns J-P. Aristolochic acid and "Chinese Herbs Nephropathy." Drug Saf. 2003;26:33–48.
3. Ju JY, Mills AM, Mahadevan MS, Fan J, Culp SH, Thomas MH, et al. Universal lynch syndrome screening should be performed in all upper tract urothelial carcinomas. Am J Surg Pathol. 2018;42:1549–55.
4. Sanguedolce F, Cormio L. The complex relationship between upper urinary tract and bladder cancer: clinical and predictive issues. Transl Androl Urol. 2018;7(Suppl 2):S248–51.
5. Toporcov TN, Wünsch FV. Epidemiological science and cancer control. Clinics. 2018;73(suppl 1):e627s–e627s.
6. Rawla P. Epidemiology of prostate cancer. World J Oncol. 2019;10:63–89.
7. Cumberbatch MGK, Jubber I, Black PC, Esperto F, Figueroa JD, Kamat AM, et al. Epidemiology of bladder cancer: a systematic review and contemporary update of risk factors in 2018. Eur Urol. 2018;74:784–95.
8. Soria F, Shariat SF, Lerner SP, Fritsche HM, Rink M, Kassouf W, et al. Epidemiology, diagnosis, preoperative evaluation and prognostic assessment of upper-tract urothelial carcinoma (UTUC). World J Urol. 2017;35:379–87.
9. Ouzzani M, Hammady H, Fedorowicz Z, Elmagarmid A. Rayyan-a web and mobile app for systematic reviews. Syst Rev. 2016;5:210.
10. Joanna Briggs Institute. Checklist for Prevalence Studies. 2017. https://joannabriggs.org/sites/default/files/2019-05/JBI_Critical_Appraisal-Checklist_for_Prevalence_Studies2017_0.pdf.
11. Rohatgi A. WebPlotDigitizer Version: 4.1. Austin, TX. 2018.
12. Mok Y, Matsushita K, Ballew SH, Sang Y, Jung KJ, Lee S, et al. Kidney Function, Proteinuria, and Cancer Incidence: The Korean Heart Study. Am J Kidney Dis. 2017;70:512–21.
13. Fernandez Aparicio T, Galan Llopis JA, Cansino Alcaide R, Pérez Fentes D, Cepeda Delgado M, Alvarez-Ossorio JL, et al. Incidence of upper tract urothelial carcinoma in Spain. Actas Urol Esp. 2020;44:512–8.
14. Visser O, Adolfsson J, Rossi S, Verne J, Gatta G, Maffezzini M, et al. Incidence and survival of rare urogenital cancers in Europe. Eur J Cancer. 2012;48:456–64.
15. Kockelbergh R, Hounsome L, Mayer E. The epidemiology of urological cancer 2001–2013. J Clin Urol. 2017;10:3–8.
16. Eylert MF, Hounsome L, Verne J, Bahl A, Jefferies ER, Persad RA. Prognosis is deteriorating for upper tract urothelial cancer: data for England 1985–2010. BJU Int. 2013;112:E107–13.
17. Almås B, Halvorsen OJ, Johannesen TB, Beisland C. Higher than expected and significantly increasing incidence of upper tract urothelial carcinoma. A population based study. World J Urol. 2021. https://doi.org/10.1007/s00345-020-03576-3.
18. Woodford R, Ranasinghe W, Aw HC, Sengupta S, Persad R. Trends in incidence and survival for upper tract urothelial cancer (UTUC) in the state of Victoria-Australia. BJU Int. 2016;117:45–9.
19. Stoyanov IS, Chernozemsky IN, Nicolov IG, Stoichev II, Petkova-Bocharova TK. Epidemiologic association between endemic nephropathy and urinary system tumors in an endemic region. J Chronic Dis. 1978;31:721–4.
20. Wang SM, Lai MN, Chen PC, Der WJ. Increased risk of urothelial cancer in young and middle aged patients with end-stage renal disease. J Formos Med Assoc. 2015;114:52–7.
21. Joung JY, Lim J, Oh CM, Jung KW, Cho H, Kim SH, et al. Current trends in the incidence and survival rate of urological cancers in Korea. Cancer Res Treat. 2017;49:607–15.
22. Cheon J, Kim CS, Lee ES, Hong SJ, Cho YH, Shin EC, et al. Survey of incidence of urological cancer in South Korea: a 15-year summary. Int J Urol. 2002;9:445–54.
23. Chow WH, Lindblad P, Gridley G, Nyrén O, McLaughlin JK, Linet MS, et al. Risk of urinary tract cancers following kidney or ureter stones. J Natl Cancer Inst. 1997;89:1453–7.
24. Hsiao PJ, Hsieh PF, Chang CH, Wu HC, Yang CR, Huang CP. Higher risk of urothelial carcinoma in the upper urinary tract than in the urinary bladder in hemodialysis patients. Ren Fail. 2016;38:663–70.
25. Nakata S, Ohtake N, Kubota Y, Imai K, Yamanaka H, Ito Y, et al. Incidence of urogenital cancers in Gunma Prefecture, Japan: a 10-year summary. Int J Urol. 1998;5:364–9.
26. Lynch CF, Cohen MB. Urinary system. Cancer. 1995;75(1 Suppl):316–29.
27. Michalek IM, Martinsen JI, Weiderpass E, Kjaerheim K, Lynge E, Sparen P, et al. Occupation and risk of cancer of the renal pelvis in Nordic countries. BJU Int. 2019;123:233–8.
28. Mellemgaard A, Carstensen B, Nørgaard N, Knudsen JB, Olsen JH. Trends in the incidence of cancer of the kidney, pelvis, ureter and bladder in Denmark 1943–88. Scand J Urol Nephrol. 1993;27:327–32.
29. Premuzic V, Gamulin M, Coric M, Jelakovic B. The incidence of urinary tract cancers is related to preserved diuresis: a single-center report. Int Urol Nephrol. 2017;49:2257–63.
30. Christensen MS, Hansen J, Ramlau-Hansen CH, Toft G, Kolstad H. Cancer incidence in workers exposed to styrene in the Danish-reinforced Plastics Industry, 1968–2012. Epidemiology. 2017;28:300–10.
31. Medunjanin D, Sonicki Z, Vena JE, Cvitkovic A, Robb SW. Geographic distribution and risk of upper urothelial carcinomas in Croatia, 2001–2011. BMC Cancer. 2019;19:950.
32. Janbabaei G, Ashrafi M, Ghazizadeh Z, Afshari M, Mousavi R-S, Jouybari M, et al. Incidence and epidemiology of urologic cancers in North of Iran. Clin Cancer Investig J. 2018;7:217.
33. Bermejo JL, Sundquist J, Hemminki K. Bladder cancer in cancer patients: population-based estimates from a large Swedish study. Br J Cancer. 2009;101:1091–9.
34. Antoni S, Soerjomataram I, Moore S, Ferlay J, Sitas F, Smith DP, et al. The ban on phenacetin is associated with changes in the incidence trends of upper-urinary tract cancers in Australia. Aust N Z J Public Health. 2014;38:455–8.
35. Noone AM, Cronin KA, Altekruse SF, Howlader N, Lewis DR, Petkov VI, et al. Cancer incidence and survival trends by subtype using data from the surveillance epidemiology and end results program, 1992–2013. Cancer Epidemiol Biomarkers Prev. 2017;26:632–41.
36. Yang J, Li S, Lv M, Wu Y, Chen Z, Shen Y, et al. Risk of subsequent primary malignancies among patients with prior colorectal cancer: a population-based cohort study. Onco Targets Ther. 2017;10:1535–48.
37. Mathew A, Devesa SS, Fraumeni JF, Chow WH. Global increases in kidney cancer incidence, 1973–1992. Eur J Cancer Prev. 2002;11:171–8.
38. Chow WH, Devesa SS, Warren JL, Fraumeni JF. Rising incidence of renal cell cancer in the United States. J Am Med Assoc. 1999;281:1628–31.
39. Holmang S, Holmberg E, Johansson SL. A population-based study of tumours of the renal pelvis and ureter: incidence, aetiology and histopathological findings. Scand J Urol. 2013;47:491–6.
40. Raman JD, Messer J, Sielatycki JA, Hollenbeak CS. Incidence and survival of patients with carcinoma of the ureter and renal pelvis in the USA, 1973–2005. BJU Int. 2011;107:1059–64.
41. Wihlborg A, Johansen C. Incidences of Kidney, Pelvis, Ureter, and Bladder Cancer in a Nationwide, population-based Cancer Registry, Denmark, 1944–2003. Urology. 2010;75:1222–7.
42. Wang SM, Lai MN, Chen PC, Pu YS, Lai MK, Hwang JS, et al. Increased upper and lower tract Urothelial carcinoma in patients with end-stage renal disease: A nationwide cohort study in Taiwan during 1997–2008. Biomed Res Int. 2014;2014:149750.
43. Cauberg ECC, Salomons MA, Kümmerlin IPED, De Reijke TM, Zwinderman AH, De La Rosette JJMCH, et al. Trends in epidemiology and treatment

of upper urinary tract tumours in the Netherlands 1995–2005: An analysis of PALGA, the Dutch national histopathology registry. BJU Int. 2010;105:922–7.
44. Munoz JJ, Ellison LM. Upper tract urothelial neoplasms: Incidence and survival during the last 2 decades. J Urol. 2000;164:1523–5.
45. Wu J, Chen S, Wu X, Mao W, Wang Y, Xu B, et al. Trends of incidence and prognosis of upper tract urothelial carcinoma. Bosn J Basic Med Sci. 2020. https://doi.org/10.17305/bjbms.2020.5345.
46. Tempo J, Logan C, O'Callaghan M, Kahokehr A, Kichenadasse G, D'Onise K, et al. Bladder, penile, renal pelvis and testis cancers: A population based analysis of incidence and survival 1977–2013. Cancer Epidemiol. 2020;65:101692.
47. Chernozemsky IN, Stoyanov IS, Petkova-Bocharova TK, Nicolov IG, Draganov IV, Stoichev II, et al. Geographic correlation between the occurrence of endemic nephropathy and urinary tract tumours in vratza district. Bulgaria Int J Cancer. 1977;19:1–11.
48. Pukkala E, Martinsen JI, Lynge E, Gunnarsdottir HK, Sparn P, Tryggvadottir L, et al. Occupation and cancer follow-up of 15 million people in five Nordic countries. Acta Oncol (Madr). 2009;48:646–790.
49. McLaughlin JK, Sonderman JS, Tarone RE, Mumma MT, Lipworth L. Cancer incidence among workers at a satellite manufacturing facility. J Occup Environ Med. 2012;54:1500–5.
50. McLaughlin JK, Malker HSR, Stone BJ, Weiner JA, Ericsson JL, Blot WJ, et al. Occupational risks for renal cancer in Sweden. Br J Ind Med. 1987;44:119–23.
51. Lynge E, Rix BA, Villadsen E, Andersen I, Hink M, Olsen E, et al. Cancer in printing workers in Denmark. Occup Environ Med. 1995;52:738–44.
52. Michalek IM, Kjærheim K, Martinsen JI, Sparén P, Tryggvadóttir L, Weiderpass E, et al. Smoking-adjusted risk of renal pelvis cancer by occupation: a population-based cohort study of Nordic men. Acta Oncol. 2020;59:112–5.
53. Ericson K, Nilbert M, Bladström A, Anderson H, Olsson H, Planck M. Familial risk of tumors associated with hereditary non-polyposis colorectal cancer: a Swedish population-based study. Scand J Gastroenterol. 2004;39:1259–65.
54. Sun LM, Lin CL, Liang JA, Liu SH, Sung FC, Chang YJ, et al. Urinary tract infection increases subsequent urinary tract cancer risk: a population-based cohort study. Cancer Sci. 2013;104:619–23.
55. Jinzaki M, Kikuchi E, Akita H, Sugiura H, Shinmoto H, Oya M. Role of computed tomography urography in the clinical evaluation of upper tract urothelial carcinoma. Int J Urol. 2016;23:284–98. https://doi.org/10.1111/iju.13032.
56. Hadkhale K, Martinsen JI, Weiderpass E, Kjaerheim K, Lynge E, Sparen P, et al. Occupation and risk of bladder cancer in Nordic countries. J Occup Environ Med. 2016;58:e301–7.
57. Golka K, Wiese A, Assennato G, Bolt HM. Occupational exposure and urological cancer. World J Urol. 2004;21:382–91.
58. Chow WH, Devesa SS. Contemporary epidemiology of renal cell cancer. Cancer J. 2008;14:288–301.
59. Crawford ED. Epidemiology of prostate cancer. Urology. 2003;62:3–12.
60. Lai MN, Wang SM, Chen PC, Chen YY, Der WJ. Population-based case-control study of chinese herbal products containing aristolochic acid and urinary tract cancer risk. J Natl Cancer Inst. 2010;102:179–86.
61. Scosyrev E, Messing J, Noyes K, Veazie P, Messing E. Surveillance Epidemiology and End Results (SEER) program and population-based research in urologic oncology: An overview. In: Urologic Oncology: Seminars and Original Investigations. Elsevier; 2012. p. 126–132.
62. World Health Organization. ICD-10. International Statistical Classification of Diseases and Related Health Problems 10th Revision. 2019;2. https://icd.who.int/browse10/2019/en#/C64-C68.
63. Siegel RL, Miller KD, Jemal A. Cancer statistics, 2017. CA Cancer J Clin. 2017;67:7–30.
64. Yu J, Lee CU, Kang M, Jeon HG, Jeong BC, Seo S II, et al. Incidences and oncological outcomes of urothelial carcinoma in kidney transplant recipients. Cancer Manag Res. 2019;11:157–66.
65. Chen J-S, Lu C-L, Huang L-C, Shen C-H, Chen SC-C. Chronic Kidney Disease is Associated With Upper Tract Urothelial Carcinoma: A Nationwide Population-Based Cohort Study in Taiwan. Medicine (Baltimore). 2016;95:e3255.
66. Balaji KC, McGuire M, Grotas J, Grimaldi G, Russo P. Upper tract recurrences following radical cystectomy: an analysis of prognostic factors, recurrence pattern and stage at presentation. J Urol. 1999;162:1603–6.
67. Kang C-H, Chen C-H, Chiang P-H. Primary urothelial carcinoma of the upper urinary tract in dialysis patients with 5-year follow-up. Jpn J Clin Oncol. 2010;40:241–46.
68. Shinka T, Uekado Y, Aoshi H, Hirano A, Ohkawa T. Occurrence of uroepithelial tumors of the upper urinary tract after the initial diagnosis of bladder cancer. J Urol. 1988;140:745–48.
69. Wright JL, Hotaling J, Porter MP. Predictors of upper tract urothelial cell carcinoma after primary bladder cancer: a population based analysis. J Urol. 2009;181:1035–9.
70. Yang M-H, Chen K-K, Yen C-C, Wang W-S, Chang Y-H, Huang WJ-S, et al. Unusually high incidence of upper urinary tract urothelial carcinoma in Taiwan. Urology. 2002;59:681–7.
71. Huguét-Perez J, Palou J, Millán-Rodriguez F, Salvador-Bayarri J, Villavicencio-Mavrich H, Vicente-Rodriguez J. Upper tract transitional cell carcinoma following cystectomy for bladder cancer. Eur Urol. 2001;40:318–23.
72. Furukawa J, Miyake H, Hara I, Takenaka A, Fujisawa M. Upper urinary tract recurrence following radical cystectomy for bladder cancer. Int J Urol. 2007;14:496–9.
73. Amar AD, Das S. Upper urinary tract transitional cell carcinoma in patients with bladder carcinoma and associated vesicoureteral reflux. J Urol. 1985;133:468–71.
74. Millán-Rodriguez F, Chechile-Toniolo G, Salvador-Bayarri J, Huguet-Perez J, Vicente-Rodriguez J. Upper urinary tract tumors after primary superficial bladder tumors: prognostic factors and risk groups. J Urol. 2000;164:1183–7.
75. Hurle R, Losa A, Manzetti A, Lembo A. Upper urinary tract tumors developing after treatment of superficial bladder cancer: 7-year follow-up of 591 consecutive patients. Urology. 1999;53:1144–8.
76. Schwartz CB, Bekirov H, Melman A. Urothelial tumors of upper tract following treatment of primary bladder transitional cell carcinoma. Urology. 1992;40:509–11.
77. Friis S, Nielsen GL, Mellemkjær L, McLaughlin JK, Thulstrup M, Blot WJ, Lipworth L, Vilstrup H, Olsen JH. Cancer risk in persons receiving prescriptions for paracetamol: A Danish cohort study. Int. J. Cancer. 2002;97:96–101.
78. Devesa SS, Silverman DT, McLaughlin JK, Brown CC, Connelly RR, Fraumeni JF Jr. Comparison of the descriptive epidemiology of urinary tract cancers. Cancer Causes Control. 1990;1(2):133–41.
79. Aragon-Ching JB, Nizam A, Henson DE. Carcinomas of the Renal Pelvis, Ureters, and Urinary Bladder Share a Carcinogenic Field as Revealed in Epidemiological Analysis of Tumor Registry Data. Clin Genitourin Cancer. 2019;17:436–42.
80. Fernandez Aparicio T, Galan Llopis JA, Cansino Alcaide R, Pérez Fentes D, Cepeda Delgado M, Alvarez-Ossorio JL, et al. Incidence of upper tract urothelial carcinoma in Spain. Actas Urol Esp. 2020;44:512–8.

32

532 nm green-light laser vaporization of upper tract urothelial carcinoma

F. Dursun[1], M. M. Pan[2], M. Morgan[1], R. R. Gonzalez[1] and R. Satkunasivam[1*]

Abstract

Background: Endoscopic management of low risk upper tract urothelial carcinoma (UTUC) may be considered in select clinical scenarios, which allows sparing the morbidity of radical nephroureterectomy while achieving acceptable oncological outcomes and preservation of kidney function. Herein, we present a case with UTUC in a solitary kidney managed with 532 nm laser vaporization through a percutaneous approach.

Case presentation: The patient in this video (Additional file 1) is an 85-year-old woman who presented with a bulky tumor in the collecting system of a congenital solitary left kidney, which was a biopsy proven low grade urothelial carcinoma. Prior to the procedure, a lower pole percutaneous nephrostomy tube was successfully placed under sedation by Interventional Radiology. The procedure was done in a prone split leg position. The mass, which was predominantly localized to the renal pelvis was efficiently vaporized with the 532 nm laser in a systematic manner with continuous irrigation of normal saline through the cystoscope. The patient was discharged home on postoperative day 2 with the nephroureterostomy catheter open to drainage. This catheter was subsequently clamped and removed two weeks later without complications. Follow up uretroscopy showed excellent treatment response and the patient remains well without complications.

Conclusion: This case report details the potential utility of 532 nm laser vaporization of UTUC, however, ongoing studies are required to demonstrate peri-operative safety and durable oncologic efficacy.

Keywords: Upper tract urothelial carcinoma, Endoscopic management, Laser ablation, Greenlight, KTP

Background

Upper tract urothelial carcinomas (UTUC) are uncommon and account for only 5–10% of urothelial carcinoma with a peak incidence in individuals aged 70–90 years [1, 2]. Nephroureterectomy with bladder-cuff removal remains the gold standard for the management of UTUC [3]. Endoscopic management may be considered in select clinical scenarios. Kidney-sparing surgery (KSS) for low risk UTUC is an option that allows sparing the morbidity of radical nephroureterectomy (RNU) while achieving acceptable oncological outcomes and preservation of kidney function. In low grade cancers it is the preferred approach, with survival being similar after KSS versus RNU [4]. In addition, it can also be considered in select patients with significant renal insufficiency or a solitary kidney.

At present, the 532 nm lithium triborate laser, also known as green-light laser, is a popular and effective surgical method for treating benign prostatic hyperplasia given its tissue affinity for hemoglobin and reduced risk of bleeding complications compared to standard resection [5]. En-bloc vapoenucleation with 532 nm laser is also reported as a feasible, safe and effective option for the management of select non-muscle invasive bladder cancer patients [6]. Given the established properties of the 532 nm laser, we sought to utilize this approach in the

*Correspondence: raj.satkunasivam@gmail.com
[1] Department of Urology, Houston Methodist Hospital, 6560 Fannin Street, Suite 2100, Houston, TX 77030, USA
Full list of author information is available at the end of the article

percutaneous management of low grade UTUC in a solitary kidney.

Case presentation

An 85-year-old woman presented with a bulky tumor in the collecting system of a congenital solitary left kidney. Her past medical history includes significant chronic obstructive pulmonary disease with a 2 pack-day smoking history more than 50 years. She has a history of recurrent low-grade non-muscle invasive bladder cancer (NMIBC) for the last 7 years for which she received intravesical BCG treatments. Her last recurrence in the bladder was 3 months prior showing non-invasive low-grade urothelial carcinoma.

Laboratory tests revealed normal renal function including serum creatinine of 0.69 mg/dl. A computerized tomography (CT) scan with a urographic phase demonstrated lobulated urothelial thickening of the left renal pelvis without hydronephrosis (Fig. 1). CT imaging of the chest did not identify metastatic disease.

The patient underwent flexible ureteroscopy and nephroscopy with ureteral washing and biopsy. A sessile tumor greater than 2 cm was visualized in the renal pelvis towards the upper pole infundibulum. Two adequate specimens were obtained in order to determine the disease grade and were consistent with low grade urothelial carcinoma.

After a detailed discussion with the patient about the risks, benefits, and possible complications of KSS, the patient elected to undergo percutaneous treatment with laser ablation of the UTUC in her solitary kidney. Prior to the procedure, a lower pole percutaneous nephrostomy tube was successfully placed under sedation by Interventional Radiology.

The patient was positioned in prone split leg position. We cystoscopically confirmed that there was no tumor recurrence in the bladder. A guidewire was passed through the nephrostomy tube, ureteroscopically grasped with a nitinol basket and was taken out to achieve through-and-through access. After placing a 12.7 French ureteral access sheath under fluoroscopy, we visualized the renal pelvis again using the ureteroscope and dilated the percutaneous tract with a balloon dilatator under direct vision and placed a 28 French Amplatz sheath, which allowed the introduction of a 24 French continuous-flow cystoscope (Richard Wolf, CITY) with normal saline for irrigation. Importantly, the ureteral access sheath was left to optimize drainage, provide low pressure in the renal pelvis, and limit any tumor seeding in the bladder.

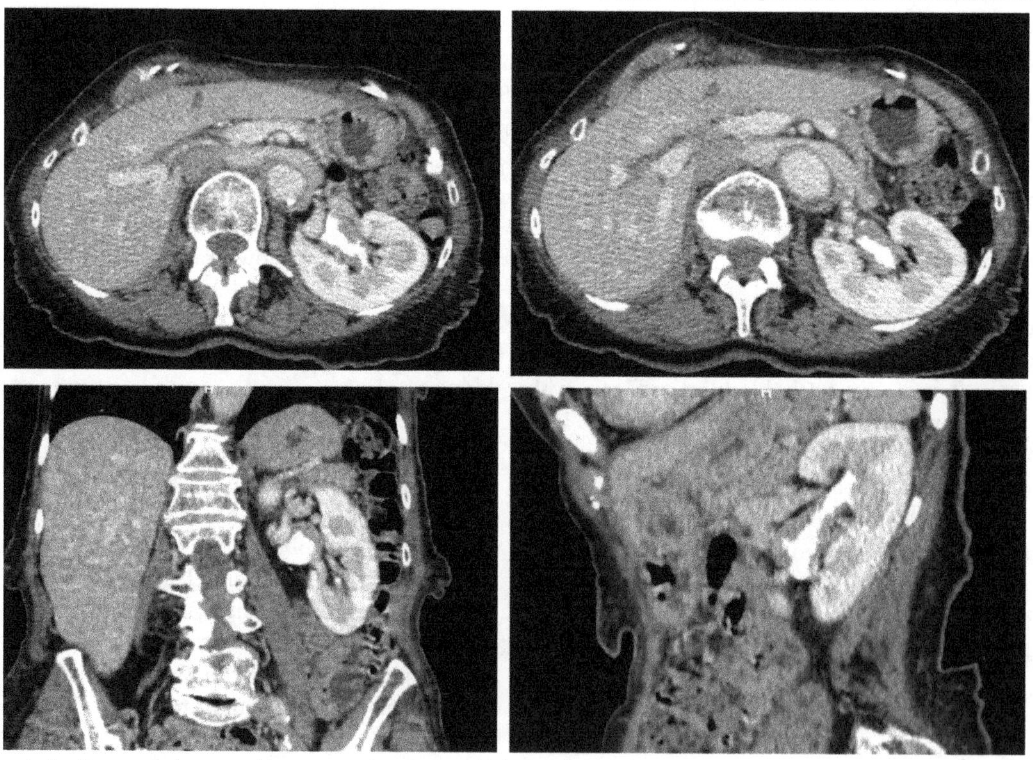

Fig. 1 A computerized tomography scan with urogram demonstrated lobulated urothelial thickening at the left renal pelvis, and infundibulum of the upper pole calyx without hydronephrosis

After systematic exploration of the collecting system, the boundaries of the large sessile tumor were visualized, and the renal pelvis mass was vaporized with the 532 nm laser in a systematic manner with continuous irrigation of normal saline through the cystoscope. GreenLight XPS LBO 180W laser console (Boston Scientific, Malborough, MA) was used with an extended application (EA) 600 micron side-fire fiber (Boston Scientific, Malborough, MA). The mass was vaporized using a setting of 40 watts; to coagulate any bleeders, the power was set at 20 watts. Care was taken to stay in near-contact with the mass during vaporization, using visible bubbles as feedback of efficient vaporization and hemostasis of the tumor bed without charring tissue. The hemostasis was achieved effectively in a very short duration at low power. Total energy used during the procedure was 39,515 J. After satisfactory tumor ablation, an 8-French nephroureteral catheter was inserted under fluoroscopic and cystoscopic guidance to maintain adequate urinary drainage.

The patient was discharged home on postoperative day 2 with the nephroureterostomy catheter open to drainage. The catheter was subsequently clamped and removed two weeks later without complications. Follow up included cystoscopy and CT urogram at 3 months. CT urogram demonstrated focal thickening in the upper pole urothelium without obvious recurrence. Ureteroscopy was performed at 6 months which demonstrated minimal residual or recurrent disease (5 mm in upper pole calyx) that was successfully ablated (thulium laser). Excellent treatment response was observed throughout the remaining collecting system. At the same time two small papillary low-grade bladder tumors were resected, followed by intravesical gemcitabine. The patient is now at 8 months of follow up and remains well, with plans for ongoing cross sectional imaging, cystoscopic and ureteroscopic follow up. Throughout the treatment, we did not observe any deleterious consequences to renal function. In the accompanying video (Additional file 1), we present our technique for KTP Green-light laser vaporization of UTUC via a percutaneous approach.

Discussion and conclusion

Upper tract urothelial carcinoma in a solitary kidney creates challenging decisions for the patient and physician. Radical nephroureterctomy is not without morbidity and the long-term quality of life and morbidity and mortality of dialysis must be considered. Endoscopic approaches are a viable option for the management of UTUC when kidney function preservation is of paramount importance. Percutaneous approaches over retrograde (ureteroscopic) approaches offer advantages with respect to better visualization and flexibility in instrumentation [7]. While laser and resection-based approaches (i.e. bipolar resectoscope) have been described, this case, to our knowledge, represents the first treatment of UTUC with 532 nm laser vaporization.

A variety of lasers have been proven to be useful for the management of superficial and low-grade UTUC without compromising oncologic outcomes or renal function [8]. The high-power 532 nm laser is selectively absorbed by hemoglobin but not by water, leading to rapid tissue vaporization with an optical penetration depth of about 0.8 mm and 2–3 mm zone of coagulation. Although the heat-affected-zone of coagulation is higher than holmium and thulium lasers, selective absorption by hemoglobin provides better coagulation and limited necrosis of the tissue below the vaporized area [9]. This 2 mm rim of coagulation zone under the vaporized area may provide a better safety profile for bleeding complications especially for patients at high risk for clinically significant bleeding [5]. The advantages of 532 nm laser vaporization through a nephrostomy tract includes better visualization as a result of both optimal coagulation and excellent irrigation flow with low intra-pelvic pressures. Limitations include lack of tissue for pathologic diagnosis (hence necessitating pre-operative confirmation of low-grade urothelial carcinoma), the lack of flexibility due to the laser fiber which may limit access to certain tumor locations, and potential perforation intraoperatively or in delayed fashion. Despite the fact that bulky tumors can be handled by this approach, our case highlights the need for ongoing close follow up as repeat ablations may be necessary. This may be particularly true in areas difficult to reach by rigid instruments.The impact on depth of penetration to normal renal tissue and potential renal functional loss as well as other renal complications remains to be carefully followed and therefore must be closely investigated in future studies. Improving outcomes for UTUC may include consideration of novel ablative technologies which have been introduced in the lower urinary tract. Overall, patient selection for endoscopic treatment remains critical and consideration must also be given to multimodal therapy with topical chemotherapeutic strategies [10].

This case report details the potential utility of 532 nm laser vaporization of UTUC, however, ongoing studies are required to demonstrate peri-operative safety and durable oncologic efficacy.

Abbreviations

UTUC: Upper tract urothelial carcinoma; KSS: Kidney-sparing surgery; RNU: Radical nephroureterectomy; NMIBC: Non-muscle invasive bladder cancer; BCG: Bacillus Calmette–Guérin; CT: Computerized tomography.

Authors' contributions

FD: Participated in manuscript design and drafted the manuscript. MP: Cared for the patient and revised the manuscript. MM: Discussed treatment options, guided in the operation. RG: Discussed treatment options, guided in the operation, revised the manuscript. RS: Diagnosed the disease, performed the operation, conceived the study, substantively revised the manuscript. All authors read and approved the final manuscript.

Competing interests
The authors declare that they have no competing interests.

Author details
[1] Department of Urology, Houston Methodist Hospital, 6560 Fannin Street, Suite 2100, Houston, TX 77030, USA. [2] Scott Department of Urology, Baylor College of Medicine, Houston, TX, USA.

References
1. Siegel RL, Miller KD, Jemal A. Cancer statistics, 2017. CACancer J Clin. 2017;67:7–30.
2. Shariat SF, Favaretto RL, Gupta A, et al. Gender differences in radical nephroureterectomy for upper tract urothelial carcinoma. World J Urol. 2011;29:481–6.
3. Margulis V, Shariat SF, Matin SF, et al. Outcomes of radical neph-roureterectomy: a series from the Upper Tract Urothelial Carcinoma Collaboration. Cancer. 2009;115:1224–33.
4. Seisen T, Peyronnet B, Dominguez-Escrig JL, et al. Oncologic outcomes of kidney-sparing surgery versus radical nephroureterecomy for upper tract urothelial carcinoma: a systematic review by the EAU Non-muscle Invasive Bladder Cancer Guidelines Panel. Eur Urol. 2016;70:1052–68.
5. Thomas JA, Tubaro A, Barber N, et al. A multicenter randomized noninferiority trial comparing GreenLight-XPS laser vaporization of the prostate and transurethral resection of the prostate for the treatment of benign prostatic obstruction: two-yr outcomes of the GOLIATH study. Eur Urol. 2016;69:94–102.
6. He D, Fan J, Wu K, et al. Novel green-light KTP laser en bloc enucleation for nonmuscle-invasive bladder cancer: technique and initial clinical experience. J Endourol. 2014;28(8):975–9.
7. Jabbour ME, Smith AD. Primary percutaneous approach to upper urinary tract transitional cell carcinoma. Urol Clin N Am. 2000;27(4):739–50. https://doi.org/10.1016/s0094-0143(05)70122-1.
8. Rouprêt M, Babjuk M, Compérat E, et al. European Association of Urology Guidelines on Upper Urinary Tract Urothelial Carcinoma: 2017 Update. Eur Urol. 2018;273:111–22.
9. Dołowy Ł, Krajewski W, Dembowski J, et al. The role of lasers in modern urology. Cent Eur J Urol. 2015;68:175–82.
10. Kleinmann N, Matin SF, Pierorazio PM, et al. Primary chemoablation of low-grade upper tract urothelial carcinoma using UGN-101, a mitomycin-containing reverse thermal gel (OLYMPUS): an open-label, single-arm, phase 3 trial. Lancet Oncol. 2020. https://doi.org/10.1016/S1470-2045(20)30147-9 (**Epub 4/29/2020**).

Permissions

All chapters in this book were first published by BioMed Central; hereby published with permission under the Creative Commons Attribution License or equivalent. Every chapter published in this book has been scrutinized by our experts. Their significance has been extensively debated. The topics covered herein carry significant findings which will fuel the growth of the discipline. They may even be implemented as practical applications or may be referred to as a beginning point for another development.

The contributors of this book come from diverse backgrounds, making this book a truly international effort. This book will bring forth new frontiers with its revolutionizing research information and detailed analysis of the nascent developments around the world.

We would like to thank all the contributing authors for lending their expertise to make the book truly unique. They have played a crucial role in the development of this book. Without their invaluable contributions this book wouldn't have been possible. They have made vital efforts to compile up to date information on the varied aspects of this subject to make this book a valuable addition to the collection of many professionals and students.

This book was conceptualized with the vision of imparting up-to-date information and advanced data in this field. To ensure the same, a matchless editorial board was set up. Every individual on the board went through rigorous rounds of assessment to prove their worth. After which they invested a large part of their time researching and compiling the most relevant data for our readers.

The editorial board has been involved in producing this book since its inception. They have spent rigorous hours researching and exploring the diverse topics which have resulted in the successful publishing of this book. They have passed on their knowledge of decades through this book. To expedite this challenging task, the publisher supported the team at every step. A small team of assistant editors was also appointed to further simplify the editing procedure and attain best results for the readers.

Apart from the editorial board, the designing team has also invested a significant amount of their time in understanding the subject and creating the most relevant covers. They scrutinized every image to scout for the most suitable representation of the subject and create an appropriate cover for the book.

The publishing team has been an ardent support to the editorial, designing and production team. Their endless efforts to recruit the best for this project, has resulted in the accomplishment of this book. They are a veteran in the field of academics and their pool of knowledge is as vast as their experience in printing. Their expertise and guidance has proved useful at every step. Their uncompromising quality standards have made this book an exceptional effort. Their encouragement from time to time has been an inspiration for everyone.

The publisher and the editorial board hope that this book will prove to be a valuable piece of knowledge for researchers, students, practitioners and scholars across the globe.

List of Contributors

Prahara Yuri, Rahmadani Puji Lestari and Firly Putri Fardilla
Division of Urology, Department of Surgery, Faculty of Medicine, Public Health and Nursing, Universitas Gadjah Mada/Dr. Sardjito Hospital, Jl. Kesehatan No.1, Yogyakarta 55281, Indonesia

Gunadi
Pediatric Surgery Division, Department of Surgery, Faculty of Medicine, Public Health and Nursing, Universitas Gadjah Mada/Dr. Sardjito Hospital, Yogyakarta, Indonesia

Ishandono Dachlan
Division of Plastic, Aesthetic and Reconstructive Surgery, Department of Surgery, Faculty of Medicine, Public Health and Nursing, Universitas Gadjah Mada/ Dr. Sardjito Hospital, Yogyakarta, Indonesia

Wei Gao, Tianying Xing and Tongwen Ou
Department of Urology, Xuanwu Hospital, Capital Medical University, Beijing 100053, China

Florian A. Schmid, Jenny A. Prange and Daniel Eberli
Department of Urology, University Hospital of Zurich, University of Zurich, Frauenklinikstrasse 10, 8091 Zurich, Switzerland

Dominic Gascho and Niklaus Zoelch
Institute of Forensic Medicine, University of Zurich, Zurich, Switzerland

Giovanni Colacicco
Institute of Anatomy, University of Zurich, Zurich, Switzerland

Zhaoyi Meng, Defu Lin, Guannan Wang, Yanchao Qu and Ning Sun
Department of Urology, Beijing Children's Hospital Affiliated With Capital Medical University, National Center for Children's Health, No. 56 Nanlishilu Rd, West District, Beijing 100045, China

Guo Nan Yin, Jiyeon Ock, Mi-Hye Kwon, Jun-Kyu Suh and Ji-Kan Ryu
Department of Urology and National Research Center for Sexual Medicine, Inha University School of Medicine, 7-206, 3rd St, Shinheung-Dong, Jung-Gu, Incheon 22332, Republic of Korea

Shuguang Piao, Zhiyong Liu and Lei Wang
Department of Urology at Changhai Hospital Affiliated with the Naval Medicine University, Shanghai 200433, People's Republic of China

Do-Kyun Kim
Korea Zoonosis Research Institute, Jeonbuk National University, Iksan, Jeonbuk 54531, Korea

Yong Song Gho
Department of Life Sciences, Pohang University of Science and Technology, Pohang, yeongsangbuk-do 37673, Korea

Maria Daniel, Hanna Szymanik-Grzelak, Agnieszka Turczyn and Małgorzata Pańczyk-Tomaszewska
Department of Paediatric Nephrology, Medical University of Warsaw, Żwirki i Wigury 63A, 02-091 Warsaw, Poland

Todd Lucas, Jonas Z. Hines, Stephanie M. Davis and Carlos Toledo
Division of Global HIV and Tuberculosis, Centers for Disease Control and Prevention, Atlanta, GA, USA

Julia Samuelson
Global HIV, Hepatitis and STIs Programmes, World Health Organization, Geneva, Switzerland

Timothy Hargreave
Department of Surgery, Edinburgh University, Scotland, UK

Ian Fellows
Fellows Statistics, Contractor, Centers for Disease Control and Prevention, San Diego, CA, USA

Amber Prainito and D. Heather Watts
U.S. Office of the Global HIV/ AIDS Coordinator, Washington, DC, USA

Valerian Kiggundu
Office of HIV/AIDS, U.S. Agency for International Development, Washington, DC, USA

Anne G. Thomas
Department of Defense, Defense Health Agency, San Diego, CA, USA

Onkemetse Conrad Ntsuape
Ministry of Health and Wellness, Gaborone, Botswana

Kunle Dare
Division of Global HIV and Tuberculosis, Centers for Disease Control and Prevention, Gaborone, Botswana

Elijah Odoyo-June
Division of Global HIV and Tuberculosis, Centers for Disease Control and Prevention, Nairobi, Kenya

Leonard Soo
U.S. Agency for International Development, Nairobi, Kenya

Likabelo Toti-Mokoteli
Ministry of Health, Maseru, Lesotho

Robert Manda
U.S. Agency for International Development, Maseru, Lesotho

Martin Kapito
Ministry of Health, Lilongwe, Malawi

Wezi Msungama
Division of Global HIV and Tuberculosis, Centers for Disease Control and Prevention, Lilongwe, Malawi

James Odek
U.S. Agency for International Development, Lilongwe, Malawi

Jotamo Come
Ministry of Health, Maputo, Mozambique

Marcos Canda
Division of Global HIV and Tuberculosis, Centers for Disease Control and Prevention, Maputo, Mozambique

Nuno Gaspar
U.S. Agency for International Development, Maputo, Mozambique

Aupokolo Mekondjo
Ministry of Health and Social Services, Windhoek, Namibia

Brigitte Zemburuka
Division of Global HIV and Tuberculosis, Centers for Disease Control and Prevention, Windhoek, Namibia

Collen Bonnecwe
National Department of Health, Pretoria, South Africa

Peter Vranken
Division of Global HIV and Tuberculosis, Centers for Disease Control and Prevention, Pretoria, South Africa

Susan Mmbando
Ministry of Health, Dar es Salaam, Tanzania

Daimon Simbeye
Division of Global HIV and Tuberculosis, Centers for Disease Control and Prevention, Dar es Salaam, Tanzania

Fredrick Rwegerera
U.S. Agency for International Development, Dar es Salaam, Tanzania

Nafuna Wamai
Division of Global HIV and Tuberculosis, Centers for Disease Control and Prevention, Kampala, Uganda

Shelia Kyobutungi
U.S. Agency for International Development, Kampala, Uganda

James Exnobert Zulu
Ministry of Health, Lusaka, Zambia

Omega Chituwo
Division of Global HIV and Tuberculosis, Centers for Disease Control and Prevention, Lusaka, Zambia

Sinokuthemba Xaba
Ministry of Health and Child Care, Harare, Zimbabwe

John Mandisarisa
Division of Global HIV and Tuberculosis, Centers for Disease Control and Prevention, Harare, Zimbabwe

Chongwen Mao, Mengjing You, Shutian Xiang and Yunshan Su
Department of Radiology, The Fourth Affiliated Hospital of Kunming Medical University, #176 Qingnian Road, Kunming 650021, Yunnan, China

Cong Peng
Department of Radiology, The Central Hospital of Wuhan, The Tongji Medical College, Huazhong University of Science and Technology, Wuhan, Hubei, China

Song Li
Department of Urology, The Fourth Affiliated Hospital of Kunming Medical University, Kunming, Yunnan, China

Liling Chen
Department of Clinical Skills Center, The Kunming Medical University, Kunming, Yunnan, China

Kewei Fang
Department of Urology, The Second Affiliated Hospital of Kunming Medical University, Kunming, Yunnan, China

Kuan-Jung Lin
Division of Urology, Department of Surgery, Taoyuan General Hospital, Ministry of Health and Welfare, Taoyuan, Taiwan
Department of Urology, College of Medicine and Shu-Tien Urological Research Center, National Yang Ming Chiao Tung University, Taipei, Taiwan

Eric Y. H. Huang, I-shen Huang, Yu-Hua Fan, Chih-Chieh Lin, Tzu-Ping Lin, Hsiao-Jen Chung, Shing-Hwa Lu, Junne-Yih Kuo, Howard Hung-Hao Wu, Yen-Hwa Chang, Alex T. L. Lin and William J. S. Huang
Department of Urology, Taipei Veterans General Hospital, No. 201, Sec. 2, Shipai Rd., Taipei City 11217, Taiwan
Department of Urology, College of Medicine and Shu-Tien Urological Research Center, National Yang Ming Chiao Tung University, Taipei, Taiwan

Shan Chen, Xiaolian Lu and Lihua Xuan
Department of Acupuncture and Moxibustion, The First Affiliated Hospital of Zhejiang Chinese Medical University, Hangzhou, China

Siyou Wang
Clinical Research Section, Shanghai Research Institute of Acupuncture and Meridian, Shanghai, China

Yunqiu Gao, Jiasheng Yan and Shenhong Wang
Department of Urology, The First Affiliated Hospital of Zhejiang Chinese Medical University, No. 54 Youdian Road, Hangzhou 310006, Zhejiang Province, China

Li-cheng Song, Hui Li, Zhi-jun Li, Ya-fei Qin and Hua-feng Zhang
Department of Orthopaedic, Tianjin Medical University General Hospital, Anshan Road No. 154, Heping District, Tianjin 300052, China

Qian Xu
School of Integrative Medicine, Tianjin University of Traditional Chinese Medicine, Tianjin 301617, China

Ya Li
Department of the Obstetrics and Gynecology, Tianjin Medical University General Hospital, Tianjin 300052, China

Bao-long Wang
Department of Urology, Tianjin Medical University General Hospital, Anshan Road No. 154, Heping District, Tianjin 300052, China

Wiwit Ananda Wahyu Setyaningsih and Nur Arfian
Department of Anatomy, Faculty of Medicine, Public Health and Nursing, Universitas Gadjah Mada, Yogyakarta, Indonesia

Jintao Hu, Cong Lai, Mingchao Gao, Kaiwen Li, Wang He, Dingjun Zhu, Wenlian Xie, Jian Huang and Jinli Han
Department of Urology, Sun Yat-Sen Memorial Hospital, Sun Yat-Sen University, 107 West Yanjiang Road, Guangzhou 510210, China
Guangdong Provincial Clinical Research Center for Urological Diseases, Guangzhou, China

Haihua Wu and Meijuan Xu
Department of Urology, Sun Yat-Sen Memorial Hospital, Sun Yat-Sen University, 107 West Yanjiang Road, Guangzhou 510210, China

Dorte Ejg Jarbøl, Peter Fentz Haastrup, Sanne Rasmussen, Jens Søndergaaard and Kirubakaran Balasubramaniam
Research Unit of General Practice, Department of Public Health, University of Southern Denmark, J.B. Winsløws Vej 9A, 2. Sal, 5000 Odense C, Denmark

Ozgu Aydogdu, Patrik Aronsson, Thomas Carlsson and Michael Winder
Department of Pharmacology, Institute of Neuroscience and Physiology, The Sahlgrenska Academy, University of Gothenburg, Gothenburg, Sweden

Pinar Uyar Gocun
Department of Pathology, School of Medicine, Gazi University, Ankara, Turkey

Guangjie Chen, Xiaohao Wang, Yijun Zhao, Linfeng Zhu and Daxing Tang
Department of Urology, The Children's Hospital, Zhejiang University, School of Medicine, National Clinical Research Center for Child Health, 57 Zhugan Xiang, Hangzhou 310053, China

Ankur Dhar
Murnaghan Urology Department, Prince of Wales Hospital, Sydney, Australia

Nicole Wen Mun Khor and Alistair Cameron-Strange
Murnaghan Urology Department, Prince of Wales Hospital, Sydney, Australia
Prince of Wales Clinical School, UNSW Medicine, Sydney, NSW, Australia

Feng Yao, XiaoLiang Jiang, Bin Xie and Ning Liu
Department of Urology, People's Hospital of Chongqing Banan District, Chongqing 401320, China

Akihiro Nakane
Education and Research Center for Community Medicine, Nagoya City University Graduate School of Medical Sciences, Nagoya, Japan
Department of Urology, Gamagori City Hospital, Gamagori, Japan
Department of Nephro-urology, Nagoya City University Graduate School of Medical Sciences, Nagoya, Japan

Hideyuki Kamisawa and Satoshi Kurokawa
Department of Nephro-urology, Nagoya City University Graduate School of Medical Sciences, Nagoya, Japan

Tetsuji Maruyama and Taiki Kato
Department of Nephro-urology, Nagoya City University Graduate School of Medical Sciences, Nagoya, Japan
Department of Urology, Nagoya City East Medical Center, 2 Wakamizu-cho, Chikusa-ku, Nagoya 464-8547, Japan

Kentaro Mizuno, Hidenori Nishio and Yutaro Hayashi
Department of Pediatric Urology, Nagoya City University Graduate School of Medical Sciences, 1 Kawasumi, Mizuho-cho, Mizuho-ku, Nagoya 467-8601, Japan

Takashi Hamakawa and Yosuke Ikegami
Department of Urology, Nagoya City East Medical Center, 2 Wakamizu-cho, Chikusa-ku, Nagoya 464-8547, Japan

Takahiro Yasui
Department of Nephro-Urology, Nagoya City University Graduate School of Medical Sciences, 1 Kawasumi, Mizuho-cho, Mizuho-ku, Nagoya 467-8601, Japan

Zhi-Wei Sun, Jian-Kang Ge, You Wu and Ye-Qing Huang
Department of Urology, Affiliated Hospital of Nantong University, No. 20 Xisi Road, Nantong, China

Margaret K. Gannon and Amy M. Pearlman
Department of Urology, Carver College of Medicine, University of Iowa, Iowa City, IA, USA

Yoshitaka Itami and Takuya Owari
Department of Urology, Hirao Hospital, 6-28 Hyobu-cho, Kashihara, Nara 634-0076, Japan
Department of Urology, Nara Medical University, 840 Shijo-cho, Kashihara, Nara 634-8522, Japan

Hitoshi Momose and Shuya Hirao
Department of Urology, Hirao Hospital, 6-28 Hyobu-cho, Kashihara, Nara 634-0076, Japan

Makito Miyake, Takashi Iwamoto, Daisuke Gotoh and Kiyohide Fujimoto
Department of Urology, Nara Medical University, 840 Shijo-cho, Kashihara, Nara 634-8522, Japan

Yongqiang Hong and Yuxin Zhang
Department of Clinical Medicine, Fujian Medical University, Fuzhou 350000, China

Shaokun Hong and Siyu Zhang
Department of General Surgery, The First Affiliated Hospital of Xiamen niversity, Xiamen 361001, China

Xiuying Kong
Xiamen University School of Medicine, Xiamen 361001, China

Yuedong Chen
Department of Clinical Medicine, Fujian Medical University, Fuzhou 350000, China
Department of Urology, The First Affiliated Hospital of Xiamen University, Xiamen 361001, China

Herik Acosta
Department of Urology, Okayama University Graduate School of Medicine, Dentistry and Pharmaceutical Sciences, 2-5-1, Shikata-cho, Kita-ku, Okayama 700-8558, Japan

Koichiro Wada, Motoo Araki, Takuya Sadahira, Shogo Watari, Yuki Maruyama, Yosuke Mitsui, Satoshi Katayama, Takehiro Iwata, Shingo Nishimura, Atsushi Takamoto, Tomoko Sako, Kohei Edamura, Yasuyuki Kobayashi, Masami Watanabe, Toyohiko Watanabe and Yasutomo Nasu
Department of Urology, Okayama University Graduate School of Medicine, Dentistry and Pharmaceutical Sciences, 2-5-1, Shikata-cho, Kita-ku, Okayama 700-8558, Japan
Okayama Urological Research Group: OURG, 2-2-7-1, Ima-cho, Kita-ku, Okayama 700-0975, Japan

Ryuta Tanimoto
Department of Urology, Kagawa Prefectural Central Hospital, 1-2-1, Asahi-machi, Takamatsu 760-8557, Japan
Okayama Urological Research Group: OURG, 2-2-7-1, Ima-cho, Kita-ku, Okayama 700-0975, Japan

Hirochika Nakajima
Department of Urology, Fukuyama City Hospital, 5-23-1, Zao-cho, Fukuyama 721-8511, Japan
Okayama Urological Research Group: OURG, 2-2-7-1, Ima-cho, Kita-ku, Okayama 700-0975, Japan

Francis Fatoye
Manchester Metropolitan University, Manchester, UK

Mahmood Ali and Ashley Jaggi
Manchester Metropolitan University, Manchester, UK
Present Address: Astellas Pharma Europe Ltd, Addlestone, UK

Margarita Landeira, Patrick J. O. Covernton and Nurul Choudhury
Present Address: Astellas Pharma Europe Ltd, Addlestone, UK

Rob van Maanen
Astellas Global Development, Leiden, The Netherlands

Qi-Feng Zhang
Department of Andrology, Guilin People's Hospital, Guilin 541002, China

Yu-Ji Zhang
Department of Medical Record Management, The First Affiliated Hospital of Hainan Medical University, Haikou 571137, China

Sheng Wang, Yu Wei, Feng Li and Ke-Jian Feng
Department of Urology, Guilin People's Hospital, Guilin 541002, China

M. G. Steffens and L. P. W. Witte
Department of Urology, ISALA Clinics, Dokter van Heesweg 2, 8025 AB Zwolle, The Netherlands

J. J. Pat, T. v. d. Aart and M. H. Blanker
Department of General Practice, University of Groningen, University Medical Centre, Groningen, Hanzeplein 1, 9713 GZ Groningen, The Netherlands

Florian H. H. Brill, Diana C. Mogrovejo, Henrik Gabriel and Jan-Hendrik Klock
Dr. Brill + Partner GmbH Institute for Hygiene and Microbiology, Stiegstück 34, 22339 Hamburg, Germany

Julia Hambach
Dr. Brill + Partner GmbH Institute for Hygiene and Microbiology, Stiegstück 34, 22339 Hamburg, Germany
Institute of Immunology, University Medical Center Hamburg-Eppendorf, Hamburg, Germany

Christian Utpatel
Molecular and Experimental Mycobacteriology, Research Center Borstel - Leibniz Lung Center, Borstel, Germany

Joerg Steinmann
Klinikum Nürnberg, Institute of Clinical Hygiene, Medical Microbiology and Infectiology, Paracelsus Medical University, Nuremberg, Germany

Andreas Arndt
Department of Research and Development, B. Braun Medical Ltd., Sempach, Switzerland

Alexander S. Somwaru
Department of Diagnostic, Molecular and Interventional Radiology, Icahn School of Medicine At Mount Sinai, 1000 10th Avenue, New York, NY 10019, USA

Stephen Metting
Valley Radiology Medical Associates, San Jose, CA, USA

Laura M. Flisnik
Department of Radiology, New York Presbyterian/ Weill Cornell Medical Center, New York, USA

Michael G. Nellamattathil
Department of Radiology, MedStar Georgetown University Hospital, Washington, DC, USA

Arjun Sharma
Department of Interventional Radiology, Brigham and Women's Hospital, Boston, MA, USA

Venkat S. Katabathina
Department of Radiology, University of Texas Health Science Center San Antonio, San Antonio, TX, USA

Ahmed Soualhi
University Hospital Hairmyres, Glasgow, UK

Elke Rammant
Translational Oncology and Urology Research, School of Cancer and Pharmaceutical Sciences, King's College London, London, UK
Department of Human Structure and Repair, Ghent University, Ghent, Belgium

Gincy George, Beth Russell, Mieke Van Hemelrijck and Cecilia Bosco
Translational Oncology and Urology Research, School of Cancer and Pharmaceutical Sciences, King's College London, London, UK

Deborah Enting
Department of Oncology, Guy's Hospital, Guy's and St Thomas' NHS Foundation Trust, London, UK

Rajesh Nair
Department of Urology, Guy's Hospital, Guy's and St Thomas' NHS Foundation Trust, London, UK

F. Dursun, M. Morgan, R. R. Gonzalez and R. Satkunasivam
Department of Urology, Houston Methodist Hospital, 6560 Fannin Street, Suite 2100, Houston, TX 77030, USA

M. M. Pan
Scott Department of Urology, Baylor College of Medicine, Houston, TX, USA

Index

www.ingramcontent.com/pod-product-compliance
Lightning Source LLC
LaVergne TN
LVHW082136200926
848484LV00008B/2063
* 9 7 9 8 8 8 7 4 0 3 3 6 6 *